DR. R.L. SCHINDLER
OAK PET CLINIC
P.O. Box 396 Hwy. 59 Bypass
Bay Minette, AL 36507
(205) 937-9158

# UPSON'S
## HANDBOOK OF
# Clinical Veterinary Pharmacology

**Dan W. Upson, D.V.M.**
Professor of Pharmacology
College of Veterinary Medicine
Kansas State University
Manhattan, Kansas

 **VM PUBLISHING, INC.**
144 N. Nettleton, Bonner Springs, Kansas 66012

**1981**

ISBN O-935078-15-0

# Preface

THE FORMAT and objectives for this handbook have evolved over
several years from my pharmacology teaching syllabus for veterinary
students and from handouts prepared for continuing education meet-
ings for practitioners. The section dealing with general principles is intended to provide a working background of those concepts that are important in the proper usage of drugs in veterinary medicine. Each drug
group is handled separately and the physiologic principles are included
where they are appropriate as a basis of understanding the drug actions. The handbook emphasizes the actions or responses of the drugs,
the mechanisms by which the drug brings about these responses, and,
where appropriate, any adverse or toxic reactions that might occur.

An attempt has been made to include the drugs most commonly used
in animals, and human drugs used in veterinary practice. Extra-label
uses of drugs are included for information and do not imply a recom-
mendation or encouragement to use these drugs in this manner. Data
on the extra-label uses of drugs provide a basis for intelligent therapeutic application of drugs in situations where the practitioner feels extra-
label use is necessary. Some drugs that are no longer available are included for historical purposes.

This handbook is in no way intended to be a textbook. An excellent
textbook is available (*Veterinary Pharmacology and Therapeutics*, 4th
edition; edited by Jones, Booth, and McDonald; and published by The
Iowa State University Press). In my opinion, this handbook, coupled
with the book *Veterinary Pharmaceuticals and Biologicals* (VPB)
edited by Aronson, Powers, and Scheidy, and published by Harwal,
would make a very useful library for the general practitioner. In an exclusive small animal practice, one might want to combine this handbook with the VPB and the *Physicians' Desk Reference* (PDR) published
by Medical Economics Company.

Emphasis throughout the handbook is on the clinical application of
the basic concepts of veterinary pharmacology. One of the values of
this handbook lies in the author's attempt to keep it current. Current
plans call for a new edition to be made available at least every two years.

*Dan W. Upson, D.V.M.*
*Manhattan, Kansas*
*April 1981*

# Table of Contents

Chapter 3
AUTONOMIC NERVOUS SYSTEM

Chapter 4
ANALGESIC and ANTI-INFLAMMATORY DRUGS

*(Continued on next page)*

## Chapter 5
## GONADOTROPINS and GONADAL HORMONES

## Chapter 6
## MUSCLE RELAXANTS

## Chapter 7
## URINARY SYSTEM

## Chapter 8
## GASTROINTESTINAL SYSTEM

## Chapter 9
## BLOOD and BLOOD-FORMING SYSTEM

## Chapter 10
## CARDIOVASCULAR SYSTEM

## Chapter 11
## ANTHELMINTICS

*(Continued on next page)*

Chapter 12
INSECTICIDES

Chapter 13
HISTAMINES and ANTIHISTAMINES

Chapter 14
DRUGS ACTING UPON THE UTERUS

Chapter 15
LOCAL ANESTHETICS

Chapter 16
LOCALLY ACTING EXTERNAL MEDICATIONS

## Chapter 17
## EXPECTORANTS and COUGH MEDICINES

## Chapter 18
## CANCER CHEMOTHERAPY

## Chapter 19
## ANTIMICROBIAL DRUGS

CHAPTER

# 1

# Principles of Pharmacology

## Introduction

Pharmacology is broadly defined as the *study of drugs*. It is a recognized discipline of biology. More-specific definitions of pharmacology include 1) changes produced in living organisms by drugs or chemical substances; 2) action of drugs upon the animal in conjunction with the action of the animal upon the drug; and 3) the interaction between chemical compounds and living organisms.

Pharmacology involves knowledge of the following aspects of a drug: 1) history; 2) source; 3) physical and chemical properties; 4) compounding; 5) biochemical and physiological effects; 6) mechanisms of action; 7) absorption; 8) distribution; 9) biotransformation; 10) excretion; and 11) therapeutic, diagnostic, and preventive uses.

The word *drug* was derived from the French word *drogue* (meaning a dry herb) and the Greek word *pharmakon* (meaning potion or poison). Classic definitions include 1) any chemical agent that affects living protoplasm, 2) chemical agents that initiate or alter responses of biological systems, 3) articles for use in the diagnosis, cure, mitigation, treatment or prevention of disease in man or other animals, 4) articles, other than food, intended to affect the structure or any function of the body of man or other animals.

**All drugs are poisons! All poisons are drugs!** Drugs are poisons that save lives and relieve disease by acting on the biological systems in living organisms. The nature of the action and the mechanism of action are major considerations. The levels of organization acted upon and the resulting responses are summarized as follows:

**Molecular pharmacology** — the pharmacology of cells, cellular components and chemical reactions involved in cellular metabolism.

**Clinical pharmacology** — pharmacology of intact animals both in health and disease.

## Major Subdivisions of Pharmacology

**Pharmacodynamics** — the response of living organisms to drugs. Pharmacodynamics occur in both healthy and diseased animals. "What the drug does to the animal", including the drug's mode of action and its effects.

**Pharmacotherapeutics** — the response of living organisms to drugs in the presence of disease.

**Pharmacokinetics**—the manner in which the living organism handles the drug. "What the body does to the drug", including absorption, distribution, metabolism and excretion.

## Pharmacological Definitions

**Alkaloid** — a chemical agent, organic in nature and containing one or more atoms of nitrogen. Many drugs, such as strychnine, atropine, eserine, epinephrine, morphine, etc., are in this category. Alkaloids have some common chemical properties such as solubility in mineral acids, insolubility in basic medium, and solubility in organic solvents.

**Analeptic** — in its broadest sense, means a drug that restores a body function. As used today, the term is used to refer to a series of more or less potent CNS stimulants; the respiratory analeptics.

**Analgesic** — causes the loss of, or dissociation from, pain.

**Anesthetic** — means without esthesia (feeling) or sensation.

**Anhydrotic** — an agent that inhibits sweating.

**Anorexic** — a drug that suppresses appetite.

**Anthelmintic** — an agent used against intestinal parasites.

**Antipruritic** — a drug that relieves itching.

**Antipyretic** — lowers an abnormally high temperature.

**Antitussive** — a drug that inhibits or controls coughing.

**Astringent** — a substance that exerts a relatively mild and reversible protein-precipitant action on tissue.

**Bactericide** — an agent that kills bacteria.

**Bacteriostat** — an agent that inhibits reproduction of bacteria.

**Cathartic** — a drug that promotes the emptying of the lower gastrointestinal tract (defecation).

**Caustic** — causes necrosis of tissue. Caustics are limited to topical use. Varying depths of penetration can be attained by different caustic agents. For example, a heavy-metal ion such as silver penetrates to a minor extent, whereas arsenic or antimony penetrates more deeply. Phenol is another chemical that penetrates deeply. The terms *corrosive* and *cauterizer* are sometimes used to mean *caustic*.

**Chemotherapy** — the use of a chemical compound in the specific treatment of a certain disease-causing agent.

**Cholagogue** — an agent that stimulates the flow of bile from the gallbladder.

**Choleretic** — increases the secretion of bile by the liver.

**Demulcent** — a soothing, inert substance used to coat an epithelial surface. (tragacanth, gum acacia, etc.). The term *protectant* is sometimes synonymously used.

**Depressant** — a drug that reduces or inhibits a body function.

**Disinfectant, germicide,** and **antiseptic** — used interchangeably. They are chemicals, toxic to microorganisms, that are applied to surfaces.

**Emetic** — a drug that induces vomiting.

**Euthanasia agent** — a drug used for humane reasons to produce quiet, painless death in animals.

**Expectorant** — a drug that increases secretions from the upper respiratory tract.

**Galactogogue** — increases the flow of milk.

**General anesthetic** — causes the total loss of sensation. Patient cannot be awakened.

**Glucoside** — a glycoside in which glucose forms the carbohydrate portion of the molecule. Among the pharmacologically important glycosides are the cardiac glycosides in the digitalis group.

**Glycoside** — a chemical compound containing a carbohydrate moiety which is attached to the main portion of the molecule via a glycosidal, or ether-like linkage.

**Hemopoietic** — a drug used to stimulate the formation of red cells or hemoglobin. *Hematinic* is a more or less synonymous term.

**Hemostatic** — an agent used to aid in the control of more serious hemorrhage.

**Hydrotic** — an agent that causes sweating.

**Hypnotic** — a sleep-producing drug, but the patient can be awakened.

**Local anesthetic** — causes the loss of sensation in localized area.

**Materia Medica** — a descriptive study that deals with the origin, preparation, dose and clinical use of drugs. An older term now replaced by the more exact sciences.

**Metrology** — the study of weights and measures.

**Narcotic** — from the pharmacological standpoint, a narcotic is a central nervous system (CNS) depressant (hypnosis and analgesia). From the older, obsolete standpoint, the term *narcotic* was used to describe an agent that had a liability for compulsive drug abuse.

**Pesticide** — an agent that controls pests on animals or crops; includes insecticides, herbicides, fungicides, rodenticides, and nematocides.

**Pharmacogenetics** — the science dealing with the interrelationships between heredity and drug response.

**Pharmacognosy** — the science concerned with the source, identification and properties of drugs of natural origin.

**Pharmacy** — the science concerned with the collection, preparation, standardization, and dispensing of drugs.

**Posology** — the study of dosages.

**Rubefacient** — an agent that causes reddening of the skin (cutaneous vasodilation). The word is used in connection with locally applied drugs, such as ether, chloroform, or alcohol.

**Sedative** — a CNS depressant used to produce a state of quietude, relaxation and relief from fear and apprehension.

**Sialogogue** — stimulates the flow of saliva.

**Soporific, somnifacient** — a sleep-producing drug.

**Stimulant** — a drug that enhances or accentuates a body function.

**Styptic** — an agent used locally to allay minor capillary hemorrhage.

**Toxicology** — the science of harmful agents (poisons).

**Vermicide** — an agent that kills worms; used interchangeably with *anthelmintic* and *vermifuge*.

**Vermifuge** — an agent that removes worms by expulsion.

## History

Pharmacotherapy developed from a mixture of religion, herbs, powders, poultices and mysticism. The first record of man's use of drugs dates back to 2800 BC when Pen T'sao rated herbs according to their effect on diseases. The use of drugs for therapeutic value was practiced by the Greeks, Hindus, Egyptians and many other societies well before the birth of Christ. Hippocrates was the first to state that diseases were an abnormal reaction of the body rather than a visitation from the gods.

# Experimental Methods
## Relating to Pharmacological Studies

**Magendie,** in 1809, identified strychnine's (Javanese arrow poison, nux vomica) site of action on the spinal cord..

**Bernard** identified the site of action of curare (South American arrow poison) at the myoneural junction.

**Withering,** in 1783, gave the clinical description of the heart-stimulating action of digitalis (purple foxglove) in human patients.

**Harvey** described the circulation of blood.

**Organic chemistry** started in the 1800s. There was a change from empirical medicine to rational therapy. Chemicals were synthesized.

# Rise of the University
## and Pharmacological Research

**Germany** — 1850, R. Buchheim and O. Schmiedeberg.

**America** — 1890s, J.J. Abel, University of Michigan and Johns Hopkins University. First full-time Professor of Pharmacology in the United States.

# Drugs and Pharmaceutical
# Preparations

A. **SOURCES OF COMPOUNDS FOR THERAPY** (with examples)

1. **Mineral**
   A) sulfur        C) iodine       E) hydrochloric acid
   B) iron          D) selenium     F) electrolytes

2. **Botanical**
   A) plants
   B) molds         E) glycosides   H) gums
   C) bacteria      F) oils         I) tannins
   D) alkaloids     G) resins       J) antibiotics

3. **Animal**
   A) insulin              C) pituitary gonadotropins   E) lanolin
   B) thyroid extract      D) conjugated estrogens

4. **Synthetic**
   A) aspirin         C) steroids     E) diuretics
   B) sulfonamides    D) procaine     F) many others

## B.  DOSAGE FORMS

1.  **Vehicles or solvents for oral medications** — used to dissolve and make drugs more palatable for oral administration.

    A) *Waters* — aqueous solutions of volatile substances, usually volatile oils; *e.g.* peppermint water (USP).

    B) *Syrups* — nearly saturated aqueous solutions of sucrose and water which may or may not contain flavoring and/or medicinal substances; *e.g.* wild cherry syrup (USP).

    C) *Elixirs* — hydroalcoholic solutions containing sweetening and flavoring substances and in some cases active medicinal agents; *e.g.* phenobarbital elixir (USP).

2.  **Vehicles or solvents for injections**

    A) *Sterile water*

    B) *Sterile saline*

    C) *Propylene glycol* — a solvent and stabilizer for many drugs; also a source of energy (5.7 C/g) when metabolized by the body. Large amounts injected in one intramuscular site are painful. Large amounts injected IV may produce hemolysis.

    D) *Polyvinylpyrrolidone (PVP-Povidone)* — a drug carrier in a loose bonding. It delays absorption in comparison to water. It has a slight anti-inflammatory effect and has been studied as a plasma expander for fluid therapy.

3.  **Solutions (primarily aqueous)**

    A) *Solutions or liquors* — liquid preparations that contain one or more substances dissolved in a liquid solvent, and which do not, because of their ingredients or method of preparation, fall into some other group of official substances.

    B) *Injections* — sterile liquids, solutions or suspensions for parenteral injection. The vehicle is important; it can alter absorption rates, duration of action, ease of administration, and patient comfort.

4.  **Suspensions**

    A) *Suspensions of insoluble powders in water*

    B) *Emulsions* — aqueous suspensions of insoluble oily or resinous drugs with an emulsifier added to increase the preparation's stability; *e.g.* cod liver oil emulsion.

    C) *Mixtures* — dispersions of insoluble solid, non-fatty substances, often with a stabilizing agent added. An example is *magmas*, mixtures having the consistency of milk or cream, *e.g.* magnesia magma, (USP) (milk of magnesia).

5.  **Solutions (alcoholic)**

    A) *Spirits or essences* — alcoholic or hydroalcoholic solutions of volatile drugs, usually of volatile oils; *e.g.* aromatic ammonia spirits.

6. **Extractive preparations**
    A) *Tinctures* — alcoholic or hydroalcoholic solutions prepared from animal, vegetable, or mineral drugs; *e.g.* tincture of digitalis.
    B) *Fluidextracts* — tinctures prepared so that 1 ml of the fluidextract represents 1 g of the air-dried drug; *e.g.* aromatic cascara sagrada fluidextract (USP).
    C) *Extracts* — obtained by evaporating the solvent from tinctures or fluidextracts. They have either a plastic or powdery consistency; *e.g.* belladonna extract.

7. **Solid dosage forms**
    A) *Vehicles* — important relative to the absorption characteristics of the preparation. Examples are: sucrose, talc, resins, PVP for sustained-release tablets or capsules.
    B) *Powders* — for oral administration in feed, water, or salt.
    C) *Capsules* — ovoid or cylindrical shells of gelatin used to administer powders or liquids *per orum*. Capsules may be coated so that they pass through the stomach without disintegrating (enteric coating), or ingredients may be compounded for timed release or sustained release.
    D) *Tablets* — granulated and dried or powdered drugs that have been compressed or molded into small disks for oral administration. They may also have an enteric coating.
    E) *Hypodermic tablets* — made under aseptic conditions. They are to be dissolved and used as an injection.
    F) *Pellets, boluses, bolettes,* and *boloids* — compressed cylinders of dried or powdered drugs used for oral administration. Different names usually denote different sizes.
    G) *Implants* — drugs prepared in a tablet-like or paste form for subcutaneous insertion using a special instrument. They are designed for extremely slow absorption.

8. **External dosage forms**
    A) *Powders for topical application* — *e.g.* wound powders.
    B) *Liniments* — liquid preparations to be applied to the skin with friction (such as a leg-brace).
    C) *Lotions* — liquid preparations intended to be soothing and applied to the skin without friction.
    D) *Ointments* — semisolid fatty or oily preparations containing medicants intended for external application. Various substances are used as a base, which may or may not be water-soluble.
    E) *Suppositories* — conical or ovoid medicated solids to be in-

serted into an orifice of the body, excluding the mouth.
They usually melt, soften, or dissolve at body temperature.
The vehicles usually used are theobroma oil (cacao butter),
glycerinated gelatin, or high-molecular-weight polyethylene glycols.

9. **Miscellaneous forms**
   A) *Gels* — suspensions of insoluble drugs in a water medium.
   The drugs are in a hydrated form in which the particle size
   approaches colloidal dimensions. If left standing, they may
   become semisolid or gelatinous.
   B) *Inhalants* — drugs which because of their high vapor
   pressure can be carried by air into the nasal passages.
   C) *Inhalations* — solutions for administration as a mist to be inhaled into the lungs.

# Drug Regulations and Standards

Drugs used in the practice of both human and veterinary medicine are
controlled by federal and state laws.

A. **HISTORY**
   1. **King John of England** — brought forth the first food and drug
   "law" in 1202.
   2. **Early U.S. laws which are no longer in effect**
      A) *1906* — Initial food and drug law. Not effective. Offered
      very little control.
      B) *1915* — Harrison Narcotic Act.
      C) *1965* — Drug Abuse and Control Amendment. More rigid
      control of CNS stimulant and depressant drugs (barbitur-
      ates, amphetamines, LSD, marijuana).

B. **DRUG LAWS APPLICABLE TO VETERINARY MEDICINE**
   1. **Federal Food Drug and Cosmetic Act** (1938) — the basic law at
   present. The law has many amendments.
   2. **Durham-Humphrey Amendment** (1951)
      A) Provided for the prescription legend on label, and separated
      drugs into two categories:
      1) Drugs that must be used by or on the order of a licensed
      veterinarian, physician or dentist. These are called *pre-
      scription drugs*. They are also called *legend drugs*, which
      refers to the prescription legend (the $R_x$).
      2) Drugs that may be sold without a prescription. These are
      called *over-the-counter drugs* (OTC). The philosophy be-

hind this amendment is that if a veterinary drug can be properly labeled to assure its safe use, it must be classified as OTC. OTC drugs must bear on the label:

a) Adequate directions for safe and effective use.
b) Warnings against misuse, and cautions relative to adverse effects.

3. **Food-Additives Amendments** (1958)
   A) Regulation of chemical substances added to food for human consumption.
   B) Contains the *Delaney Clause*. Provides that no additive shall be deemed safe if, by tests appropriate for evaluating the safety of food additives, the substance is shown to induce cancer in man or animal.

   With reference to veterinary drugs, this means that if the drug is suspected of causing cancer in man or animals, then *no residue* (zero tolerance) of such drug is allowed in any edible portion of, or in any food derived from, the treated animal.

4. **Kefauver-Harris Drug Amendment** (1962)
   A) Provided for:
      1) Registration of pharmaceutical manufacturing firms
      2) Drug manufacturing controls
      3) Factory inspection
      4) Proper labeling
      5) Generic names
      6) Control of advertising used by drug companies
      7) Reporting of adverse effects of drugs
      8) Withdrawal from the market of a previously approved drug by FDA

   B) Provided for approval of new drugs with a defined step-by-step protocol.
      1 )*First step* — Investigational New Animal Drug Application. (INADA)
      2) *Second step* — New Animal Drug Application. (NADA)
      3) Sponsoring company *must prove:*
         a) *Safety*
            (1) To animal being medicated (target species)
            (2) No human health hazard if given to food-producing animals or from handling the drug
         b) *Efficacy* — The drug must do what the label claims.

    4) Feed additives are handled in same way as other drugs. An NADA must be filed for approval. This document will state the exact level of the drug in feed and its specific purpose. A veterinarian may prescribe a drug(s) to be used in a feed as an additive only if the feed mill has an *approved* NADA *on file*. Form 1900 (effective in 1981) is needed to comply with this requirement.

C) Drugs approved after 1938 and before 1962 are handled as follows:

    1) Have been and are being reviewed for *efficacy*, or had already been deemed *safe (grandfather clause)*

    2) Reviewed by a committee under National Academy of Science, National Research Council (NAS/NRC)

    3) Judgment is rendered that drug(s) is:

        a) not effective

        b) probably not effective

        c) probably effective

        d) effective

    4) FDA usually concurs with recommendation of the review committee.

5. **Animal Drug Amendment** (1968)

A) Consolidated provisions of the Act with respect to the regulation of new animal drugs

6. **Comprehensive Drug Abuse Prevention and Control Act of 1970.** Became law May 1, 1971. Established the Drug Enforcement Administration (DEA).

A) This act (Public Law 91-513) supersedes the Harrison Narcotic Act and the Drug Abuse Control Act and any amendments to the two.

B) Any veterinarian using and/or prescribing controlled substances must register with the DEA. Forms for submitting new and renewal applications, and information can be obtained from:

      United States Department of Justice
      Drug Enforcement Administration
      P.O. Box 28083, Central Station
      Washington, D.C. 20005
      Telephone: (202) 724-1013

    (See chart on next page for regional offices.)

C) Ordering of controlled drugs

    1) Schedule II drugs must be ordered on a special order form in triplicate. Order forms may be obtained using requisition form DEA-222D.

## DEA REGIONAL OFFICES and STATES SERVICED

### Effective October 1, 1978

| Northeastern | Southeastern | North Central | South Central | Western |
|---|---|---|---|---|
| 555 West 57th Street | 8400 N.W. 53rd Street | 219 South Dearborn | 1880 Regal Row | 350 S. Figueroa |
| New York, New York 10019 | Miami, Florida 33166 | Chicago, Illinois 60604 | Dallas, Texas 75235 | Los Angeles, Calif. 90071 |
| (212) 399-5131 | (305) 591-4880 | (312) 353-7889 | (214) 767-7248 | (213) 688-2650 |
| New York | Florida | Illinois | Texas | California |
| New Jersey | Georgia | Indiana | Oklahoma | Nevada |
| Pennsylvania | Maryland | Wisconsin | New Mexico | Guam |
| Delaware | Washington, D.C. | Michigan | Arizona | Alaska |
| Massachusetts | Virginia | Ohio | Colorado | Washington |
| Connecticut | North Carolina | Kentucky | Utah | Oregon |
| Rhode Island | South Carolina | West Virginia | Wyoming | Idaho |
| New Hampshire | Louisiana | Missouri | | Montana |
| Vermont | Arkansas | Iowa | | Hawaii |
| Maine | Alabama | Minnesota | | |
| | Mississippi | North Dakota | | |
| | Tennessee | South Dakota | | |
| | Virgin Islands | Nebraska | | |
| | | Kansas | | |

      2) A DEA number is necessary for ordering drugs in schedules III, IV, and V.

D) A prescription order:
      1) Must be signed by the prescriber when it is written.
      2) Must have prescriber's name, address and DEA registration number.
      3) Must have full name and address of the client.

E) Drug security
      1) Schedule II controlled substances must be kept in a locked cabinet. Schedule III, IV, and V controlled substances may be kept in a locked cabinet or dispersed throughout the noncontrolled stock in a way that will discourage theft.
      2) An inventory of all controlled drugs should be kept along with records of receipt and dispensation.

F) Controlled substances are divided into five schedules:
      1) **Schedule I** — Substances with high potential for abuse, no currently accepted medical use, and a lack of accepted safety for use. (Not available to practitioners.)
      2) **Schedule II** — Substances with high potential for abuse, accepted medical use with severe restrictions, and their use may lead to severe psychological or physical dependence.
      3) **Schedule III** — Substances with less potential for abuse than those in Schedules I or II, accepted medical use, and

may lead to moderate or low degree of physical dependence, but high psychological dependence.

4) **Schedule IV** — Substances with low potential for abuse,
accepted medical use, and limited physical or psychological dependence in comparison to those in Schedule III.

5) **Schedule V** — Substances that have accepted medical
uses, low potential for abuse, and limited physical or
psychological dependence in comparison to those in
Schedule IV.

G) The letter C has been used on drug-abuse control substances
with the $R_x$ symbol in its center. The C will be retained, but
the schedule number will be used instead of the $R_x$ symbol. All
controlled-substance labeling must have on it Ⅽ, ⅭⅡ, ⅭⅢ, ⅭⅣ,
or ⅭⅤ to indicate the drug's schedule.

H) Records of acquisition and disposition must be kept for two
years.

I) Substances in Schedule II must be recorded separately. No
prescription for Schedule II substances may be refilled.

J) Schedules III, IV, and V prescriptions may be refilled five
times within a 6-month period if so specified when the prescription is written or any time interval less than 5 in 6 months
if specified. If times of refill are not specified, then the prescription may not be refilled.

K) Thefts should be reported immediately to local police and
nearest DEA office, and physical inventories should be taken
immediately. Special forms are available from DEA.

L) Controlled substances used on patients in the office should
be recorded on the patient-record card. Also, any item dispensed should be recorded on the patient-record form and
accountability records.

M) If any substance in Schedule II, III, or IV is dispensed, the
following must appear on the label: "Caution: Federal Law
prohibits transfer of this drug to any person other than the
patient for whom it was prescribed".

N) A physical inventory must be made every two years.

O) Institutions and individuals performing experimental research with domestic or imported substances subject to the
law should contact the nearest DEA office for special provisions.

P) A well-established client-practitioner relationship should exist before any of these substances are dispensed, either directly or by prescription.

Q) A veterinarian may delegate authority to an assistant to give
a controlled drug to an animal, provided that the assistant is
under the practitioner's direct supervision. It is, however, il-

legal for a student or other individual to use or have in his or her possession, a controlled drug, without the direct supervision of a licensed veterinarian. (*See* guidelines, number 12.)

---

# Schedule of Controlled Substances

Partial listing of drugs important to veterinary medicine

## Schedule I

Benzylmorphine
Codeine methylbromide
Heroin
'Morphine methylbromide
Lysergic acid diethylamide
Marihuana

Tetrahydrocannabinol
 (from marihuana)
Peyote
Psilocybin
Psilocyn

## Schedule II

Opium extracts
Opium fluid extracts
Tincture of opium
Codeine
Ethylmorphine
Hydrocodone
Hydromorphone
Metopon
Meperidine (Demerol®)
Phenmetrazine (Preludin®)
Morphine
Oxymorphone (Numorphan®)
Amphetamine

Methylphenidate (Ritalin®)
Coca leaves
Cocaine
Anileridine
Dihydrocodeine
Diphenoxylate (Lomotil®)
Fentanyl (Innovar®)
Methadone
Methaqualone (Somnafac®)
Methamphetamine
Pentobarbital sodium
Secobarbital sodium
Phencyclidine

Etorphine (M-99): Now available to veterinarians engaged in zoo and exotic animal practice, wildlife management programs and research.

## Schedule III

Nalorphine (Nalline®)
Surital®
Bio-Tal®

Kemithal®
Pentothal®
Dipentol®

## Schedule IV

Chloral hydrate
Methohexital
Meprobamate (Equanil®)
Diazepam (Valium®)

Methylphenobarbital
Phenobarbital
Propoxyphene (Darvon®)
Chlordiazepoxide (Librium®)

## Schedule V

Designated small amounts of codeine (less than 1 mg/ml), ethylmorphine (less than 1 mg/ml), morphine (less than 15 mg/100 ml)

## GUIDELINES FOR
## PRESCRIBERS OF CONTROLLED DRUGS

1. Keep prescription blanks in a safe place where they cannot be easily stolen. Minimize the number of prescription pads in use.

2. Write prescriptions for Schedule II drugs in ink or indelible pencil or use a typewriter. Such prescriptions must be signed by the veterinarian.

3. Write out the actual amount prescribed as well as using an Arabic or Roman numeral, in order to discourage alterations in written prescriptions.

4. Avoid writing prescriptions for large quantities of controlled drugs unless you determine absolutely that such quantities are needed.

5. Maintain a minimal stock of controlled drugs in the pharmacy or car.

6. Be cautious when a client states that another veterinarian had been prescribing a controlled drug. Consult the other veterinarian or examine the patient thoroughly to determine for yourself whether a controlled drug should be prescribed.

7. On the patient's case record, record the administration of controlled substances.

8. Use prescription blanks only for writing prescriptions—not for memos. A drug-abuser could easily erase the message and forge a prescription.

9. Never sign prescription blanks in advance.

10. Keep an accurate record of controlled drugs dispensed—as required under the Controlled Substances Act of 1970.

11. Assist the pharmacist by verifying information about any prescription you have written. A corresponding responsibility rests with the pharmacist who dispenses the prescriptions.

12. The Drug Enforcement Administration (DEA) has stated that necessary amounts of commercial pentobarbital preparations, in a solution of any strength, may be stored and used for euthanasia on the premises of humane organizations and animal shelters without violation of federal regulations controlling Schedule II substances, pro-

vided that the attending veterinarian holds a valid controlled-substances registration at the location of the humane organization, and orders the schedule drugs on official order forms for delivery to that address. The drugs may be used only at the direction of the attending veterinarian, but the veterinarian need not be present to receive shipments of drugs nor at the time of administration. A veterinarian should hold a separate registration at every address at which he or she practices or expects to store and use controlled drugs, including all humane organizations or animal shelters for which he or she is the attending veterinarian. Adequate records must be maintained at each location. Those records must show amounts received, amounts used, and purposes for which used. The drugs must be stored in securely locked cabinets. This interpretation of the law was stated by DEA in response to inquiries by AVMA at a DEA/Prescribers Working Committee meeting in Washington, DC on November 18, 1974.

13. Phone the nearest office of the Drug Enforcement Administration to obtain or to report information. Your call will be held in the strictest confidence.

## REGULATORY REQUIREMENTS
### (Consult regulations for specific requirements.)

| Schedule | Registration | Recordkeeping | Distribution Restrictions | Dispensing Limits | Security |
|---|---|---|---|---|---|
| I | Required | Separate | Order forms | Research use only | Vault/safe |
| II | Required | Separate | Order forms | Rx: written; no refills | Vault/safe |
| III | Required | Readily retrievable | Records required | Rx: written or oral; with medical authorization, refills up to 5 times in 6 months | Secure storage area |
| IV | Required | Readily retrievable | Records required | Rx: written or oral; with medical authorization, refills up to 5 times in 6 months | Secure storage area |
| V | Required | Readily retrievable | Records required | OTC (Rx drugs limited to M.D.'s order) | Secure storage area |

7. **Poison Prevention Packaging Act** (1970) — Federal laws require special packaging for human drugs that could be dangerous to children. The required packaging is a container that cannot be readily opened by a child under 5 years of age, but can be opened and properly reclosed by most adults. Several manufacturers now produce childproof containers that have met the requirement of the FDA.

   This law technically applies only to drugs for human patients, but it should also apply when veterinarians dispense drugs. The law has been a life saver.

8. **Adminstration of federal regulations.** The Congress of the United States enacts the laws. The laws relative to drugs are administered by:
   A) U.S. Department of Health and Human Services (HHS), Food and Drug Administration (FDA). Bureau of Veterinary Medicine (BVM) administers Food, Drug and Cosmetic Act and its amendments relative to animal drugs.
   B) U.S. Department of Justice, Drug Enforcement Administration (DEA), enforces Comprehensive Drug Abuse Prevention and Control Act.
   C) U.S. Department of Agriculture, Food Safety and Quality Service (FSQS); Animal and Plant Health Inspection Service (APHIS); and Meat and Poultry Inspection (MPI).

9. **1947 Federal Insecticide, Fungicide and Rodenticide Act** — provides for the proper labeling, efficacy and safety of pesticides. USDA administers this act.

10. **Miller Pesticide Residue Amendment** — gave FDA the authority and responsibility for assuring safe pesticide residues on or in raw agricultural commodities.

# EPA Announces Pesticide
# Policy for Veterinarians

The Environmental Protection Agency's (EPA) Office of Pesticide Programs and Office of Enforcement have clarified the legal responsibilities of veterinarians who use or dispense pesticides in their practices (*Federal Register*, November 1, 1979). Specifically, if a veterinarian using or dispensing pesticides follows safety precautions described in the policy statement, then EPA will excuse the veterinarian from meeting certain procedural requirements imposed by the Federal Insecticide, Fungicide, and Rodenticide Act (FIFRA), as amended.

The EPA has clarified the legal responsibilities of veterinarians using restricted-use pesticides (RUPs). Ordinarily, only a certified applicator, or a person "under direct supervision" of a certified applicator, may use RUPs. However, federal regulations exempt from the certification requirement veterinarians who use RUPs in the "normal course of their practice." This exemption extends also to employees of a veterinarian using RUPs under the direct supervision of the veterinarian. Veterinarians are not, however, authorized to dispense RUPs to clients who are not certified applicators. In addition, veterinarians must use every pesticide according to label directions.

The EPA also described specifically the legal responsibilities of veterinarians who repackage registered pesticides, or who mix special pesticide blends and dispense them to clients. Usually, persons engaged in such practices must register the product and their establishment with EPA and comply with labeling, packaging, and recordkeeping requirements imposed by FIFRA. However, a veterinarian who repackages these products will not be subject to the requirements if:

1) the repackaged pesticide is registered by EPA for a use consistent with the use for which the pesticide is prescribed;
2) the pesticide is not a RUP (unless it is dispensed to an appropriately certified client);
3) the veterinarian supplies the client with labeling carrying specific safety precautions and other essential information;
4) the dispensed container meets federal child-resistant packaging requirements if children might gain access to the pesticide;
5) the pesticide is prescribed by the veterinarian on a case-by-case basis to meet a specific pest problem.

Similarly, veterinarians who mix and dispense their own special blends will not be subject to registration, labeling, packaging, and recordkeeping requirements if:

1) the special blend is produced by the addition of ingredients to, or mixing of, pesticides registered by EPA;
2) none of the ingredients is a RUP (unless the blend is dispensed only to an appropriately certified client;
3) the use prescribed is consistent with uses authorized by the labeling of the registered ingredients, and the labeling does not prohibit the mixture;
4) the veterinarian supplies the client with labeling carrying specific safety precautions and other essential data;

5) the pesticide is prescribed on a case-by-case basis for a specific pest problem;

6) the special blend is formulated and dispensed in accordance with recognized clinical practices and is not to be used for experimentation; and

7) the dispensed container meets federal child-resistant packaging requirements if the pesticide is likely to come within the reach of children.

In addition, when applying or dispensing a special pesticide blend for treatment of food animals, the veterinarian must ascertain that residue tolerances or clearances for the pesticide are specified under the Federal Food, Drug and Cosmetic Act.

The EPA policy encourages voluntary compliance with federal standards for child-resistant packaging whenever dispensed pesticides could fall into the hands of children.

EPA's policy does not affect state and local requirements for veterinary practice.

# Veterinarians May Obtain
# Ethyl Alcohol Tax-Free

The Bureau of Alcohol, Tobacco, and Firearms (ATF), Department of the Treasury, has ruled that veterinary hospitals and charitable veterinary clinics may obtain ethyl alcohol, tax-free, for treating animals.

For some time, veterinarians have requested that they be included among those permitted to purchase ethyl alcohol tax-free for nonbeverage purposes. AVMA and AAHA, among others, had urged the Bureau to allow veterinarians the same priority as physicians in procuring ethyl alcohol. The main veterinary use of ethyl alcohol is to treat ethylene glycol poisoning. Injection of 20% ethyl alcohol and 5% sodium bicarbonate is recommended for treating such poisoning.

Veterinary practitioners requesting tax-free ethyl alcohol must obtain an application (Form 4326) for limited industrial use and limited withdrawal permits. Practitioners who want to use not more than 120 proof-gallons of tax-free alcohol during a calendar year may file Form 4326 if (1) the alcohol is obtained from one supplier, (2) the maximum quantity of such alcohol to be on hand, in transit, and unaccounted for at any one time will not exceed 14 proof-gallons, and (3) the alcohol will not be recovered (re-used).

Neither a fee nor the posting of bond is required, a use inventory must be kept and is subject to audit by ATF at any time. Applicants must supply evidence establishing their authority to obtain the tax-free ethyl alcohol. Application forms and other details are available from the regional offices of the ATF:

| Region | Toll-Free Phone |
|---|---|
| 1) *Central* (Indiana, Kentucky, Michigan, Ohio, West Virginia) | Ohio: 800-582-1880<br>All others: 800-543-1932 |
| 2) *Mid-Atlantic* (Delaware, District of Columbia, Maryland, New Jersey, Pennsylvania, Virginia) | Pennsylvania: 800-462-1650<br>All others: 800-523-0677, |
| 3) *Midwest* (Illinois, Iowa, Kansas, Minnesota, Missouri, North Dakota, South Dakota, Wisconsin) | Illinois, 800-572-3178<br>All others: 800-621-3211 |
| 4) *North-Atlantic* (Connecticut, Maine, Massachusetts, New Hampshire, New York, Rhode Island, Vermont, Puerto Rico, Virgin Islands) | New York: 800-442-8275<br>All others: 800-223-2162, |
| 5) *Southeast* (Alabama, Florida, Georgia, Mississippi, North Carolina, South Carolina, Tennessee) | Georgia: 800-282-8878<br>All others: 800-241-3701 |
| 6) *Southwest* (Arkansas, Colorado, Louisiana, New Mexico, Oklahoma, Texas, Wyoming) | Texas: 800-422-7251<br>All others: 800-527-9380 |
| 7) *Western* (Alaska\*, Arizona, California, Hawaii\*, Idaho, Montana, Nevada, Oregon, Utah, Washington) | All others: 800-277-4176, |

\*Service not yet available

# Sales of
# Veterinary Prescription Drugs

Concern over possible improper sales of veterinary prescription drugs by laymen has been expressed by veterinary groups and FDA officials. Veterinarians have certain legal and professional responsibilities when dispensing drugs. These responsibilities and a current list of veterinary drugs requiring the prescription legend   *To be used by or on the order of a licensed veterinarian*   are included in this discussion.

## A. LEGAL AND PROFESSIONAL RESPONSIBILITIES

1. **A veterinarian may use (administer and prescribe) any drug he or she can legally purchase.** A licensed veterinarian can prescribe and dispense without limitations so long as only the veterinarian and the client are involved. The veterinarian

assumes professional and legal responsibilities for prescribing and dispensing. The FDA assumes that the veterinarian knows and follows current recommendations for new drugs. The FDA also expects the veterinarian to prescribe only final-dosage forms of drugs for which a New Animal Drug Application (NADA) has been approved. Generally, only approved-dosage forms are available to the practitioner because the manufacturer may not legally sell a new product without previous approval of the product from the FDA. Thus, new drug preparations, including premixes for addition to medicated feeds, are not generally available to individual veterinarians or to feed manufacturers because they do not have NADAs approved by the FDA. A licensed veterinarian can buy an approved drug preparation (the final-dosage form) for dispensing to a client. However, without an approved NADA the veterinarian cannot buy a drug in pure form or as a feed premix for repackaging and routine product marketing.

2. **A veterinarian is responsible for the purity, safety, identity, and dosage of any dispensed drug he or she compounds.** The veterinarian is also responsible if the product differs in any way from the form in which it was originally marketed. If the package is dispensed unopened, the manufacturer shares responsibility with the veterinarian.

3. **Adequate directions must be provided for correct and effective use of a dispensed drug.** Specific, *written* directions should always be given; an original copy of the directions should be handed to the client and a copy kept for the practitioner's record and protection. As the public becomes more aware of residue problems, the provision of written directions assumes greater legal and professional importance.

4. **Oral directions are considered acceptable by the FDA.** However, a practitioner could seldom prove in court that adequate oral directions had been provided, except through favorable testimony by a witness to the event. A practicing veterinarian should *never* rely on oral directions.

5. **Directions for the use of drugs must be accurate so that a patient may be treated safely and effectively.** Consumers must be protected from drug-contaminated edible animal products and not be subjected to any hazard.

6. **Veterinary prescription drugs** — used only by or on the order of a *licensed veterinarian*; a summary:
   A) All tranquilizers, except those in animal feeds
   B) All controlled substances (Schedules I, II, III, IV, V)

C) Anticonvulsants

D) Muscle relaxants

E) Anesthetics in addition to barbiturates
   1) General anesthetics
   2) All injectable, local anesthetics (but not topical anesthetics used on the skin, in the eye, etc.)

F) Hormones
   1) *Corticosteroids* — when in injectable, ophthalmic, otic, and oral preparations, but *not* the intramammary topical, and intrauterine preparations
   2) *Estrogens* except when in feed
   3) *Anterior pituitary hormones*
   4) *Thyroid preparations or extracts,* except those used in feeds

G) Drugs that act on the autonomic nervous system. All injectables and oral preparations, but *not* the topical and ophthalmic products.

H) CNS stimulants

I) Certain antibiotics and antimicrobials

J) Certain anthelmintics

K) Drugs limited to prescription, based upon how they are administered
   1) Those labeled for intravenous administration to dogs, cats and other small animals
   2) Those labeled for intraarticular, intrathecal, epidural paravertebral, subconjunctival, or retrobulbar administration
   3) Those labeled for intraperitoneal injection in horses

## B. WHERE TO FILE COMPLAINTS OF ILLEGAL PRESCRIPTION-DRUG USE AND OTHER COMPLAINTS

Complaints should be lodged with the Compliance Officer at the nearest FDA office. These offices are listed in the telephone directory under "United States Government."

Current list of veterinary drugs requiring the prescription legend — the drugs listed are to be used only by or on the order of a *licensed veterinarian*. (List furnished by Dr. F. Edward Sterner, Regional Veterinary Medical Officer, Denver, Colorado and dated 6-9-78.)

## Veterinary Prescription Drugs
### (Alphabetical Listing of Specific Drugs)

A-H
Acepromazine
Adrenomone
Albamast
Albaplex
Albon
Amforol
Amoxi-Drop
Amoxi-Tabs
Amoxicillin*
Amp-Equine
Amphicol-V
Ampi – Tab
Ampi-Bol
Ampi-Ject
Anacetin
Anaprime
Anocol
Aquachel
Aquamycin
Aristovet
Arquel
Arsenamide Sodium
Azimycin
Azium
Azra-Bute
Bac-Neo-Poly
Bac-Neo-Polymyxin
　　Hydrocortisone
Bactrovet
Banamine
Bemacol
Benza-Pen
Betasone
Betavet
Bicillin
Bio-Delta
Bio-Mycin
Bio-Mycin-C
Bio-Tal

Biocycline
Biosol Sterile Solution
Bizolin
Bo-Se
Boviclox
Brevane
Buta-Phen
Butamed
Butatron
Butazolidin
Camvet
Canopar
Cap-O-Mycin
Caparsolate Sodium
Carbocaine HCL with
　　Suprarenin
Carcide
Caytine
Centrine
Chemichloro
Chlora-Tabs
Chloral-Mycin
Chloramphenicol
Chlorasol
Chlorasone
Chlorbiotic
Chloricol
Chloromycetin
Chloropent
Chorionic Gonadotropin*
Chortropin
Combi Pen
Combisteroid
Combot
Combuthal
Conofite
Conderm
Cortaba
Corti-Fluorosone
Cortisate-20

Crystiben
Crysticillin 300 A.S.
Curecal-Feline
Cyclaine
Cypip
Cystorelin
Cytobin
D. N. P.
D. E. C.-Sol
Dantafur
Darbazine
Debrin
Dec
Delta Albaplex
Delta-Cortef
Depo-Medrol
Depo-Penicillin
Dermathycin
Dix-A-Vet
Dexa P/S
Dexa Sone-Biotic
Dexa-Di-Pen
Dexa-Pen-Mycin
Dexam-2
Dexameth-A-Vet
Dexamethasone*
Dexamycin
Dexasone
Dexate
Di-Pen
Diathal
Dicloxin
Dilantin
Dinz
Diquel
Dirocide
Disomer Chronotabs
Diuril
Dizan
Domoso

* Generic

Dopram-V
Dornavac
Dry-Clox
Dui-Pen
Duracillin AS
DV-202
DV-201
Dyrex
E-SE
Ectoral
Elanone-V
Entromycin
Equi Bute
Equi-Thesin
Equigel
Equipoise
Equiproxen
Equizole
F.S.H.-F.
Ferti-Cept
Filaramide
Filaribitis
Filaricide
Flo-Cillin
Flucort
Flucorticin
Fluosmin
Fluothane
Follutein
Formula 888
Freed
Fulvicin U/F
Fulvidex
Furadantin
Gastrografin
Gecolate
Gentocin
Glo-Vet
Glycodex
Golden-Bute
Grysio
Hanazone
Hanomycin
Hava-Span
Havidote
Hetacin K
Histavet-P
Histosol
Hycholin
Hydeltrone
Hydrozide
Hypaque-VM
Innovar-Vet

Instilin 10 X
Intragel
Jenotone
Kanfosone
Kantrim
Kay-Cycline-V
Keflex
Keflodin
Kemithal
Ketaset
Ketaset Plus
Kymar
L-SE
Lactate
Lasix
Lincocin
Liquamycin Injectable for
    Anaplasmosis or Anthrax
Liquamycin Intramuscular
Liquamycin 100 for
    Anaplasmosis or Anthrax
Liquichlor
Liquisone F
Longicil
Longipen
Loridine
Maolate
Medacide SDM
Medi-Pets of Primidone
Medichol
Medrol
Mesulfin
Methagon
Meticillin-S
Meticortelone
Meticorten
Metimyd
Metofane
Midicel
Mikedimide
Milibis-V
Mu-Se
Mychel-Vet
Mylepsin
M50-50 Diprenorphane
M99 Etorphene
Nalline
Naloxone
Naquasone
Narcan
Neo Predef
Neo-Aristocort
Neo-Aristovet

Neo-Cartef with Tetracaine
Neo-Darbazine
Neo-Delta Cartef
Neo-Delta-Cartef with Tetracaine
Neo-Predef with Tetracaine
Neo-Synalar
Neobacimyx
Neobacimyx-H
Neobiotic
Neomyxin-F
Nolvapent
Nortran
Numorphan
Omnipen
Ophthaine
Optiprime Opthakote
Optisone
Orbenin
Orbenin DC
Osborn Butatron
Osborn Viceton
Osteum
Ovaban
Oxyject 50
Oxyject 100
Oxysteclin
P.L.H.
P.O.P.
P/M Brand Dexamethone
P/M Chloramphenicol
P/M Pen B&G
P/M Sterociotic
P/M Tetracycline
Palosein
Panacur
Panolog
Panmycin
Parvex Plus
Parvex Suspension
Penicillin VK
Pentosol
Pharmatran
Phen-Buta-Vet
Phenyl-B
Phenylbutazone*
Phenyzone-E
Polyflex
Polyotic Oblets
Predef
Prednis-A-Vet
Prednisolone*
Predsem
Primidone

* Generic

Princillin
Pro Pen G
Pro Pen G in Dihydrostrep
    Sol with Dex & Chl Mal
Proban Cythioate
Procaine Penicillin in
    Dihydrostreptomycin*
Promazine
Prostin F2 Alpha
Protamone-D
Protopam
Psymod
Pyraminth
Quartermaster Dry Cow
Ramosone
Rea-Cil
Recovr
Renazide
Renografin-76
Renovist
Rheaform
Ripercol L-Piperazine
Robaxin
Robaxin-V
Robinul-V
Robizone-V
Rompun
S.E.Z.
Scolaban
Sel-E-Vit B
Sel-E-Vit O
Seleen Suspension
Seletoc
Sernylan
Serpasil
Sodium Pentobarbital*
Sodium Thiopental*
Solu-Delta Cortef

Somnopentyl
Sparine
Spectam
Spectinomycin Injectable*
Spectinomycin Tablet*
Stiglyn
Strekacin
Strongid T
Styrid Caricide
Sudine
Sul-Thi-Dine
Suldixine
Spanbolet II
Sulfamylon-N
Sulfixine
Sulmet Sterile Solution
Supra-Sulfa
Surital
Symbio
Synalar
Sychrocept
Synotic
Synsac
T-61 Euthanasia
Task
Telmin
Temaril-P
Terramycin Injectable for
    Anaplasmosis or Anthrax*
Terramycin Potentiated*
Terramycin Vet Capsules*
Tetra-D
Tetra-Drops
Tetrachel-Vet
Tetracycline Capsules*
Tetracyn Ointment
Tevcocin
Tevcodyne

Therazone
Thorazine
Tinavet
Topical Tritop
Toptic
Toxital
Tranvet
Tresaderm
Tri-Optic S
Tribodine
Tribrissen
Tylocine
Tylocine Sulfa
Unitop
Uteracon
Utonex
V-Cillin-K
Veesyn Covotab
Veesyn Granules
Vet-Kem T-113
Vetalar
Vetalog
Vetame
Vetamethasone
Vetamox
Veticol
Vetisulid
Vetocin
Vetrachloracin 1%
Vetropolycin
Voren Suspension
Westazon
Whipcide
Winstrol-V
Xytoxin
Yomesan
Zenadrid
Zonometh

---

* Generic

# Responsibility in the Use of Drugs

In summary, the veterinarian's responsibility in the use of drugs falls into three categories:

1. **The legal category.** A veterinarian may be prosecuted for violating the law under the Federal Food, Drug and Cosmetic Act and its amendments, the Controlled Substances Act, and any applicable state drug laws. The veterinarian may also encounter legal problems and be sued for malpractice as a result of improperly using a drug on a patient.

2. **Safety of the patient.** Of primary concern for the veterinarian is the health of the animal being treated. In addition, the veterinarian must be concerned about whether the drug actions might influence the animal's productivity. Last, the veterinarian must be concerned about the possibility of a drug altering the value of an animal as a companion.

3. **Human health hazards.** This broad category includes such things as drug residues in meat, milk and eggs, and accidents related to administering drugs to the animals—such as being bitten, scratched, kicked, or fallen on. Does the way these drugs are used on animals have an impact on the environment? For example, a controversy exists over the widespread use of feed-additive levels of antibiotics. Does that practice constitute a potential human health hazard via the transfer of resistance from animal bacteria to human pathogens?

A. **FOLLOW LABEL INSTRUCTIONS.**

1. **Labeling for new drugs is approved by FDA — the product must be approved for** *safety* **and** *efficacy* according to information reported by the manufacturer.

2. **Manufacturer will not accept responsibility — the product** must be used as specified or for the condition covered when approved new-drug labeling was submitted to FDA. (Same would apply to other drugs.)

B. **INFORM CLIENT OF PROPER WITHDRAWAL TIMES.**

1. **In meat, milk or egg producing animals**
2. **When drug is administered by veterinarian**
3. **When drug is administered by owner — as follow-up and** original treatment
4. **When drugs are used in feed or water**
5. **Animal I.D. tape may be used**

The Michigan Veterinary Medical Association has devised a way to identify animals treated with drugs requiring a preslaughter withdrawal or milk-discard period. The yellow-and-black tag is pictured here.

| | | |
|---|---|---|
| **PLACE AROUND TAIL OR LEG** | **WARNING          WARNING          WARNING**<br>THIS ANIMAL HAS BEEN TREATED WITH A MEDICATION THAT PRODUCES<br>A TEMPORARY RESIDUE<br><br>**DO NOT SELL MILK UNTIL AFTER:**_____<br><br>**DO NOT SLAUGHTER UNTIL:**_____<br><br>SUPPLIED BY MICHIGAN VETERINARY MEDICAL ASSOCIATION | **AFFIX ADHESIVE SIDES TOGETHER** |

The Association recommends using a waterproof marking pen to record the appropriate date. The tag should be affixed to an area of the tail or leg where it will not be obscured by mud or dirt.

The idea of supplying the tags on a continuous tape was conceived by Dr. Arnold F. Hentschl, DVM, Harbor Beach, Michigan. An 80-tag roll of tape and a dispenser are available from the Association for $2.25; a box of 12 rolls is $24.00 plus postage. Contact: Mrs. Pat Loomis, c/o The Michigan Veterinary Medical Assn., 1314 Waukazoo Drive, Holland. Michigan 49423.

C. **WHEN USING DRUGS OTHER THAN AS LABELED** (*e.g.*, a drug labeled for human use; a veterinary drug used other than as labeled, or "no label" [the veterinarian's own compounded mixture]):

 1. **You have a responsibility to your client** — use the best possible therapy available.

 2. **Use sound professional judgment** — you alone are responsible.

 3. **Assure sufficient withdrawal time if the drug is used in food-producing animals.** Base your decision on scientific pharmacokinetic data and not on hearsay.

 4. **Observe animal closely for any unexpected side reactions.**

D. **KNOW MEDICAL HISTORY OF ANIMALS TREATED.**

 1. **What drugs or chemicals has the animal been given for at least one week?**

    2. What medications are in animals' feeds — low levels for feed efficiency, estrus regulation, etc.?

    3. Any treatment for parasites within the prior week?

E. **KNOW THE PHARMACOLOGICAL ACTIONS OF ALL DRUGS USED IN COMBINATION.**

    1. If several drugs are given, know if they are compatible or counteracting; *e.g.*, penicillin-streptomycin are compatible and synergistic; phenothiazine-derivative tranquilizers and organophosphate wormers used simultaneously are potentially toxic.

    2. Know if drugs will potentiate or have no effect on each other.

    3. Some drugs are incompatible when mixed together; *e.g.*, sulfonamides and calcium solutions.

F. **BEWARE OF POSSIBLE SIDE REACTIONS.**

    1. Inform owner or lay assistants of what to look for.

    2. Know what antidote might be used to alleviate a reaction. Dispense the antidote to the owner whenever appropriate; *e.g.*, epinephrine for anaphylaxis.

G. **REPORT ADVERSE REACTIONS OR LACK OF EFFICACY.**
Report to the FDA via "Alert to Adverse Reaction" card, and to manufacturer via detail person or supplier or direct by phone if:

    1. Animal has reaction not listed in labeling

    2. Drug does not give the proper effect when used as directed

    3. Drugs are not compatible and the label has no warning

H. **ADVISE CLIENT ON PROPER USE OF DISPENSED DRUGS.**

    1. Assure yourself that client has been properly instructed.

    2. Alert client to possible side reactions.

    3. Inform client to observe withdrawal times.

I. **RESPECT THE PRESCRIPTION AND CONTROL DRUG LEGENDS.**

    1. Do not dispense a prescription drug unless you have properly diagnosed the conditions for which the drug is to be used — make sure the client is capable of using the drug properly.

    2. Keep records of purchase and use of Schedule II drugs.

# References for
# Veterinary Pharmacology

A. **COMPENDIA**

**United States Pharmacopeia** (USP) and **National Formulary** (NF) are now combined. They provide official standards for quality and purity and are reference standards for assay and testing. They are not particularly useful to practitioners as reference but indirectly are important because they set up standards of drug quality for the pharmaceutical industry.

B. **REFERENCE SOURCES**

1. **Merck Index of Chemicals and Drugs;** Merck and Company.
   Gives chemistry information such as structural and empiric formulae and nomenclature, and medicinal uses (where applicable) with key references to both.

2. **Physicians Desk Reference** (PDR); Medical Economics Co.
   Published annually for human drugs. Lists drugs under the name of each pharmaceutical company, giving indications, dosages, contraindications, warnings and how supplied.

3. **Facts and Comparisons;** Facts and Comparisons, Inc.
   Revised pages issued each month. Human drugs are grouped by system usage. Same type of information as PDR but adds a comparison of the cost of similar compounds. Human drugs.

4. **Handbook of Veterinary Drugs;** Rossoff; Springer Publishing Co.
   A) Lists and discusses some 1800 drugs
      1) Generic and trade names
      2) General action(s)
      3) Use, doses (all species), warnings

5. **The Complete Desk Reference of Veterinary Pharmaceuticals and Biologicals;** Aronson; Harwal Publishing Co.
   Drugs are cross-referenced and listed by name and by manufacturer. Product information section: Composition, Indications, Therapeutic Activity, Pharmacology, Dosage, Precautions, How Supplied. Patterned after PDR. An excellent source of information.

C. **SELECTED BOOKS**

1. **Veterinary**
   A) **Veterinary Pharmacology and Therapeutics, 4th ed.** Jones; Iowa State University Press.
   B) **Current Veterinary Therapy VI.** Kirk; W.B. Saunders Co.

      C) **Drug Dosage in Laboratory Animal.** Barnes; University of California Press.

      D) **Principles of Drug Disposition in Domestic Animals.** Baggot; W.B. Saunders Co.

      E) **Veterinary Applied Pharmacology and Therapeutics.** Brander; Williams and Wilkins Co.

  2. **Human**

      A) **The Pharmacological Basis of Therapeutics.** Goodman and Gillman; Macmillan Publishing Co.

      B) **Medical Pharmacology.** Goth; C.V. Mosby Co.

      C) **Review of Medical Pharmacology.** Myers; Lange Medical Publications.

      D) **Handbook of Pharmacology.** Cutting; Appleton-Century-Crofts.

# Marketing of Pharmaceuticals

The trend in industry is to large parent companies with separate divisions based upon their sales policies or marketing areas.

| Parent Company (Human Sales) | Sales to Graduate Veterinarians* | Animal Health (Over-the-Counter Sales) |
|---|---|---|
| Burroughs Wellcome | Wellcome/Jen Sal | Cooper/Rocking R |
| Upjohn | Upjohn | Tuco |
| SmithKline & French | Norden | SKF |
| American Home Products | Fort Dodge | Wyeth |

*The statement *Sales to Graduate Veterinarians Only* on the label is not a legal requirement but is only a statement of the company's sales policy.

A. **SOURCES OF DRUGS** — veterinarians can buy drugs from many sources, depending upon the company that manufactures the product.

  1. **Direct from the company** — detail person or salespersons

  2. **Company branches** — situated in major cities

  3. **Distributors** — usually carry the products of several different companies

  4. **Companies that sell generic drugs, or mail-order houses**

B.  NOMENCLATURE
   1.  **Drug names**
       A) *Code* — pharmaceutical company identification term; usu-
          ally letters plus a number. SKF525A is an example.
       B) *Chemical* — based upon chemical structure; *e.g.*, sodium
          5-ethyl, 5-(1-methyl butyl) barbiturate.

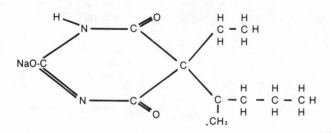

       C) *Generic or nonproprietary name* — picked by the company
          but is not exclusive; *e.g.* pentobarbital sodium.
       D) *Trade or proprietary name* — picked by the company and
          when registered is the company's exclusive property; *e.g.*
          Nembutal®, Diabutal®, Napental® (several manufac-
          turers).
   2.  **Patented drugs** (proprietary drugs or trade-name drugs). A com-
       pany that develops a new drug usually patents the chemical
       compound. Then, for 17 years, the compound is protected
       by law and the company has exclusive marketing rights.
       Those rights may be negotiated to allow another company to
       market the compound by paying the original company a
       royalty.
   3.  **Generic drugs.** These are compounds that either were never pa-
       tented or for which the patent has expired. Such drugs may
       be marketed under their generic names by other companies.
       Those companies may register trade names of their own but
       may not use the original trade name.

# Administering, Prescribing, and Dispensing Drugs

A. **PHARMACOTHERAPY MUST BE BASED UPON:**
   1. **An accurate diagnosis**
   2. **An understanding of the way the disease has altered the animal's anatomy and physiology;** *i.e.* the form and function of a diseased animal.
   3. **A thorough understanding** — an ability to apply the basic principles of pharmacology to set up a treatment regimen.

B. **SPECIFIC THERAPY** — This is the ultimate, but it is not always possible. Symptomatic and supportive treatments are important when used judiciously.
   1. **Harm never** — "Above all, do no harm" (Hippocrates).
   2. **Cure when possible**
   3. **Relieve often**
   4. **Comfort always**
   5. **Remember how much you do not know** — "Do not pour strange medicines into your patient" (Sir William Osler).

C. **FIXED DRUG COMBINATIONS** — tend to polypharmacy. Some of the problems are:
   1. **The practitioner did not select the ingredients and their concentrations** — the company has set these for its products (fixed-dose combinations).
   2. **Relative dose of each ingredient is fixed.**
   3. **Practitioners tend to use "name" drugs rather than selecting the most beneficial drug(s),** based upon knowledge of medicine and clinical pharmacology.
   4. **FDA takes a dim view of fixed drug combinations** . However, some are beneficial and pharmacologically rational; *e.g.* trimethoprim/sulfonamide combinations.

D. **INCOMPATIBILITY** — some drugs must not be used together because one of the following types of incompatibilities may arise.
   1. **Chemical** — the ingredients may react when brought together; a new and different compound results.
   2. **Physical or pharmaceutical** — the ingredients may change their physical state when combined; *e.g.* cloudy, precipitate, etc.
   3. **Therapeutic** — the actions of the drugs are antagonistic.

4. **Toxic** — combinations may be toxic even though each drug is safe when given alone and in the same dose.

E. **DISPENSING OF DRUGS**

1. Respect prescription drug laws.

2. Respect controlled drug laws.

3. Give written directions; *i.e.* dose, how given, how often, dangers, and withdrawal times for food-producing animals.

F. **WRITING THE PRESCRIPTION**

1. Write legibly.

2. Keep a copy.

3. Include DEA number when needed.

4. When desirable, make sure that either the number of doses, the label directions, or both, dictate the duration of therapy.

5. Make sure the species appears on the prescription — present knowledge of comparative pharmacology dictates this.

6. State your refill policy.

7. State whether drug name is to appear on dispensed label.

8. Proofread.

9. Latin words and phrases — commonly used in prescription writing are listed below.

| Abbreviation | Latin | English Meaning |
|---|---|---|
| ad lib. | *ad libitum* | as desired |
| b.i.d. | *bis in die* | twice a day |
| ft. | *fiat* | make |
| h. | *hora* | hour |
| m. | *misce* | mix |
| q.i.d. | *quater in die* | four times a day |
| q.s. | *quantum sufficit* | as much as needed |
| sig. or S. | *signa* | label |
| sol. | *solutio* | solution |
| tab. | *tabella* | tablet |
| t.i.d. | *ter in die* | three times a day |
| o.d. | *omnie die* | daily |
| s.i.d. | *semel in die* | once a day |
| cap | | capsule |

10.**Format for writing prescriptions.** (*See* below.)
  A) Heading
    Name and address of doctor, date issued
    Name and address of client
    Species of animal
  B) Superscription is the recipe (you take): Rx.
  C) Inscription contains a message or the ingredients: names of drugs and amounts.
  D) Subscription or the directions to the pharmacist: how to prepare; usually not necessary as you will prescribe a prepared product.
  E) Label (Sig)"you write": directions to patient; what the pharmacist puts on the label.
  F) DEA No.____. Signature (name and degree).
11.**A typical prescription:**

---

Telephone   123-4567                date _____

DAN W. UPSON, D.V.M.
    201 Cedar Drive                Manhattan, Kansas

Client's Name_____Address_____
Species_____Age_____Sex_____

Rx                                                       g or ml

  Sig.

Refill____times
Label____(yes or no)

_____        _____ D.V.M.
DEA No.

---

12.**Pharmaceutical arithmetic and metrology**
  A) Metric system is based upon the meter (metre)
    1) 1 centimeter = 1/100 meter (0.01 m)
    2) 1 gram (g) = 1/1000 of the mass of 1 liter of water
    3) 1 liter = the volume of 1 kilogram of pure water
    4) 1 cubic centimeter (cc) = a cube; 1 cm is the length of each edge. The cube will hold 1 g of water.
    5) 1000 cc = 1 liter and 1/1000 of a liter = 1 ml; thus 1 cc = 1 ml = 1 g water

B) Mass

| 1000 | $10^3$ g | = | kilogram (kg) |
|---|---|---|---|
| 1.0 | $10^0$ g | = | gram (g) |
| 0.001 | $10^{-3}$ g | = | milligram (mg) |
| 0.000001 | $10^{-6}$ g | = | microgram (μg) |
| | | | gamma |
| | $10^{-9}$ g | = | nanogram (ng) |
| | $10^{-12}$ g | = | picogram (pg or μμg) |

C) Capacity—Volume

| 1000 | cc = liter (l) |
|---|---|
| 1.0 | cc = milliliter (ml, cc) |
| 0.001 | cc = microliter (μl) lambda |

13. **Percentage solutions** — some authorities insist that the weight-weight (w/w) method is the only way to make accurate percentage solutions. Other authorities prefer the weight-volume (w/v) method. The USP prescribes a practical method of making the pharmacy practice uniform. In defining standards, the expression *percent* is used, according to circumstances, with one of three different meanings:

A) Percent weight in volume (w/v) expresses the number of grams of a constituent in 100 ml of solution.

B) Percent weight in weight (w/w) expresses the number of grams of a constituent in 100 g of solution.

C) Percent volume in volume (v/v) expresses the number of milliliters of a constituent in 100 ml of solution.

The USP specifies: "The term *percent* used in prescriptions without qualification means . . . for solutions or suspensions of solids in liquids, *percent weight in volume*; for solutions of liquids in liquids, percent volume in volume; and for solutions of gases in liquids, percent weight in volume."

14. **To prepare a weight-in-volume (w/v) percentage solution:**

A) Multiply the desired number of milliliters of solution by the percent expressed as a whole number.

B) Divide the product by 100. The quotient will be the number of grams of drug required.

C) To the required number of grams of drug, add enough solvent to make the desired number of milliliters of finished solution.

15. Solution concentration

| Percent | mg/ml | Solution |
|---------|-------|----------|
| 100.0 | 1000.0 | 1-1 |
| 10.0 | 100.0 | 1-10 |
| 1.0 | 10.0 | 1-100 |
| 0.1 | 1.0 | 1-1,000 |
| 0.01 | 0.1 | 1-10,000 |
| 0.001 | 0.01 | 1-100,000 |
| 0.0001 | 0.001 | 1-1,000,000 |

16. **Concentrations of drug in percentage solutions**
    1 g drug / 1 ml water  =   100% solution
    1 g drug / 100 ml water  =    1% solution
    1000 mg drug / 100 ml water  =    1% solution
    10 mg drug / 1 ml water  =   1% solution

17. **Problems involving ratio** — to make a ratio solution (1:20, 1:500, 1:2,000, etc.) with metric measures:
    A) Divide the desired number of milliliters of solution by the larger number of the ratio. The quotient will be the number of grams of drug to be used.
    B) Add to the required number of grams of drug enough solvent to make the desired number of milliliters.

18. **Parts per million (PPM)**
    1 PPM = 1 mg/liter or 1 mg/1000 g
    1 PPM = 1 $\mu$g/ml
    1 PPM = 0.0001%
    1 oz of sand in 31¼ tons of cement is 1 PPM
    A book 1/16 in. is 1 PPM of a stack 1 mile high
    1 minute is 1 PPM of 1.9 years

19. **Parts per billion (PPB)**
    1 PPB = 1 $\mu$g/liter or 1 ng/ml or 1 ng/g
    1 PPB = 0.0000001%

20. **Approximate equivalents**

| 1 Quart | 1 liter | 1000 ml |
|---|---|---|
| 1 Pint | 16 ounces | 1 lb(HOH)500 ml |
| 1 Glass | 8 fluid oz | 240 ml |
| 1 Teacup | 4 fluid oz | 120 ml |
| 1 Tablespoon | 0.5 ounce | 15 ml |
| 1 Teaspoon | 1 fluid dram | 5 ml |
| 15 Drops (water) | 15 minims | 1 ml |
|  | 2.2 lb | 1 kg |
|  | 1 grain (gr) | 65 mg |
|  | 1 ounce | 30 ml |

21. **HAVE and NEED** — conversion system for pharmaceutical calculations.
   A) Set down and label:

   | HAVE | NEED |
   |---|---|

   B)                                   Convert to workable units

   C) Convert to units to match NEED
   D) Solve

   1) Example:
      a) 5 gr tab          ?_____HOH to give a 3.25% sol.
      b)                   3.25% sol. = 32.5 mg/ml
      c) 5 gr = 325 mg
      d) 325 mg ÷ 32.5 mg/ml = 10 ml HOH

22. **Reduction of stock solutions.** To make a more dilute solution from a concentrated one, the following equation is useful.

$$\frac{\% \text{ Desired} \times \text{Volume Desired}}{\% \text{ Available}} = \text{Volume of Concentrate Needed}$$

# Medication for Individual or Herd Treatment

A. **FACTORS INFLUENCING WATER CONSUMPTION**
   1. **Environmental temperature and humidity**
   2. **Character of feed** — high protein content, high proportion of fiber, or dryness increases water consumption.
   3. **Illness** — can markedly increase or decrease water intake.

## B. AVERAGE DAILY WATER CONSUMPTION

### 1. Chickens                 Gallons/100 Birds

| | |
|---|---|
| 4 weeks old. | 2.0 |
| 8 weeks old. | 4.1 |
| 12 weeks old. | 5.5 |
| Non-laying hens. | 5.0 |
| Laying hens (moderate temperatures). | 5.0-7.5 |
| Laying hens (90 F). | 9.0 |

### 2. Swine                 Gallons/Head

| | |
|---|---|
| 30 lb body weight | 0.6-1.2 |
| 60-80 lb body weight. | 0.84 |
| 75-125 lb body weight. | 2.00 |
| 200-230 lb body weight. | 1.4-3.6 |
| Pregnant sows. | 3.6-4.5 |
| Lactating sows. | 4.8-6.0 |

### 3. Cattle                 Gallons/Head

| | |
|---|---|
| Dairy calves (4-8 weeks old). | 1-1.5 |
| Dairy calves (12-20 weeks old). | 2-4.5 |
| Dairy calves (26 weeks old). | 3-6 |
| Dairy heifer (pregnant). | 7-10 |
| Stress or feeder calves (maintenance). | 4-6 |
| Steer (fattening ration). | 8-10 |
| Range cattle. | 10-12 |
| Dairy cow (maintenance or low production). | 12-15 |
| Dairy cow (lactation). | 15-25 |

### 4. Turkeys                 Gallons/100 Birds

| | |
|---|---|
| 4 weeks old. | 3.0 |
| 8 weeks old. | 7.1 |
| 12 weeks old. | 10.6 |
| 18 weeks old. | 14.0 |

### 5. Sheep                 Gallons/Head*

| | |
|---|---|
| Lambs (on hay or pasture and grain ration trace). | 0.8 |
| Ewes. | 1.0 |
| Lactating ewes. | 1.5 |

*Sheep on good pasture may drink little or no water.

## C. AVERAGE DAILY WATER CONSUMPTION

1. **Swine, horses and poultry** — consume about 2 to 3 lb water/lb dry feed eaten.
2. **Cattle and sheep** — drink 3 to 4 lb water/ lb dry matter eaten.

## D. TO CALCULATE CAPACITY OF TANKS AND TROUGHS IN GALLONS

**CIRCULAR TANK:**

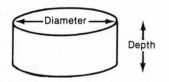

Diameter x Diameter x Depth x 5.86 = No. Gals.

**RECTANGULAR TANK:**

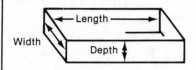

Width x Depth x Length x 7.46 = No. Gals.

**ROUND-END TANK:**

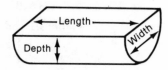

Width x Depth x Length x 2.93 = No. Gals.

**V-END TROUGH:**

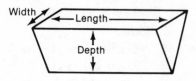

Width x Depth x Length x 3.73 = No. Gals.

---

**STOCK TANK CAPACITIES**
**Height: 2 Feet**

| CIRCULAR TYPE | | ROUND-END TYPE | | |
|---|---|---|---|---|
| Dia (Ft) | Cap (Gal) | Width (Ft) | Length (Ft) | Cap (Gal) |
| 3 | 100 | 2 | 4 | 95 |
| 3½ | 140 | 2 | 5 | 120 |
| 4 | 185 | 2 | 6 | 140 |
| 4½ | 235 | 2 | 7 | 185 |
| 5 | 290 | 2 | 8 | 195 |
| 5½ | 350 | 2 | 10 | 250 |
| 6 | 420 | 3 | 5 | 175 |
| 6½ | 495 | 3 | 6 | 220 |
| 7 | 570 | 3 | 7 | 260 |
| 7½ | 660 | 3 | 8 | 300 |
| 8 | 750 | 3 | 10 | 385 |
| 9 | 950 | 3 | 12 | 475 |
| 10 | 1170 | 3 | 14 | 560 |

# Routes of Drug Administration

Many factors influence the choice of route by which a drug is given.

1. **Therapeutic considerations**
   A) Rapidity of onset of desired action
   B) Duration of desired action
   C) Site of action the drug must reach in animal's body in order to be effective

2. **Physical-chemical properties of the drug are important considerations** — *e.g.*, irritation to tissues, solubility, and whether the drug is a weak acid or a weak base.

A. **ORAL** (*per os, per orum*, by mouth)

1. **Usually slower onset of action than by injection**
2. **Gives longer duration of action**
3. **Requires a larger dose than by injection because**
   A) of species variation in digestive tracts. For example, the oral dose in a ruminant animal is subject to dilution (40-50 gal. vat) and bacterial degradation.
   B) oral dose is absorbed into the blood from the gut, then goes through the liver before entering the general circulation. Intraperitoneal injections are also absorbed by this system and must pass through the liver. In the liver, drugs may be inactivated by drug-metabolizing enzymes; hence less drug in the active form enters the general circulation.
   C) of loss of nonabsorbed drug with the feces.
4. **Relatively safer because of slower absorption**
5. **Limitations** — vomiting, diarrhea, and destruction by digestive juices greatly reduce the amount of drug absorbed.
6. **A common route of administration in veterinary medicine**

B. **PARENTERAL** (all forms of injection)

1. **Intravenous (IV) (venoclysis)**
   A) High initial blood levels
   B) Fastest onset of action of any route commonly used
   C) Usually shortest duration of action
   D) Should be given slowly
   E) Irritating drugs can be given by this route
2. **Intraperitoneal (IP)**
   A) Variable onset and duration. The drug enters portal circulation and passes through the liver before entering general circulation.

   B) May be detrimental to best interests of the animal and owner. IP injection may cause tissue damage and adhesions, leading to illness and/or excessive carcass trimming. It may cause electrolyte imbalance and peritonitis, may enter other organs, and may be very painful—all of which can lead to a shock-like condition.

3. **Intramuscular** (IM)
   A) Relatively rapid onset
   B) Duration longer than IV
   C) Duration may be altered by the choice of vehicle, by altering the particulate make-up of the drug, or by adding organic groups to the drug molecule.

4. **Subcutaneous** (SC) (hypodermoclysis)
   A) Slightly slower in onset than IM
   B) Duration may be a little longer than IM because of slower absorption.

5. **Intraarterial**
   A) Injection may be made into an artery leading directly to a specific organ or tissue site.
   B) Extra-fast action
   C) Gives high levels in the specific site; usually gives lower systemic levels
   D) May happen by *mistake*. For example, intracarotid injection instead of intrajugular. Drug goes straight to brain in high concentration.

6. **Epidural**
   A) Used for spinal anesthesia in animals
   B) Intrathecal or intraspinal for injection into spinal fluid

7. **Intrapleural and Intrapulmonary**
   A) Rapid blood levels are reached.
   B) Tissue damage may result (controversial).
   C) Cats and debilitated small animals may require this route.

8. **Intramedullary** (bone marrow injection)
   A) Injection sites are sternum in man, femur in dog and cat.
   B) Rapid blood level
   C) Not common in veterinary medicine

9. **Intradermal**
   A) Injection is made between the dermis and epidermis.
   B) Slow release into blood, and blood levels are low.
   C) Action may be prolonged because of slow absorption.

10. **Subcutaneous implantation**
    A) Slow release
    B) Long duration

    C) Low blood levels

11. Parenteral solutions

    A) Injection should be carefully handled and, before using, should be carefully checked.

    B) Must be sterile.

    C) Must not have any precipitate. Suspensions may be given IM or SC, but not IV.

    D) For all parenteral routes except IV, solutions must not be irritating, unusually acid, or unusually alkaline.

    E) Should not be at extreme of temperature when given.

C. **INHALATION** — many drugs may be given via inspired air.

    1. **Anesthetics**

    2. **Bronchodilators**

    3. **Antibiotics**

    4. **Therapeutic gases**

    5. **May provide very rapid blood levels**

    6. **May also be important toxicologically**

D. **TOPICAL** — applies to drugs put on the skin and mucous membranes. Local action is usually intended. Some must be non-irritating. Some are irritating or caustic in order to produce a desired action. Some absorption of certain drugs is possible. Absorption depends not only on the active substance and site of application, but also on the vehicle used.

    1. **Skin** — important site of application. Oily vehicles increase absorption, whereas water vehicles tend to diminish absorption. Most drugs are not well absorbed through intact skin.

    2. **Mucosa** — the drug is put in contact with mucous membranes.

        A) *Sublingual* — the drug (tablet) is placed under the tongue, but not swallowed.

            1) Important difference in route of absorption into the general circulation. Skips the portal system and hence the drug-inactivating enzymes of the liver.

            2) May be rapid. Nitroglycerin is used sublingually for angina in man. The action begins as soon as 20 seconds.

        B) *Rectum* — certain drugs are absorbed readily into blood through the rectal mucosa.

        C) *Nasal septum* — certain drugs are absorbed readily into blood.

        D) *Urethra* — little drug is absorbed into the blood.

        E) *Uterus* — with some drugs (sulfonamides and antibiotics) absorption into the blood may be considerable.

F) *Vagina* — variable absorption, some drugs may be absorbed.
G) *Bladder* — some absorption into blood occurs.
H) *Intramammary* — many drugs are well absorbed into blood by back-diffusion.
I) *Ophthalmic* — rapid absorption may occur when drugs are placed on the surface of the eye and/or reach the conjunctival membranes.

# Absorption and Distribution of Drugs

In order to reach its site of action, a drug must move across a succession of membranes. In the process of being metabolized and/or excreted the drug must pass another succession of membranes. Example: an orally administered tranquilizer crosses the gastrointestinal epithelium (*absorption*); the blood-brain barrier, the individual brain cell membrane, the subcellular membrane boundaries (*action*); the subcellular membrane, the brain cell membrane, the liver cell membrane, the endoplasmic reticulum membrane (*inactivation*); the liver cell membrane, glomerular membrane of kidney and/or the kidney tubule cell membrane (*excretion*).

A. **ACTION** — directly related to the *concentration* of *free* (nonprotein-bound) drug at the site of action. The concentration of free drug at the site of action is directly related to the *dosage* regimen, but it also depends upon:

1. **Extent and rate of absorption from site of administration into blood**
2. **Distribution to various tissues of the body**
3. **Plasma binding and tissue binding** (localization)
4. **Rate of biotransformation and/or excretion**

B. **PRINCIPLES OF MEMBRANE TRANSPORT**
1. **Passive transport**
   A) Two methods
      1) Filtration through pores in the membrane
      2) Dissolving into the membrane. These membranes have a high lipid content. *Most* drugs move by this route. They dissolve into one side of the membrane, then move through and out the other side.
   B) Transfer is proportional to:
      1) Concentration gradient across the membrane

        2) Lipid solubility of the drug, or how readily it dissolves into the membrane

        3) Degree of ionization—ratio of ionized to non-ionized drug

  2. **Active transport**

    A) *Uphill* — the drug moves against a concentration gradient.

    B) *Facilitated diffusion* — the drug moves with the concentration gradient but at a rate faster than could be accomplished with passive diffusion.

      1) Selective

      2) Mediated by carrier systems and enzymes

      3) Requires energy

      4) May be inhibited by low body temperature

      5) May be inhibited by metabolic poisons

      6) May be competitively inhibited by chemically similar compounds

      7) May be saturated by high concentrations of drug

C . **VARIABLES INFLUENCING DRUG MOVEMENT ACROSS MEMBRANES**

  1. **Physiochemical properties of the drug** — important attributes influencing drug movement are:

    A) Size and shape of molecule

    B) Lipid solubility

    C) Degree of ionization

  2. **Most drugs are in the non-ionized form when they cross membranes.**

  3. **Ionized or non-ionized status of drug molecule depends upon two factors:**

    A) the pKa of the drug

    B) the pH of the environment in which the drug is located

  4. **pKa of drug** — a mathematical representation of its ability to ionize. It is relative to whether a *drug* is a weak or strong acid or base. The pKa values are computed by the Henderson-Hasselbach equation.

$$pKa = pH + \log \frac{\text{non-ionized acid}}{\text{ionized acid}}$$

$$pKa = pH + \log \frac{\text{ionized base}}{\text{non-ionized base}}$$

5. **Acidic drugs** — donate hydrogen ion ($H^+$) and are thus ionized.
   A) This ability to donate $H^+$ is quantitated by the term pKa.
   The lower the pKa, the stronger the acid.
   The higher the pKa, the weaker the acid.

6. **Basic drugs** — accept hydrogen ion ($H^+$) and are thus ionized.
   A) The ability to accept $H^+$ may also be designated by pKa by manipulating the Henderson-Hasselbach equation.
   The higher the pKa, the stronger the base.
   The lower the pKa, the weaker the base.

7. **Drugs are considered in terms of their ability to dissociate as acids** — hence, in terms of their pKa.
   A) *Strong acids* — high degree of $H^+$ donation
   B) *Weak acids* — lesser degree of $H^+$ donation
   C) *Weak bases* — even less ability to donate $H^+$. Actually they weakly accept $H^+$.
   D) *Strong bases* — practically no ability to donate $H^+$. Instead, they strongly accept $H^+$.
   Most drugs are weak acids or weak bases.

8. **pH of the environment** — a mathematical representation of the $H^+$ ion concentration of the medium in which the drug is placed. It is relative to whether the *medium* will donate or accept $H^+$. The medium or environment refers to the solution (blood, urine, gastric juice, milk) the *drug is in* at a given time.

   *Ion trapping* — if a drug is found in an environment in which it readily *ionizes* (examples: a weak base in the acid stomach or a weak acid in an alkaline urine) it will not diffuse or move across membranes. Hence it remains "trapped" in the medium where it was originally found. (*See* schematic and table on facing page.)

9. **Guidelines**
   $$A) \text{ Relative ratio of } \frac{\text{NON-IONIZED}}{\text{IONIZED}} \text{ is the important factor.}$$

   B) Drugs follow concentration gradients and usually move downhill.
   C) This is not an all-or-none movement situation; it only governs the *rate* of movement.
   D) There are exceptions. Differences in the lipid solubilities of drugs can alter the passive transport rates.

# ION-TRAPPING EXAMPLE

At *Equilibrium*—the concentration of non-ionized drug is the same on both sides of the membrane. More TOTAL DRUG is on the side of the greatest degree of ionization.

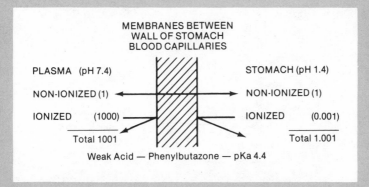

MEMBRANES BETWEEN
WALL OF STOMACH
BLOOD CAPILLARIES

| PLASMA (pH 7.4) | STOMACH (pH 1.4) |
|---|---|
| NON-IONIZED (1) | NON-IONIZED (1) |
| IONIZED (1000) | IONIZED (0.001) |
| Total 1001 | Total 1.001 |

Weak Acid — Phenylbutazone — pKa 4.4

## Summary of Schematic

Phenylbutazone is a weak acid. When placed in a highly acid medium in the stomach, it cannot readily ionize. Therefore, it remains non-ionized (ratio of 1000:1 more molecules non-ionized) and hence *moves* across membranes into blood. When the phenylbutazone reaches the plasma, which is slightly alkaline, the drug can donate $H^+$ and ionize; it then is "trapped" in the plasma.

|  | Acidic Drugs | Basic Drugs |
|---|---|---|
| Stomach | Are non-ionized<br>Good absorption | Are ionized<br>Poor absorption |
| Intestine | Are ionized<br>Poor absorption | Are non-ionized<br>Good absorption |

10. Examples of stomach and intestine absorption

| WEAK ACIDS | WEAK BASES |
|---|---|
| $PKa - pH = \log \dfrac{\text{NON-ION}}{\text{ION}}$ | $Pka - pH = \log \dfrac{\text{ION}}{\text{NON-ION}}$ |
| ASPIRIN pKa = 3.5 | AMINOPYRINE pKa = 5 |
| STOMACH pH = 2<br><br>$3.5 - 2 = \log \dfrac{N}{I}$<br><br>$1.5 = \log \dfrac{N}{I}$<br><br>$N = \dfrac{30}{I}$<br>RATIO FAVORS ABSORPTION | STOMACH pH = 2<br><br>$5 - 2 = \log \dfrac{I}{N}$<br><br>$3 = \log \dfrac{I}{N}$<br><br>$I = \dfrac{1000}{1}$ |
| INTESTINE pH = 6<br><br>$3.5 - 6 = \log \dfrac{N}{I}$<br><br>$-2.5 = \log \dfrac{N}{I}$<br><br>$\dfrac{N}{I} = \dfrac{1}{300}$ | INTESTINE pH = 6<br><br>$5 - 6 = \log \dfrac{I}{N}$<br><br>$-1 = \log \dfrac{I}{N}$<br><br>$\dfrac{I}{N} = \dfrac{1}{10}$<br><br>RATIO FAVORS ABSORPTION |

## D. VARIABLES INFLUENCING DRUG ABSORPTION

1. **Circulation of blood** — absorption of a drug from a particular site is directly related to blood flow to that site. Greater blood flow increases absorption of drug from that area.

   A) The following will increase the blood flow:
   1) *Fear, rage* and *adrenergic drugs* — increase the blood flow to site of IM injections.
   2) *Heat* and *massage* — increase blood flow to parenteral sites.

   B) The following will decrease the blood flow:
   1) *Shock* — intravenous administration is the only reliable route. Intramuscular route of injection is possible.
   2) *Edema* — poor circulation.
   3) *Cooling parenteral site* — constricts vessels in the area.
   4) *Fear, rage* and *adrenergic drugs* — reduce blood flow to the gastrointestinal tract and SC sites.

    5) Systemic drop in blood pressure

   C) *Anatomic* — degree of vascularity differs in different sites; *e.g.*, relatively poor blood supply to joint capsule.

2. **Solubility of drug in water**
   A) Drugs in solution are usually absorbed faster.
   B) The rate at which solids are absorbed depends upon the rate of dissolution.

3. **Concentration of drug at the site of absorption** — the drug must contact the membranes. A greater downhill gradient is created.

4. **Absorbing surface area**
   A) The larger the area of the absorbing surface, the greater the absorption.
   B) May use a spreading factor such as hyaluronidase (an enzyme).

5. **Route of administration may alter the absorption of drugs.**

E. **VARIABLES IN DRUG ABSORPTION AFTER ORAL ADMINISTRATION**

1. **Status of gastrointestinal tract**
   A) Greater motility (diarrhea) reduces absorption of drugs.
   B) Reduced motility (constipation) increases absorption.
      1) *Horse* — phenothiazine toxicity may result from constipation and increased absorption of the drug.

2. **Interaction of drug with other substances**
   A) *Cyclamate* — inhibits absorption of lincomycin.
   B) *Antacids* — decrease the absorption of: phenylbutazone, Furadantin®, pentobarbital, iron.
   C) *Milk, calcium, aluminum, magnesium* — decrease the absorption of tetracyclines.
   D) *Antacids* — increase the pH in the stomach, which increases the amount of penicillin G absorbed.
   E) *Mineral oil* — decreases the absorption of fat-soluble vitamins and highly fat-soluble drugs.
   F) *Food* — increases the protein binding of many drugs in the gut, which decreases their absorption.
   G) *Dilantin*® — decreases the absorption of folic acid, which may lead to anemia.

3. **Decrease in blood flow to mucosae of the intestinal tract because of shock and adrenergic stimulation** — decreases the absorption of orally administered drugs.

4. **Biological variation** — absorption varies from animal to animal, possibly to a greater degree than is generally thought.
   A) Variable and erratic absorption of digoxin in dogs

B) "Slow absorbers" and "fast absorbers" in man
C) Experimentation with oral phenylbutazone in horses:
  1) 900-lb male, peak blood levels in 10 hours; maximum concentration was 28 μg/ml
  2) 850-lb female, peak blood levels in 2 hours; maximum concentration was 55 μg/ml

5. **Low pH of stomach may precipitate some drugs** — may inactivate and/or prevent their absorption.

# Drug Distribution

Refers to the movement of drugs after they are absorbed into the blood. Where does the drug go, and how rapidly does it go there?

1. **Across membranes and into cells,** a schematic of sequences:

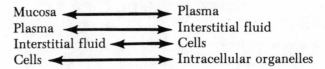

Mucosa ⟷ Plasma
Plasma ⟷ Interstitial fluid
Interstitial fluid ⟷ Cells
Cells ⟷ Intracellular organelles

A. **STORAGE DEPOTS IN THE ANIMAL'S BODY:**

1. **Plasma protein binding** — may act as a drug reservoir.
  A) Free drug reaches a dynamic equilibrium with bound drug.
  B) Bound drug is *not active* and is *not metabolized.*

2. **Cell storage** — drug may be protein bound within cell.

3. **Fat, liver, kidney, connective tissue, bone and muscle may act as tissue storage depots** — they are important in residue studies.

B. **PLACENTAL TRANSFER**

1. **Drugs move primarily by simple diffusion from maternal blood into fetal blood.**
  A) Non-ionized, highly-lipid soluble compounds move rapidly into fetal circulation from the mother's blood.

C. **TRANSFER OF DRUGS INTO THE CENTRAL NERVOUS SYSTEM**

1. **Crossing the "blood-brain barrier"**

2. **Brain constitutes a small portion of body by weight but receives a generous blood supply (14% of cardiac output in man and 8% in the dog).**

3. **Drugs enter CNS from blood via two routes:**
  A) Via cerebrospinal fluid which comes from choroid plexus

B) Via capillaries to extracellular fluid to cells

4. **Variables related to drug passage into the** CNS:
   A) Drugs tend to pass more readily into brain of neonates because membranes are more permeable.
   B) Highly ionized, polar compounds penetrate poorly.
   C) Highly lipid-soluble, non-ionized compounds penetrate readily.
   D) Pathologic changes may alter the permeability of the CNS membranes. Traumatic injury, inflammation and allergic reactions all *increase* the permeability; hence drugs enter the brain more readily.
   E) A drop in blood pressure or a lack of oxygen to the brain, or both, will increase the permeability of the CNS membranes. This will *increase* the movement of drugs into the brain.

D. **REDISTRIBUTION**
   1. **The movement of drugs into storage from active sites** — ends drug action by pulling the drug from the site of action.
   2. **From storage back into circulation** — the drug may or may not reach active sites in concentrations sufficient to give an action. If the storage sites (fat, for example) are saturated, a subsequent dose may give an exaggerated or prolonged effect. This is the case when a second dose of Surital® or Dipentol® is given to an animal while the fat stores are full from the first dose.

### Schematic Summary
### of Drug Absorption and Distribution

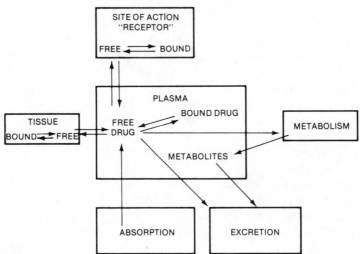

# Biotransformation

**Biotransformation** may be defined as *any chemical alteration of the drug molecule by the cells of the animal.* Mammalian enzyme systems in many different tissues can biotransform drugs. Older terms are *drug inactivation* or *drug detoxification.*

If drugs had to be excreted in their original form, many would remain in the body for extended periods of time. In order to move across membranes to reach active sites, the drugs are of necessity lipid-soluble, non-polar compounds. In this form they are not readily excreted, because they are resorbed into the blood in the kidney. Polar compounds are less readily absorbed, more water-soluble and more readily excreted.

A. **TWO MAJOR RESULTS OF BIOTRANSFORMATION:**

1. **Metabolites** are more polar, more water-soluble and more easily excreted in urine and bile. This is because they are:
   A) More ionized
   B) Less able to bind to plasma protein and cellular protein
   C) Less likely to store in tissues, fat, muscle, kidney
   D) Less able to pass membranes

2. **Change in activity of drug**
   A) Metabolites are usually less active or are inactive
   B) Metabolites may be more active

B. **BIOTRANSFORMATION SITES IN THE BODY**

1. **Principal site is liver** — the *hepatic endoplasmic reticulum* is a canal or pipeline-like organelle within the cytoplasm. *Microsomes* is the term denoting this functional entity.
   A) *Smooth endoplasmic reticulum*—drug metabolism takes place. Features of *hepatic microsomal enzyme systems:*
   1) They most probably are lipid receptors and lipoproteins.
   2) High lipid-soluble compounds can serve as substrates. Most drugs are in this category.
   3) They lack substrate specificity. They metabolize substances of widely different chemical make-up if they are *lipid*-soluble.
   4) Resulting compounds (metabolites) are more *water*-soluble.
   5) Biotransform mainly foreign compounds, with the exception of steroids, bilirubin and fatty acids.
   6) Involves: NADPH, cytochrome c reductase, non-heme iron, cytochrome P-450, supply of reduced NADP.
   B) *Rough endoplasmic reticulum* — protein synthesis takes place.

2. Relatively small degree of biotransformation takes place in extrahepatic tissues — some occurs in the brain, kidney, small intestine, and plasma.

3. Some drugs are metabolized by intermediary metabolism enzyme systems within the cells.

C. **DRUG GIVEN ORALLY** — may in some cases be inactivated before it reaches systemic blood. This is also true of IP injections. The drug travels through the liver before entering the systemic blood supply.

D. **CHEMICAL CLASSIFICATION OF BIOTRANSFORMATION:**

1. **Oxidation** — microsomal and nonmicrosomal
   A) Hydroxylation
   B) Removal of hydrogen
   C) Deamination
   D) Dealkylation
   E) Sulfoxide formation

2. **Reduction** — microsomal
   A) Nitrogen reduction
   B) Addition of hydrogen

3. **Hydrolysis** — plasma, nonmicrosomal and microsomal
   A) Splitting of ester and amide bonds

4. **Conjugation** — synthetic reactions, microsomal. Drug plus endogenous substance yields a conjugated drug. Examples of endogenous substances used to conjugate drugs:
   A) Glucuronic acid
   B) Amino acids — glycine
   C) Acetate
   D) Methyl group
   E) Sulfate

5. **May require a combination of reactions** — such as hydroxylation and then conjugation.

E. **FACTORS THAT DELAY OR ENHANCE BIOTRANSFORMATION**

1. **Protein binding in plasma delays biotransformation** — the drug is not as available to enzyme systems in the liver cells if it is bound to protein in the plasma.

2. **Localization of drug in tissue sites** such as adipose tissue delays biotransformation.

3. **Hepatic pathology may delay biotransformation.**

4. **Age**
   A) Newborns are deficient in drug-metabolizing enzymes; they

usually are fairly mature by one month of age.

    B) Older animals are less able to metabolize drugs because of a decreased ability to synthesize the protein enzymes used in biotransformation.

5. **Poor nutritional status may inhibit biotransformation.**

6. **Species differences in biotransformation** — the slower the biotransformation, the more prolonged the action.

    A) *Cat* — biotransforms salicylates with much difficulty.

    B) Species differences relative to succinylcholine biotransformation:

        1) Plasma esterase levels are high in *man* and *horse*, low in *cattle*. *Man* and *horse* biotransform succinylcholine rapidly, *cows* very, very slowly.

    C) *Man* versus *dog* — meperidine biotransformation:

        1) *Man* — 17 % /hour

        2) *Dog* — 90 % /hour

    D) Hexobarbital half life:

        1) *Mouse* — 19 minutes

        2) *Rat* — 140 minutes

        3) *Man* — 360 minutes

        4) *Dog* — 260 minutes

7. **Genetic and strain differences**

    A) Deficiency or lack of enzymes necessary for biotransformation may be inherited.

    B) *Pharmacogenetics* is the science that deals with these differences.

8. **Lower body temperature results in decreased biotransformation rate.** Shock or anesthesia are examples where body temperature may drop and thereby lower biotransformation rates.

9. **Sex differences.** Female rats sleep four times as long as male rats given hexobarbital, because females have slower inactivation rates.

10. **Route of administration can affect metabolism.**

    A) Drugs administered orally and IP pass through the liver (some metabolized) before they become systemic. Apomorphine given IM to the dog produces vomiting in 2 to 5 minutes. Same dose administered IP gives no response.

    B) Orally administered drugs — the intestinal wall can biotransform some drugs; hence small amounts may be inactive when they reach the blood.

11. **Inhibition of enzymes by other drugs**

    A) Decreased inactivation occurs and hence the drug acts longer.

B) Dogs given SKF-525A, then given hexobarbital, sleep eight hours instead of 90 minutes.

C) Chloramphenicol prolongs anesthesia under pentobarbital by inhibiting hepatic microsomal enzyme systems in the liver, thus slowing the inactivation of the pentobarbital.

12. **Stimulation of enzymes by other drugs**
    A) Many drugs may stimulate hepatic microsomal enzymes to greater activity. Examples of drugs that enhance hepatic biotransformation are phenobarbital, phenylbutazone, and chlorinated hydrocarbon insecticides.
       1) Increased enzyme activity may give greater inactivation, which leads to a shorter duration of drug action.
       2) Reported increases in liver weight result from increased enzyme protein synthesis.
    B) Enhanced inactivation may be a mechanism for the development of tolerance or resistance to a drug after continued use.
    C) May have some therapeutic use. In the human infant, phenobarbital has been shown to reduce hyperbilirubinemia by enhancing bilirubin conjugation and hence its excretion.

    Phenobarbital given daily in the feed of dairy cattle has been shown, under field conditions, to reduce the body load of DDT by enhancing its biotransformation and hence its excretion. One must also be aware that when two or more drugs are administered simultaneously, if one of them is capable of microsomal enzyme induction, the duration of action of the others may be changed (usually shortened).

## Examples of Biotransformation and Metabolite Activity

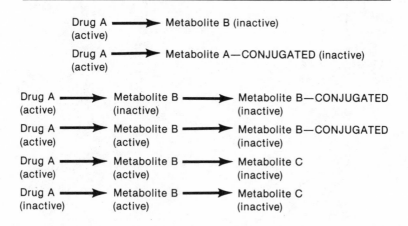

**NEPHRON**

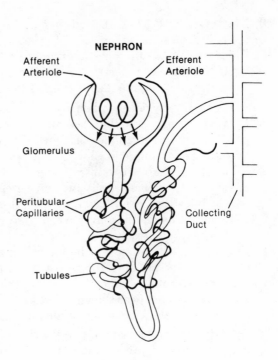

Afferent Arteriole

Efferent Arteriole

Glomerulus

Peritubular Capillaries

Collecting Duct

Tubules

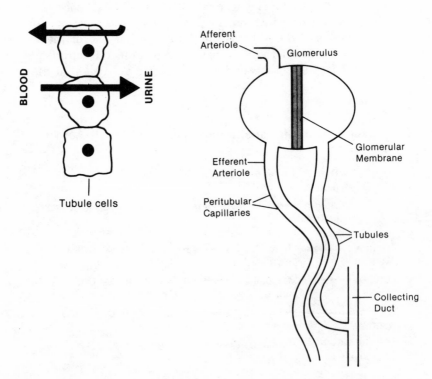

BLOOD

URINE

Tubule cells

Afferent Arteriole

Glomerulus

Glomerular Membrane

Efferent Arteriole

Peritubular Capillaries

Tubules

Collecting Duct

# Excretion

A. **KIDNEY** — the organ system responsible for excreting the greatest amounts of most drugs. Kidneys excrete drugs by one or more of the following means:

1. **Glomerular filtration** — most drugs are filtered at the glomerular membrane. Rate of filtration is governed primarily by physiological processes such as the filtration rate, and by the degree of binding of the drug to plasma proteins. The filtrate (with dissolved drugs) moves to the tubule cells. Protein-bound drugs do not pass through the glomerular filtrate.

2. **Tubular resorption** — certain drugs and forms of drugs are resorbed from the tubular fluid into the blood.
   A) Lipid-soluble drug is quite readily resorbed into blood from filtrate.
   B) Un-ionized drug is resorbed into blood from filtrate.
   C) Ionized drug and water-soluble, polar compounds are *not* resorbed into the blood from the filtrate and are excreted with the urine. This is a form of *ion-trapping*.
   D) More acidic urine enhances excretion of a weak base (more ionized).
   E) More basic urine enhances excretion of a weak acid (more ionized).

3. **Secretion by tubule cells**
   A) This system moves drugs from the blood into the urine.
   B) *Active transport* — a carrier-mediated, energy-using system.
   C) Utilizes endogenous-compound, active-secretion schemes that are physiologically important.
      Penicillin and uric acid share the same active-secretion scheme for excretion.
   D) For proper excretion of drugs, it is important that the kidney be functioning properly and that the animal be in a state of proper water balance.

B. **INTESTINE** — drugs appear in the feces by one or more of the following means:

1. **Unabsorbed, orally administered drug** — remains in gastrointestinal tract and is excreted.

2. **Hepatic secretion of drugs into bile and hence into the intestine.** Many of these drugs are resorbed into the blood and then excreted via the kidney (enterohepatic circulation).

3. **Active secretion from plasma across the intestinal wall into the feces.**

C. **LUNGS** — any volatile substance in the plasma will be excreted in expired air. Gaseous or inhalation anesthetics are examples.

D. **MILK** — many drugs pass readily from the blood to the milk. This is important to nurslings and as a residue problem in dairy cattle.

E. **SWEAT** — not quantitatively important but some drugs do appear in sweat.

F. **SALIVA** — important in forensic (diagnostic) veterinary medicine; a means to detect drugs that may be in blood.

# Mechanisms of Drug Action

No drug has a single action in the animal's body. Nevertheless, the selectivity of most drugs is remarkable.

A. **STRUCTURAL ACTIVITY RELATIONSHIPS**
1. **The molecular structure and spatial configuration of a drug** — determines its ability to "fit" or interact with a corresponding active site or "receptor substance" in or on certain cells. Lock-and-key fit brings about *action*. (*See* schematic.)
2. **Receptors** — areas on or adjacent to cell membranes which have a geometric, three-dimensional form. They are most likely protein in nature, and are enzyme or enzyme-like.
3. **DRUG** — may have two parts or segments of its molecule.
   A) The part that attaches the drug to the receptor area results in *affinity*.
   B) The part of the molecule that has exact fit results in *efficacy*.
   C) A drug with both affinity and efficacy is called an *agonist* and will give action when it reaches a receptor.
   D) An agonist with a smaller degree of efficacy is called a *partial agonist*.
   E) A drug with affinity but no efficacy (reacts with and fills the receptor site but does not elicit action) is called a *competitive antagonist* and thus is a receptor blocker.
   F) *Partial agonist* and *agonist* at the same site at the same time:
      1) May be additive and fill more sites, hence giving more action.
      2) May lead to antagonization of the agonist by the partial agonist. The latter may compete for a primary receptor site and keep the more-active agonist off of the receptor. The action of the partial agonist is very weak and not clinically noticeable. Morphine and nalorphine (Nalline® —

Merck) are examples; Nalline®, a partial agonist, reverses the action of morphine.

4. **Drug-receptor binding** — bond types
   A) *The Van der Waals* — London forces, weak bonds
   B) *Hydrogen bonds* — oxygen and nitrogen, through water
   C) *Ionic bonds*
   (A, B and C are reversible at body temperature.)
   D) *Hydrophobic bonds* — alter structure of receptor
   E) *Covalent bonds* — strong, difficult to reverse

5. **Schematic of Important DRUG-RECEPTOR Interactions**

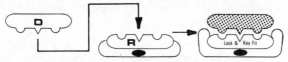

A) *Drug* (D) and *Receptor* (R) interact — changes characteristics (stimulus) of the cell membrane and brings about an action.

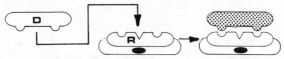

B) *Drug* and *Receptor* interact — no stimulus, causing no action. Receptor is covered up, but no lock-and-key fit. The receptor is blocked.

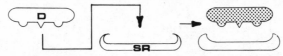

C) *Drug* interacts with *receptors* that are not capable of exciting action. *Silent receptors* (SR) are a form of binding, such as plasma protein binding.

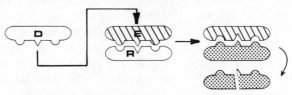

D) *Drug* interacts with *receptor* of a drug-destroying enzyme (E) in the liver or plasma. The drug is inactivated.

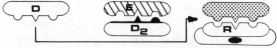

E) *Drug* interacts with the *receptor* of the drug, destroying enzyme in example D. The enzyme is blocked and effect of the drug is prolonged because it is more slowly inactivated.

B. **DRUGS USED MEDICINALLY MODULATE THE INTENSITY OF A SPECIALIZED ORGAN SYSTEM** — the animal is now operating with drug-altered physiological processes which may either enhance or interfere with metabolism.

1. **Drug action classified by overall action**
   A) Stimulation
   B) Depression
   C) Irritation
   D) Replacement
   E) Chemotherapy

2. **The different modes or mechanisms of drug action**
   A) Drugs may interfere with the schemes by which cells are maintained in a functional state.
      1) Alter the passage of substances into and out of cells by changing permeability or by altering transport mechanisms
      2) Alter cellular enzyme activity, either enhancing or inhibiting cell metabolism
      3) Alter physiochemical make-up of cells, such as changing osmotic, colloidal, or surface forces
   B) *Chelation* — the loose binding of a substance by a drug; for example, EDTA chelates calcium and lead.
   C) Drugs may influence bound forms of physiologically active substances. For example:
      1) Displace a hormone from plasma protein, making it more active
      2) Displace a hormone from tissue sites, making it more active
      Example: Ephedrine causes release of norepinephrine from storage and deposition onto active site.
   D) *Biological antagonism* — drugs may act as antimetabolites.
      1) Drugs may act as chemical analogues. Foreign compound (drug) is mistakenly taken into an intermediary metabolism scheme of a cell. The drug later inhibits the scheme and thereby changes the cell function. Examples:
         a) *Sulfonamides* — inhibit the multiplication of bacteria by substituting for PABA, resulting in inhibition of protein synthesis in the bacteria.
         b) *Anticancer drugs* — inhibit rapidly multiplying cancer cells by substituting for vital substances in cellular metabolic schemes that result in protein synthesis called antimetabolites.
   E) Drugs may block receptors.
      1) A drug may compete with another drug or an endogenous

substance for an active site on a receptor.

2) Receptor blockade represents an *agonist* versus an *antagonist*. The antagonist has a greater affinity and hence wins out. The receptor is now blocked; no action.

3) Acetylcholine *versus* curare or atropine — atropine or curare blocks acetylcholine off of receptors and prevents its action.

F) Drugs may influence biological control systems.

1) May activate enzymes. For example, by influencing cyclic AMP (a vital cellular-function control factor).

2) Examples:

a) Epinephrine triggers conversion of glycogen to glucose via an action upon cyclic AMP.

b) Corticosteroids activate hepatic transaminases which convert certain amino acids to glucose.

3) May cause the release of nervous-system chemical messengers from their inactive form to their active form.

G) *Replacement* — drugs may be used to restore the proper levels of endogenous substances. Endocrine therapy may be an example.

H) A drug may be a neurotransmitter or may mimic or influence the action of a neurotransmitter.

# Factors that Modify Drug Response and Dose

Drug response is a function of the amount of free drug (not protein bound) at the proper receptor-active site. This amount of drug is, of course, related to the *dosage* and *frequency* of administration, but is also affected by many other factors. The total of all the factors so far discussed must be considered when a proper drug *therapeutic regimen* is set up. Following is an outline of those considerations.

A.  **DRUG REGIMEN**

1.  **In setting up a treatment regimen one must decide:**

A. Drug or drugs to be used

B. Route of administration

C. Dose: how much? how often? how long will the regimen be continued?

B.  **ROUTE OF ADMINISTRATION**

1.  **Dosage varies with different routes of administration** — as a guide only: oral  = 1; subcutaneous = ½; intravenous = ¼; *i.e.* a larger oral dose is required to achieve the same blood levels obtained intravenously.

2. **Drug action may be altered by route or administration.**
   A) Magnesium sulfate in hot packs will reduce swelling.
   B) Magnesium sulfate, orally, has a laxative action.
   C) Magnesium sulfate IV has a CNS depressant action, causing muscle relaxation.

3. **Onset and duration of action depend upon route of administration.**
   A) IV — quicker onset but shorter duration
   B) Oral — slower onset but longer duration

C. **TIMING OF ADMINISTRATION**

   1. **Time of day** — hypnotics are more potent at night. Stimulants are more potent during the day.

   2. **Relation to season** — interaction of the drug with the animal's biological clock. Hormone levels and enzyme activities have been shown to vary rhythmically during a 24-hour period.

   3. **Relation to environment** — influence of such factors as ambient temperature, humidity, and oxygen supply on the animal's response to drugs. May be partly responsible for the variability seen from day to day in the response of animals to anesthetics.

   4. **Oral administration of drugs relative to time of feeding in simple-stomached animals** — have different emptying times, rate of passage of food, binding of drug to food.

D. **SPECIES VARIATION** — extremely important in veterinary pharmacology

   1. **Differences in cell and organ responses that may result in different clinically observable responses and/or toxic reactions:**
      A) Morphine produces CNS depression in the dog but produces CNS stimulation and even mania in the cat.
      B) Diethylstilbestrol can induce abortion in cattle but will not induce abortion in women.
      C) Horses appear to be sensitive to the phenothiazine-derivative tranquilizers. In some cases such tranquilizers may even produce CNS excitation.
      D) The Greyhound appears to handle certain drugs in an individual fashion, possibly because of a difference in responding systems or possibly because of a minimal amount of body fat. The drugs tend to stay in the animal's system for longer periods. This may create special requirements for care in administering anesthetics to Greyhounds. The Greyhound may sleep for extended periods when given barbiturates. These dogs may also be predisposed to an inherited

overheating syndrome; the halogenated anesthetics are known to precipitate this severe condition.

E) There are also great differences among the animals in sensitivity to the digitalis glycosides. For example, the $LD_{50}$ of digitoxin in the rat is 670 times that for the cat.

F) Response to drugs that cause emesis is extremely variable. There is no drug that will induce vomiting in mice, rats, rabbits, horses, or ruminants, because these animals either cannot vomit or they vomit with extreme difficulty.

2. **Plasma level and active-site level of free drug.**
   A) Differences in biotransformation and/or excretion rates depend on the concentration of active, free drug at the active sites. For example, the plasma half-life of salicylate varies greatly among species because of a marked difference in the rate of biotransformation. Plasma half-life in the cat is 38 hours, in the dog 8 hours, in swine 6 hours, in the horse 1 hour, and in the goat 0.8 hour. The half-life of salicylate in man, as a comparison, is about 5 hours. This means that the dosage and dosage interval must be based upon the kinetics of the drug in each species, and recommendations for one species may not be proper for another.
   
   B) Differences in binding — plasma and tissue. Plasma proteins vary from species to species. The antibiotic cloxacillin is 93% plasma-protein bound in man but only 30% plasma-protein bound in horses. It is obvious, then, that with cloxacillin at a similar *total* plasma concentration in the horse, a great deal more free antibiotic will be present to act in the plasma.

3. **Differences in digestive tract** — simple-stomached omnivores, simple-stomached herbivores, and ruminants

## E. INDIVIDUAL VARIATION

1. **Body weight**
   A. It is the primary determining factor of dosage; is stated as mg/kg or mg/lb.
   B. Is only an *approximation*, and a guide.
   C. Has many limitations — fat *versus* lean animal, status of fill of GI tract, a severely dehydrated animal, old animal or newborn.

2. **Age.** Problems in arriving at a proper dose and dosing schedule for the very young or very old. These animals usually require smaller and less frequent doses because they biotransform and excrete drugs more slowly. Also there is less muscle mass for

distribution of volume in young and old.

3. **Sex**
   A) There is considerable evidence for response differences between male and female animals.
   B) Drug use must also take into account the status of the reproductive tract, and whether the animal is lactating.

4. **Temperament of individual animal needs to be considered.**
   A) Particularly important for drugs affecting the CNS.
   B) Tranquilizer responses may differ among animals, depending on whether the animal is calm or agitated.
   C) Placebo effect in man may be another example. After taking prescribed medication, which in reality is nothing but sugar, the patient feels better.

5. **Biochemical individuality and variability**
   A) No two individuals react the same way to the same drug.
   B) There is no "normal". The individuality of each patient must be considered, where possible.
   C) Genetic factors. Pharmacogenetics is the study of these factors related to drug responses.
   1) Quantitative (degree of) and qualitative (nature of) response differences are due to inherited characteristics.
   2) Differences of cellular make-up are governed by the genetic make-up of the animal.

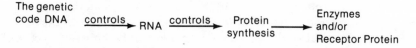

The genetic code DNA $\xrightarrow{\text{controls}}$ RNA $\xrightarrow{\text{controls}}$ Protein synthesis $\longrightarrow$ Enzymes and/or Receptor Protein

6. **Biochemical individuality may be involved in the following:**
   A) *Idiosyncrasy* — an extraordinary drug reaction that is qualitatively different from the expected response.
   B) *Drug Allergy* — hypersensitivity (drug fever)
   1) Prior exposure is necessary. Owner may not be aware of a drug that the animal has been given previously.
   2) Drug allergy is a function of the immune response.
      a) Drugs or their metabolites may be antigens or may combine with a body protein to form an antigen (hapten).
      b) Antigen stimulates antibody production by the animal. The animal must be genetically capable of producing the antibody.
      c) *Antibody* and *antigen* react and a toxic substance(s) is released. The released substances then bring about the allergic (toxic) reaction.
   3) Requires only a small amount of drug to trigger hypersen-

sitivity — *not dose-related.*
4) Allergic reactions may be:
   a) *Acute* — anaphylactic—occur within 3 or 4 minutes or up to an hour.
   b) *Subacute* — occur within 1 to 24 hours.
   c) *Delayed* — may not appear until 10 days later.
C) *Hyperreactive*
   1) The nature of the animal's response is as predicted.
   2) The quantitative response is exaggerated. The animal gives a greater than usual response to the normal dose.
D) *Hyporeactive*
   1) The nature of the animal's response is as predicted.
   2) The quantitative response is less. The animal gives a lesser response, or no response, to the normal dose.
C and D are based upon the "average" of a population.
E) *Tolerance* — drug resistance
   1) Unusual resistance to the ordinary dose of a drug. A larger dose is needed to achieve the usual effect.
   2) Except when congenital, tolerance develops after *continuous exposure* of the animal to a drug.
   3) Mechanisms that may bring about tolerance:
      a) Cells may increase biotransformation of a drug, and hence the drug is inactivated faster and less drug is available to bring about the desired response.
      b) Cells may adapt and become acclimatized. Some cells may incorporate the drug into their metabolic schemes, which may help to explain *dependence* and withdrawal symptoms that occur with certain CNS drugs.
      c) Increased excretion or decreased absorption of drug.
      d) Tachyphylaxis is the rapid development of tolerance.
   4) Ephedrine example of tachyphylaxis:
      a) Ephedrine causes release of the neurotransmitter norepinephrine from nerve endings.
      b) Released norepinephrine acts on cell(s) supplied by the nerve ending.
      c) Repeated ephedrine dosing depletes norepinephrine released from nerve endings.
      d) Depleted stores of norepinephrine are less able to give action because less of the neurotransmitter is released to act on target cell(s).
   5) May have cross tolerance
      a) An animal becomes tolerant to one drug and thus may also be tolerant to another drug.
      b) Drugs are usually of same chemical grouping.

    c) Drugs of the same activity. Human alcoholics may be very tolerant of general anesthetics and hence difficult to anesthetize using usual dosage regimens.

E. **PATHOLOGICAL CONDITIONS**

1. **Altered absorption, biotransformation and excretion** — disease may alter the plasma levels and hence the drug response.

2. **Diarrhea** — drugs spend less time in the gastrointestinal tract, which decreases their absorption.

3. **Constipation may increase drug absorption.**

4. **Hepatic pathology** — impairs biotransformation.
    *Hepatitis* — barbiturates act longer. Pathologic changes in the liver may be chemically induced.

5. **Kidney pathology** — usually accompanied by decreased drug excretion or increased glomerular filtration.

6. **Inflammation of central nervous system** (meningitis, encephalitis) — enhances the entry of certain drugs into the CNS.

F. **DRUG AUGMENTATION**

1. **Cumulative effect** — the sum of two or more doses brings about a gradual increase in the plasma level of a drug because the dose is repeated before the administered drug is totally biotransformed and/or excreted.

G. **DRUG INTERACTIONS** — more than one drug acting in the animal's body at the same time.

1. **May be desirable and have therapeutic value**

2. **May be undesirable therapy and cause treatment failure or adverse reactions.**

3. **Examples of drug interactions:**
    A) *Synergism* — two or more drugs, given at the same time, enhance a pharmacologic response.
        1) The term *summation* means that the effects are additive ($2 + 3 = 5$).
        2) The term *potentiation* means that the response is greater than the sum of the actions of the drugs ($2 + 3 = 7$).
    B) *Clinical synergism* — the drugs do not act at the same site or even induce the same response, but one drug enhances the therapeutic effect of the other drug. Example: when epinephrine and procaine are mixed and injected for local anesthesia, the epinephrine slows the absorption of the procaine from the site and hence prolongs its duration of action locally.
    C) *Antagonism* — two or more drugs, given at the same time,

**An Example of the Accumulation of a Drug at
Half-Life of Four Hours and When Half-Life is Doubled**

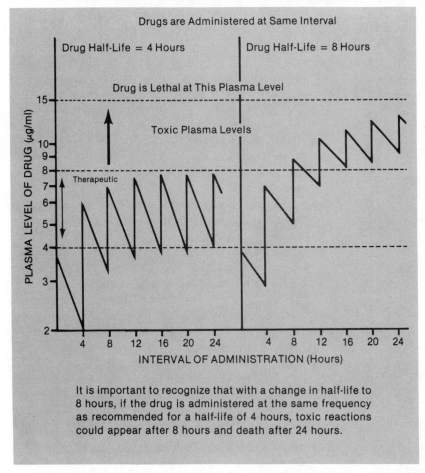

Drugs are Administered at Same Interval

Drug Half-Life = 4 Hours    Drug Half-Life = 8 Hours

Drug is Lethal at This Plasma Level

Toxic Plasma Levels

Therapeutic

PLASMA LEVEL OF DRUG (μg/ml)

INTERVAL OF ADMINISTRATION (Hours)

It is important to recognize that with a change in half-life to
8 hours, if the drug is administered at the same frequency
as recommended for a half-life of 4 hours, toxic reactions
could appear after 8 hours and death after 24 hours.

inhibit or decrease the pharmacologic response. Four types
of antagonism:

1) *Combination* — drugs form a chemical bond which inactivates the drugs.
   a) Chelation is an example.
      (1) BAL chelates arsenic, mercury.
      (2) EDTA chelates lead.
      (3) Sulphur (thiocyanate) chelates the cyanide radical
          and is thus effective in treating cyanide (prussic
          acid) poisoning.

2) *Opposite effects* — drugs act upon the same organ system
   and produce a physiological type of antagonism. For ex-

ample, epinephrine has an effect opposite that of histamine on blood pressure and size of bronchioles. Pentobarbital depresses the respiratory center and Dopram-V®
(Robins) stimulates the respiratory center.

3) *Competitive*

    a) Drugs compete with a normal substrate or another
drug for active site on an enzyme or receptor site.

    b) Examples:

        (1) Antihistamines block the action of histamine by
keeping the histamine off of its receptors.

        (2) Atropine blocks the action of acetylcholine at cer-
tain receptors. More of the inhibited substance
must be administered to counteract or reverse the
antagonism.

    c) *Biological antagonism* — a special type of competitive
antagonism; the drug competes with an endogenous
substance for a spot in an enzymatic scheme and takes
the place of the normal substance. Thus, an abnormal
new product is created. The scheme then shuts down
and loses its normal function. Examples:

        (1) The action of sulfonamides on certain bacterial
cells by competing for PABA

        (2) The action of many anticancer drugs in rapidly
multiplying cells

4) *Noncompetitive*

    a) Forms a chemical bond with active site on enzyme or
receptor site

        (1) Mercury and sulfhydryl group, attaching to en-
zymes, inactivates the enzyme

        (2) Some organophosphates and the enzyme cholines-
terase

    b) For all practical purposes the union is *nonreversible.*

D) *Alteration of absorption* — one drug may inhibit or enhance
the absorption of another drug from the gastrointestinal
tract. Examples:

1) Antacids, calcium, aluminum or iron may complex the
tetracyclines and thus decrease their absorption.

2) A change in the environmental pH alters the ratio of
ionized to non-ionized drug, hence increasing the amount
of drug absorbed.

3) Mineral oil decreases the absorption of fat-soluble drugs
and fat-soluble vitamins.

4) An increase in the pH of the stomach protects acid-labile
drugs from destruction in the stomach.

E) *Alteration of binding*
1) Competition between drugs for binding sites on plasma proteins
2) General example — Drug A is 90% protein-bound (90 mg/100 ml plasma) plus 10% free drug (10 mg/100 ml), and 10 mg/100 ml Drug A gives *action*.

   If Drug B is given, it will displace Drug A from plasma protein binding sites because Drug B has a greater affinity for the binding sites. As a result, we have 100 mg free Drug A/100 ml, which will enhance the effects of Drug A or may even be high enough to be toxic.
3) Specific examples:

| Strongly-bound drug | Weakly-bound drug that will be *displaced* and its action potentiated |
|---|---|
| Phenylbutazone | Sulfonamide |
| Phenylbutazone | Penicillin |
| Phenylbutazone | Corticosteroid |
| Salicylates | Sulfonamide |
| Salicylates | Methotrexate |

4) May bring about release of an endogenous substance from its inactive bound state so that the substance becomes an active free compound. Many drugs cause the release of histamine bound in the cells. The free histamine becomes *active* and toxic.
F) *Alteration of biotransformation*
1) Many drugs inhibit the hepatic microsomal enzymes, causing a reduced biotransformation of certain other drugs. Example: chloramphenicol inhibits the biotransformation of pentobarbital and prolongs pentobarbital-induced anesthesia.
2) Many drugs bring about the stimulation (induction) of hepatic microsomal enzymes and hence an increase in biotransformation of some drugs. Barbiturates, DDT, alcohol, and phenylbutazone are examples of microsomal enzyme inducers.
3) Some drugs inhibit or block the action of other enzyme systems that inactivate drugs. Example: phenothiazine-derivative tranquilizers and organophosphates inhibit cholinesterases. Thus they greatly delay the inactivation of succinylcholine chloride — Sucostrin® (Squibb), Anece-

tin® (Burroughs-Wellcome), Quelicin® (Abbott).

G) *Alteration of excretion*

   1) A change in the pH of urine can alter tubular resorption of drugs by altering the ratio of ionized to non-ionized drug in the tubular fluid.

   2) Certain drugs compete for carrier systems in tubular secretion, thus delaying active secretion of one of the substances by saturating the carrier system.

Specific drug interactions, where known in veterinary medicine, will be included with the discussions of different drugs or drug groups.

H. **SIDE EFFECTS**

  1. **Usually a predictable additional response**

  2. **May be tolerated in order to achieve the desired effect.** However, the client should be advised of the side effects.

I. **CONTRAINDICATIONS**

  1. **For some predictable reason, a drug should not be given.**

   A) Diethylstilbestrol should not be given to a pregnant brood cow.

   B) Penicillin should not be given to an animal known to be hypersensitive to that antibiotic.

# Quantitation of Drug Response

It is important to have a means for measuring the relationship between the amount of a drug administered and the action produced by that amount of drug. The two such drug-response relationships are:

  1. The magnitude of the actions

  2. The time to onset of action and the duration of action

A. **DOSE** — response relationships relative to the *magnitude* of the action. A given dose produces an observable degree of action; *e.g.* a 10 mmHg change in mean blood pressure, or a 60 ml/hr increase in urine flow.

  1. **Graded response** — measured in individuals. Data from several individuals are collected. An increase in dose produces an increase in response up to a maximum plateau or ceiling. These data may be quantitated by means of a *Dose-Response Curve*. Four characterizing parameters of a dose-response curve are:

   A) *Potency* — location of the curve along the dose axis. Potency is not necessarily correlated to clinical superiority; *e.g.* effective dose may be 1 μg or 100 mg, as long as it can be administered *safely*.

B) *Slope* — more important in theory. A steep slope for a CNS depressant would mean little margin between sedation, hypnosis, anesthesia and even respiratory paralysis.

C) *Maximum efficacy* or ceiling effect — not necessarily related to potency. Larger doses do not enhance response. Dosages above this level should not be given.

D) *Variability*—range of effects at a given dose, or the vertical range. Range of doses needed to give a specified response is the horizontal range.

## Dose-Response Curve

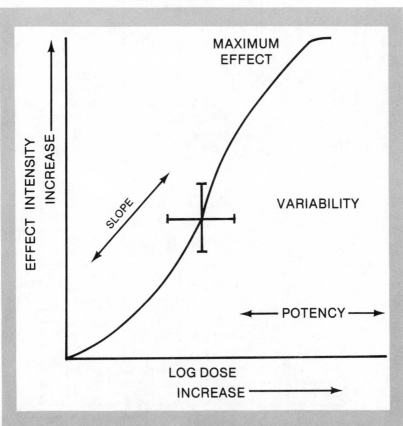

2. **Quantal response**
   A) Quantitated drug responses in a population of individuals usually follow a normal distribution curve.
   B) All-or-none response, such as yes *versus* no, live *versus* dead, paralyzed *versus* nonparalyzed or asleep *versus* awake
   C) Vary the dose and observe the frequency of a fixed effect (such as paralysis, convulsions or death) at each dose level.

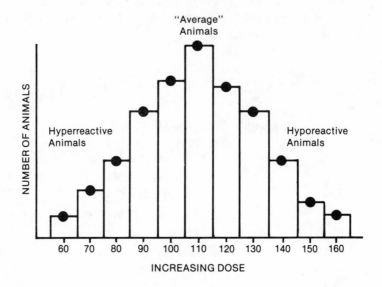

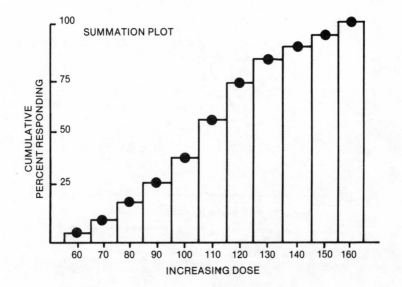

3. **Example of a normal distribution curve**
   A) Same dose is given to all test animals.
   B) Increased intensity of response (5 to 35 mmHg rise) is plotted against the number of individuals giving that response.
   C) This is called by several names:
      1) Normal frequency distribution curve
      2) Normal curve
      3) Gaussian curve

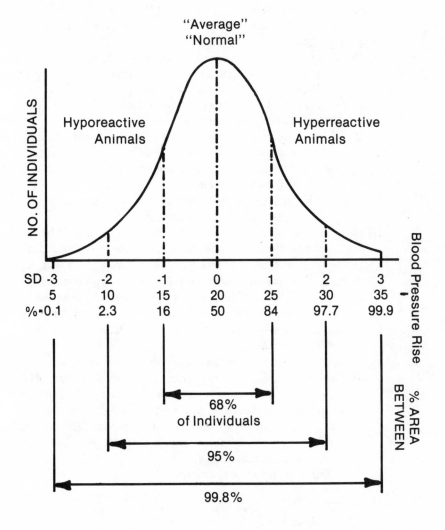

B.  **TIME-RESPONSE RELATIONSHIPS** — onset and duration.

1.  **Onset of drug response** — the time after a drug is administered until the proper concentration (threshold) of the drug reaches and interacts at active site(s), thus giving action.

    A) Quantitation is called the *latent period.*

    B) Is a function of dose and route of administration

    C) Intravenous injections have a shorter latent period than oral doses; a larger dose may shorten the latent period.

2.  **Duration of drug response** — the length of time that the threshold concentration of drug interacts at receptor sites, thus maintaining action.

    A) Drug action may be stopped by several means:

    1) Drug may be inactivated and/or eliminated as follows:

       a) Eliminated unchanged via the lungs, kidney, sweat or

       b) Converted to another compound and eliminated or

       c) Converted to an inactive form

    2) Action may be terminated without the elimination of drug, as follows:

       a) Redistribution of drug to inactive sites in the body, such as fat and muscle

       b) Tolerance to the drug develops at the cellular level

       c) Administration of an antagonist

    B) Quantitation of duration of action may be estimated by using a *plasma disappearance curve.* The rate at which a drug in the animal's body leaves the plasma may be shown by plotting the plasma concentration of the drug *versus* time. (*See* curves 1 & 2.) The drug's rate of entry into the plasma from an intramuscular, subcutaneous or oral dose may also be included. (*See* curve 4.) These curves assume an excess of drug-biotransforming enzyme sites.

    C) Important principles of these curves:

    1) The drop in plasma concentration follows an exponential curve; *i.e.*, the change in concentration per unit of time is a function of the concentration of the drug in the plasma. The greater the concentration of drug, the greater the amount that leaves the plasma in a given period of time (first-order kinetics).

    2) Because of the above principle:

    $$\frac{\text{drug concentration at any hour}}{\text{drug concentration at previous hour}} = \begin{array}{l}\text{a number which}\\ \text{is a constant}\end{array}$$

    3) Because of the principles just cited, it follows that the plasma halftime ($t\frac{1}{2}$), which is the time required for the

## Schematic Plasma Disappearance Curves

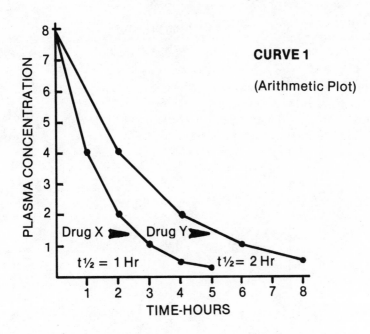

CURVE 1

(Arithmetic Plot)

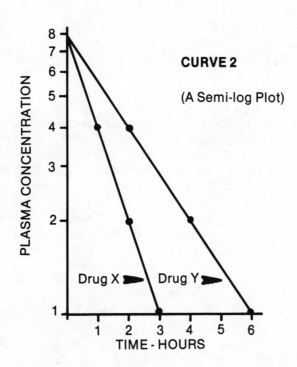

CURVE 2

(A Semi-log Plot)

## CURVE 3

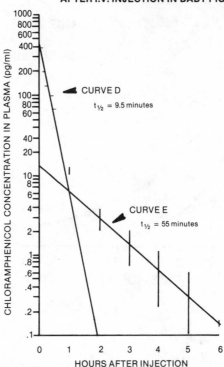

**PLASMA DISAPPEARANCE CURVE
AFTER I.V. INJECTION IN BABY PIGS**

plasma concentration of a drug to decrease by one-half of a former value, is also a constant. In Curves 1 and 2, drug × plasma concentration drops from 4 to 2 and from 2 to 1 in 1 hour; therefore, its $t\frac{1}{2}$ is 1 hour. Drug Y requires 2 hours for the same decreases; therefore, its $t\frac{1}{2}$ is 2 hours.

4) There may actually be two or three separate curves or components of a plasma disappearance curve if samples are drawn frequently enough over a long enough period of time. In Curve 3, Curve D represents the rapid distribution of chloramphenicol from plasma into the tissues. Curve E represents the biotransformation and/or excretion of the drug.

5) Usually a dynamic equilibrium can be assumed between the concentration of active drug at action sites in the tissues and the concentration in the plasma; therefore, plas-

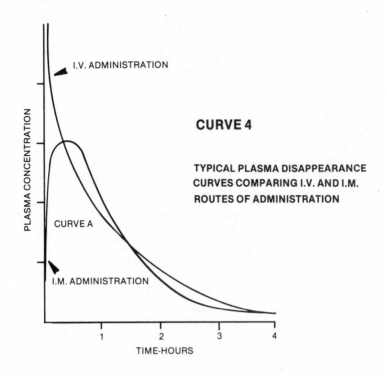

I.V. ADMINISTRATION

**CURVE 4**

**TYPICAL PLASMA DISAPPEARANCE
CURVES COMPARING I.V. AND I.M.
ROUTES OF ADMINISTRATION**

CURVE A

I.M. ADMINISTRATION

PLASMA CONCENTRATION

TIME-HOURS

ma concentrations and disappearance curves can usually
(not always) be used as a guide to estimate duration of
drug action. For example, an IV injection of chloramphenicol as shown in Curve 3 will give a plasma level
greater than 2 $\mu$g/ml for approximately 3 hours.
D) With some drugs, the disappearance is not exponential. A
constant amount is metabolized per hour because there is
more drug than biotransforming enzyme sites (zero-order
kinetics). Ethyl alcohol is an example.
3. **An important principle to be noted**: if you have a *short-dura-
tion drug*, doubling the dose will not double its duration of action, because the greater the plasma concentration, the faster
the drug disappears.
4. **To increase duration of action:**
A) Choose another drug with a longer t$_{1/2}$.
B) Use a route of administration by which the drug is absorbed
more slowly.
C) Use a drug prepared in a vehicle that is absorbed more slowly.
D) Repeat the dosage.
E) Inhibit metabolism or excretion of the drug.

# Evaluation of Drug Safety

You can never study a whole population of animals. You can only examine a sample from a population and estimate the parameters of the population that are useful; *e.g.* $ED_{50}$, $ED_{99}$, $LD_1$, $LD_{50}$.

A. **ESTIMATE THE RELATIONSHIP BETWEEN EFFECTIVE DOSES AND TOXIC OR LETHAL DOSES.**

   1. **Administer the drug to groups of animals at different doses.**
   2. **Plot percent of animals giving response and percent of deaths or toxic reactions against dose.** This is using the principle of dose-response curves.
   3. **Read across from the percent axis and down to find the dose for that percent.** By this means find the *effective dose* for 50% of animals ($ED_{50}$) or the least dose that caused death of 1% of the animals = ($LD_1$). The $LD_{50}$, $ED_{99}$, etc. are plotted in the same way.

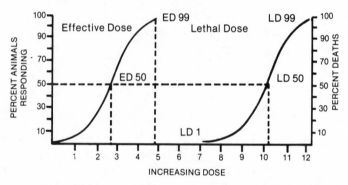

EXPERIMENTAL DATA — 20 ANIMALS / GROUP

| DOSE | RESPONSE | | DEATH | |
|---|---|---|---|---|
| | Number of Animals | % | Number of Animals | % |
| 1 | 1 | 5 | | |
| 2 | 4 | 20 | | |
| 3 | 12 | 60 | | |
| 4 | 18 | 90 | | |
| 5 | 20 | 100 | | |
| 6 | | | | |
| 7 | | | 1 | 5 |
| 8 | | | 2 | 10 |
| 9 | | | 4 | 20 |
| 10 | | | 8 | 40 |
| 11 | | | 18 | 90 |
| 12 | | | 20 | 100 |

B. **COMPARE THE MARGIN BETWEEN THE EFFECTIVE DOSE AND THE LETHAL DOSE.**

1. **The THERAPEUTIC INDEX may be used.**

   A) Therapeutic index $= \dfrac{LD_{50}}{ED_{50}}$

   B) The larger the number, the greater the safety.
   C) This index alone is not a true assessment of a drug's margin of safety.

2. **The standard safety margin (SSM) is a more accurate method.** This value expresses the percentage dose-increase between the $ED_{99}$ and the $LD_1$.

$$SSM(\%) = (\dfrac{LD_1}{ED_{99}} - 1) \times 100$$

Obviously, the wider the margin between the $ED_{99}$ and the $LD_1$, the safer the drug. There may be exceptions to strict application of this principle, but it holds true for most drugs used in veterinary medical practice.

# Inferences in Efficacy and Safety

In evaluating drugs, certain judgments must be made relative to a drug or its comparison to another drug. The use of the terms "good", "poor", "moderate", "useful", "effective", "not effective", "probably effective", "better", "superior", "routinely indicated", or "effective" in a majority of instances substantiates that there are some problems in drug evaluation. A tool that may provide useful information upon which judgment can be based is the application of statistical methods to the variables of biological events (*biostatistics*).

**Biostatistics** — a way to derive generalizations from variable phenomena.

A. **GENERALIZATIONS TO BE DERIVED FROM STATISTICS:**

1. **Are the data usual or unusual** (from same population)? A permissible range may be established for considering the data usual or "normal."
2. **Significant difference** — is there a real difference or might the difference be due to chance alone?
3. **Is there a demonstrable relationship** — *i.e.*, how closely are events related?

B.  **BIOSTATISTICS WILL NOT DEMONSTRATE CAUSE.**

C.  **DEMONSTRATE RELATIONSHIPS** — between treated and nontreated animals (nontreated controls).

   1. **Collect data from properly performed controlled experimentation for which the protocol has been carefully designed** — sampling, control groups, same handling and conditions, etc.

   2. Assume the null hypothesis which states that there is *no difference* between the control and the treatment groups, under the conditions of the experiment, other than by chance.

   3. **Use proper statistical evaluations of the data from both groups.**

   4. **Use the results of the statistics to:**
      A) Accept the null hypothesis that no difference exists and any noted difference represents chance; or
      B) Reject the null hypothesis and state that the observed difference varied too greatly to represent chance alone. Said another way: the difference between the treatment group and the control group is real or significant.

D.  **STUDENT'S t-TEST** — an often used biostatistical tool to determine the significance of the observed differences between drug treatment groups and controls.

   1. **The t-value** — a computed number from given formulae using the experimental data from both the treatment and control groups.

   2. **The t-value represents:**
      **The number of standard deviations on either side of the mean, or a measure of the** *standard score,* **or**

$$t = \frac{\text{observed differences in means}}{\text{estimated standard deviations of means}}$$
$$\text{(how groups differ)}$$

   3. **The probability of t** — written p(t), is an estimation of the probability that a t-value would occur as the result of chance alone.

   4. **The relationship of t and probability of chance is read from a table of t in which the degrees of freedom** (number of animals or samples on the test group) **are taken into account.**

   5. **The interpretation of this computed value is:**
      A) p(t) less than 0.01 means that a *t-value* of this size would occur from chance alone less than 1 time in 100 if the compared differences were the same. The null hypothesis would

be rejected, which means that the differences between groups were significant.

B) Levels of significance are decided on the basis of many factors related to a study, such as the number of animals or type of tests used. The following is a general guide used for pharmacological testing:

    1) $p(t)$ greater than 0.05 — *Not significant* (NS). The difference is not great enough to rule out **chance alone.**

    2) $p(t)$ less than 0.05 — *Significant.* May need more animals or more data to clearly establish significance.

    3) $p(t)$ less than 0.01 — *Highly significant*

    4) $p(t)$ less than 0.001 — *Very highly significant*

C) Small numbers of animals or samples need great differences (**larger t values**) to be significant. With large numbers of animals or samples, smaller differences can be significant.

D) A sample section from a table of t is shown below. The table takes into account the concepts discussed above.

### Table of Probability of t

| Degrees of Freedom | Probability of t | | | |
|---|---|---|---|---|
| | 0.1 | 0.05 | 0.01 | 0.001 |
| 1 | 6.31 | 12.71 | 63.66 | 636 |
| 5 | 2.02 | 2.57 | 4.03 | 6.87 |
| 10 | 1.81 | 2.23 | 3.17 | 4.59 |
| 15 | 1.75 | 2.13 | 2.95 | 4.07 |
| 20 | 1.72 | 2.09 | 2.85 | 3.85 |
| 30 | 1.70 | 2.04 | 2.75 | 3.65 |
| 60 | 1.67 | 2.00 | 2.66 | 3.46 |
| 100 | 1.66 | 1.98 | 2.62 | 3.39 |
| 1000 | 1.64 | 1.96 | 2.58 | 3.30 |

## F. PROBLEMS IN EVALUATING EFFICACY

1. **The distinction of difference** (statistical difference) — does not necessarily imply meaningful clinical difference.

2. **Pharmacologic versus therapeutic efficacy** — the ability of a drug to cause a significant change in some parameter in a given organ system may not necessarily mean the drug has therapeutic efficacy. Properly performed clinical trials are needed but are difficult to evaluate.

3. **Trials and comparisons of new drugs** — may be done using only closely related, healthy animals under ideal conditions. The

proof of the pudding is how well the drug performs in sick animals under field conditions; *i.e.*, model studies as opposed to clinical studies.

4. **Multiple responses to a single therapeutic agent are difficult to evaluate** — it is even more difficult to evaluate the responses of fixed drug combinations.

# Summary Scheme:
# General Principles of Drug Actions

The following scheme is an attempt to summarize the principles involved in the introduction of a drug into the animal's body, movement of the drug to the proper site of action, mechanics of the drug's action, and elimination of the drug from the animal's body. An attempt is made also to include the many variables involved in these processes, together with the important points for biological variations. This scheme is intended for use as a means of reviewing the relationships of all of the principles discussed up to this point.

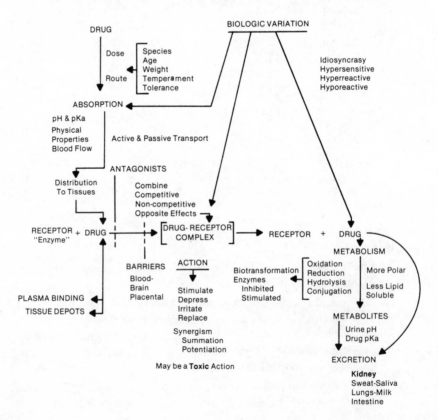

# Drug Toxicity

A. **GENERAL PRINCIPLES**
  1. **"All substances are poisons.** The right dose differentiates a poison from a remedy"—Paracelsus (1493-1541).
     A) No drug is entirely free from hazard.
     B) The toxic reaction may be an extension or exaggeration of the desired effect, or it may be a different type of reaction.
  2. **Variables or predisposing factors related to drug toxicity**
     A) Drug-related variables:
        1) *Chemical make-up of the compound* — certain groups of chemicals are potentially more toxic than others. Additional chemical groups many times can cause a problem. Example: the procaine in procaine penicillin G.
        2) *Route of administration* — A parenteral route is more likely than the oral route to cause adverse reactions. Higher blood levels are reached, and more quickly.
        3) *Quality of drug* affects bioavailability.
           a) Purity, sterility
           b) Stability or degree of deterioration, and expiration dates are important.
           c) Degradation products may be toxic.
           d) All drugs should receive proper care and handling. For example, refrigeration may be essential.

     B) Animal-related variables:
        1) *Age* — young and old animals are most susceptible.
        2) *Pregnancy* — female is more susceptible to adverse drug reactions. For example, some antibiotics are more hepatotoxic to a pregnant animal.
        3) *Congenital*
           a) Biological variation and biochemical individuality
           b) Some animals are more susceptible and may exhibit exaggerated responses. These are hyperreactive individuals that are obviously more susceptible to a toxic exaggeration of the drug effect.
        4) *Allergic history* — unfortunately this is not always known.
        5) *Simultaneous illness* — particularly liver and/or kidney diseases can alter the biotransformation and elimination of a drug.
        6) *Organ-to-organ interactions.* Example: increased levels of gonadal steroids and corticosteroids may have a detrimental influence on liver function.

3. **Causes of adverse drug reactions:**
   A) Frank overdose — *i.e.*, too high a dose, for too long, or too frequently.
   B) Relative overdose — simply means that the usual dose is too much. General causes of a relative overdose:
      1) Animal may be extremely hyperreactive
      2) Drug may be absorbed too quickly from the site of administration. A change of vehicle could increase absorption.
      3) Impaired inactivation and/or excretion of the drug
         a) In very young or very old animals
         b) In cases of liver and/or kidney disease
         c) With interference by other drugs
         d) In cases of a genetic deficiency of biotransforming enzymes
      4) Improper route of administration. Examples:
         a) With an accidental intracarotid injection, a large bolus of drug goes, undiluted, directly to the brain.
         b) A suspension, such as procaine penicillin G, given IV, can cause serious circulatory problems.
   C) Side effects or nontherapeutic effects — may have to be tolerated, but the client should be made aware of them.
   D) Accidental exposure or contact
      1) Ingestion of contaminated feed or water
      2) Contact with skin
      3) Inhalation
      4) Error in medication. Many therapeutic agents are so potent that dosage regimens must be precisely calculated.
   E) Interaction with other agents
      1) There is a tendency toward *polypharmacy*.
      2) Some drugs must not be given, or must be given very carefully when certain other drugs are in the animal's body. Example: phenothiazine-derivative tranquilizers and organophosphate drugs.
   F) Instituting incorrect therapy. For example: digitalis glycosides may be very toxic when given to an animal with a normal heart.

4. **Precautions against drug toxicities:**
   A) Use proper dosage, frequency and duration of administration.
   B) Avoid drug combinations where possible.
   C) Avoid mixing drugs, unless you are thoroughly familiar with the mixture or it has been clinically tested.
   D) Avoid a toxic drug if a less toxic one will suffice.

     E) Be aware of potential hazards and the precautions listed in package inserts.

     F) Use only drugs of high quality
       1) Proper dating
       2) Proper handling, storage, refrigeration if necessary
       3) No contamination or precipates

     G) Follow label directions. If you use a drug for an animal or a condition other than cited on the label, be sure you know the pharmacology and toxicology relative to this use of the drug.

     H) Obtain a good history of drug(s) given previously and of any prior adverse drug reactions.

5. **Treatment of drug toxicities**
     A) Remove source of offending substance(s).
     B) Enhance removal from animal's body.
       1) Induce vomiting in dogs and cats. Warm sodium chloride solution is an excellent emergency emetic. Apomorphine is the most reliable emetic for dogs. Be careful to prevent aspiration pneumonia.
       2) Speed up removal from intestines.
         a) Enema or gastrointestinal lavage is rapid and effective. In treating an unconscious or semiconscious animal, use care to prevent inhalation of foreign matter.
         b) Laxatives may be used but are rather slow acting.
       3) Speed metabolism and/or excretion of the drug.
     C) Counteract the toxic reactions.
       1) Specific treatments or antidotes:
         a) Chelation or competitive antagonism
         b) Physiological antagonism (opposite effects)
       2) Symptomatic treatment — attend to the animal's physiological needs: fluids, glucose, oxygen.
     D) Proper care and nursing
       1) Keep patient warm if in shock.
       2) Maintain open airways.

6. **Human health hazards of veterinary drugs**
     A) Guard against accidental ingestion of veterinary drugs, especially by children. Veterinarians should warn clients to take the same precautions as taken with human drugs relative to the availability of drugs to children. Label toxic drugs **Poison.** Use child-proof containers.

B) Tissue storage (tissue residues)
   1) A drug residue is simply an amount of a drug that is being temporarily stored in a certain tissue.
   2) The tissues of most importance to the livestock industry are meat, milk and eggs.
   3) The sophistication of modern instrumentation and research techniques make possible the identification and quantitation of drugs in amounts so small that they defy the imagination.
      a) Picogram = 0.000,000,000,001 g
      b) It is now possible to quantitate parts per trillion.
         1 part per trillion = 1 picogram/g or ml of material tested.
   4) Significance of drug residues in animal-food products
      a) *Potential* danger to human health
         (1) Toxic to man if large enough amounts are ingested.
         (2) May be toxic to certain organs.
         (3) May have an inhibitory effect on fertility.
         (4) May have adverse effects on fetus.
         (5) May be carcinogenic.
         (6) May initiate a drug allergy.
             During the days of high doses of penicillin in mastitis infusion products, some human cases of allergy to milk contaminated with penicillin were reported. With that exception, *no* case has ever been reported of an adverse reaction in man resulting from residue of a drug given to a food-producing animal.
      b) Residues may also be economically important to the livestock producer.
         (1) If samples of animal-food products are found to contain unlawful amounts of a drug, the product will be condemned and destroyed.
         (2) If samples of the same animal-food products continually contain unlawful amounts of a drug, a valuable medication or feed additive may be taken off the market. Examples are sulfonamides in swine and diethylstilbestrol in cattle.
   5) Veterinarian and/or livestockman may be prosecuted under the law if the drugs were wrongfully used.
   6) Veterinarian *might* be held liable for financial losses suffered by a client due to condemnations caused by residue if the residue resulted from the veterinarian's negligence in using the drug.

7) Problem areas that may lead to unlawful amounts of drugs or chemicals in tissues:
   a) Not following proper dosage regimens
   b) Not following proper withdrawal procedures, such as:
      (1) Withdrawing medication before slaughter
      (2) Discarding milk after mastitis therapy
   c) Using drug-contaminated equipment to mix ration during withdrawal period
   d) Feeding accidentally contaminated feeds, such as:
      (1) Pesticide-contaminated grain
      (2) Pesticide-contaminated hay
   e) Using wrong insecticides on or around the animals
   f) Using medications or medicated feeds in an unauthorized manner

# The Drug-Residue Problem

The following report from an FDA, BVM *Drug Memo* gives an overview of the residue problem.

Inadequate cleaning of feed equipment was the leading probable cause of illegal drug residues in food-producing animals, primarily sulfamethazine in swine, during 1977. A Food and Drug Administration (FDA) report cited failure to properly clean feed mixers, storage bins, and delivery trucks in 44 per cent of the residue violations where a probable cause could be found. Failure to observe pre-slaughter withdrawal times was the second leading probable cause (41 per cent of the cases).

Medicated feed was the most common route of administration involved in illegal residues, accounting for 74 per cent of the violations where a route of administration could be determined.

Figures from 1977 cannot validly be compared with figures from other years, because of the preponderance of residue violations involving sulfamethazine in swine in 1977; 328 of the 436 investigations made during the year involved sulfa residues in swine.

|  | Total 1977 | Second half 1977 |
|---|---|---|
| Number of investigations included in report | 436 | 267 |
| Number in which producer was identified | 366 (84%) | 221 (83%) |
| Number in which probable cause was found | 251 (69%) | 152 (69%) |
| Inadequately cleaned feed equipment | 44% | 54% |
| Withdrawal time not observed | 41% | 26% |
| Feeding or feed mixing error | 8% | 12% |
| No withdrawal time on drug label | 3% | 3% |
| Unapproved use of drug | 2% | 2% |
| Other | 1% | 4% |
| Number in which route of administration was found | 327 (74%) | 192 (71%) |
| Medicated feed | 74% | 95% |
| Injectable | 20% | 1% |
| Water medication | 3% | 4% |
| Direct oral dosage | 2% | — |

**RESULTS OF FIELD INVESTIGATION
OF ILLEGAL DRUG-RESIDUE REPORTS**

|  | Second Half 1976 | First Half 1976 | 1976 Total | 1975 Total |
|---|---|---|---|---|
| Number of investigations | 130 | 156 | 286 | 165 |
| Premises of origin determined | 117 (90%) | 139 (89%) | 256 (90%) | 157 (95%) |
| Probable cause of residue determined | 62 (53%) | 82 (59%) | 144 (56%) | 118 (75%) |
| Withdrawal time not observed | 79% | 61% | 69% | 67% |
| Inadequate cleaning— mixers, bins, trucks, feeders, water tanks | 10% | 12% | 11% | 12% |
| Unapproved usage of drug | 5% | 17% | 6% | 3% |
| Feed mixing, feeding or delivery error or accident | 5% | 11% | 8% | 14% |
| Use of drug with no withdrawal information on label | 1% | 7% | 5% | 3% |
| Route of drug administration determined | 101 (78%) | 108 (69%) | 209 (73%) | 130 (79%) |
| Injectable | 72% | 47% | 59% | 36% |
| Medicated feed | 21% | 41% | 31% | 51% |
| Water medication | 1% | 5% | 3% | 4% |
| Direct oral dosage | 2% | 5% | 3% | 9% |
| Mammary infusion | 4% | 2% | 2% | — |
| Implant | — | 1% | 1% | — |

A.  **KEY POINTS FOR THE PREVENTION OF UNLAWFUL RESIDUES**

1. Comply strictly with withdrawal requirements before marketing animals. (*See* charts beginning on page 89.)
   A) Do not assume that the required withdrawal time will pass between sale and slaughter of animals. Be safe. Take the animals off medication sufficiently ahead of sale.
   B) Thoroughly clean equipment before mixing drug-free rations.
2. Use medications only for purposes and species of animal indicated on the label.
3. Be careful when giving other drugs to animals receiving medicated feeds — a different withdrawal time may be indicated.

4. Give written instructions for proper use of drugs.

5. Carefully study and heed all warning statements on the label.

6. Encourage clients to be careful — feeds may become contaminated with other drugs, chemicals, or pesticides.

7. Never recommend mixing a drug or chemical into a feed — unless so authorized under state and federal laws.

8. Use, dispense or prescribe only specifically recommended insecticides for animals and premises.

## B. TRANSFER OF RESISTANCE TO ANTIBIOTICS FROM ANIMAL BACTERIA TO HUMAN PATHOGENS

Scientists working in microbiology have clearly shown that resistance to antibiotics can be transferred from one bacterial population to another. This is a transfer other than to daughter cells. The theory is well documented. Therefore, if this resistance were transferred from animal bacteria to bacteria pathogenic to man, a potential for a human health hazard is clearly involved. However, after many years of antibiotic use there has been no documentation that widespread use of antibiotics in animals has contributed to a human health hazard. Both veterinarians and livestockmen should concentrate on using antibiotics only where they are appropriate and eliminate indiscriminate use of antibiotics. This would do two things:

1. Diminish the likelihood of creating a human health hazard

2. Be more economical for livestockmen — in the minds of many veterinarians and livestockmen, antibiotics are often used when they are unnecessary.

## Food—Animal Drug Withdrawal Times*

### BEEF—CATTLE DRUG LIST

| Active ingredients | Withdrawal (days) |
|---|---|
| **INJECTABLES** | |
| Dihydrostreptomycin sulfate | 30 |
| Erythromycin | 14 |
| Levamisole phosphate | 7 |
| Oxytetracycline | 15 - 22 |
| Procaine penicillin G | 5 |
| Procaine penicillin G and dihydrostreptomycin sulfate | 30 |
| Sulfadimethoxine | 7 |
| Sulfamethazine | 10 |
| Sulfamerazine and sulfathiazole sodium | 10 |
| Sulfathiazole sodium and sulfapyridine sodium | 10 |
| Tylosin | 8 |
| **ORAL USE** | |
| Amprolium | 1 |
| Chlormadione acetate | 28 |
| Chlortetracycline | 2 - 10 |
| Chlortetracycline and sulfamethazine | 7 |
| Crufomate | 7 |
| Diethylstilbestrol | 14 |
| Famphur | 4 |
| Haloxon | 7 |
| Levamisole | 2 |
| Melengestrol acetate | 2 |
| Ronnel | 10 |
| Sulfabromomethazine | 10 |
| Sulfadimethoxine | 7 |
| Sulfamethazine | 10 |
| Sulfaquinoxaline | 10 |
| Thiabendazole | 3 |
| Tetracycline hydrochloride | 5 |
| **TOPICALS** | |
| Famphur and xylene | 35 |
| Fenthion | 35 - 45 |
| | (add 45 days if retreated) |
| N-(mercaptomethyl) phthalimide S-phosphorodithioate | 21 |
| **IMPLANTS** | |
| Diethylstilbestrol | 120 |
| Progesterone and estradiol benzoate | 60 |
| Estradiol benzoate and testosterone proprionate | 60 |
| Zeranol | 65 |

* From: Bureau of Veterinary Medicine *MEMO*, June 1978.

## BEEF—CALF DRUG LIST

| Active ingredients | Withdrawal (days) |
| --- | --- |

**INJECTABLES**

| | |
| --- | --- |
| Ampicillin trihydrate | 9 |
| Sodium sulfachlorpyridazine | 5 |
| Sulfadimethoxine | 7 |
| Dihydrostreptomycin | Withdrawal times |
| Erythromycin | for these drugs |
| Levamisole | are listed in |
| Oxytetracycline | the Beef Cattle |
| Tylosin | section. |
| Procaine penicillin G | |
| Procaine penicillin G and dihydrostreptomycin | |
| Sulfamethazine | |

**ORAL USE**

| | |
| --- | --- |
| Ampicillin tryhydrate | 7 |
| Chlorhexidine dihydrochloride and dihydrostreptomycin sulfate | 3 |
| Chlortetracycline hydrochloride | 1 - 3 |
| Chlortetracycline hydrochloride and chlortetracycline bisulfate | 3 |
| Chlortetracycline and neomycin | 1 |
| Dihydrostreptomycin | 30 |
| Streptomycin | 2 |
| Sulfachlorpyridazine | 7 |
| Sulfamethazine, streptomycin and phthalysulfathiazole | 10 |
| Tetracycline hydrochloride | 12 |
| Amprolium | Withdrawal times |
| Chlortetracycline sulfamethazine or vitamin B | for these drugs |
| Famphur | and drugs for |
| Haloxon | topical use in |
| Levamisole | calves are listed |
| Ronnel | in the Beef |
| Sulfabromethazine | Cattle section. |
| Sulfamethazine | |
| Sulfadimethoxine | |
| Tetracycline | |
| Thiabendazole | |

**IMPLANTS**

| | |
| --- | --- |
| Zeranol | 65 |

## DAIRY—CATTLE DRUG LIST

| Active ingredients | Withdrawal (days) | Milk discard milkings (hours) |
|---|---|---|
| **NON-LACTATING COWS** | | |
| **INJECTABLES** | | |
| Oxytetracycline | 15 - 22 | |
| **ORAL USE** | | |
| Famphur (feed) | 4 | |
| Ronnel (feed) | 10 | |
| (before slaughter, or freshening) | | |
| Sulfadimethoxine | 7 | |
| **TOPICALS** | | |
| Famphur & xylene | 35 | |
| Fenthion | 35 | |
| (add 45 days if retreated) | | |
| N-(mercaptomethyl) phthalimide | | |
| S-(O-O-dimethyl phosphordithioate) | 21 | |
| **LACTATING COWS** | | |
| **INJECTABLES** | | |
| Erythromycin | -- | 6 (72) |
| Furosemide | 2 | 4 (48) |
| Procaine penicillin G | 5 | 4-6 (48-72) |
| Procaine penicillin G and dihydrostreptomycin | 30 | 4-6 (48-72) |
| Sulfadimethoxine | 5 | 5 (60) |
| Sulfamethazine | 10 | 8 (96) |
| Tylosin | 8 | 8 (96) |
| **ORAL USE** | | |
| Dexamethasone and trichlormethiazide | -- | 6 (72) |
| Furosemide | -- | 4 (48) |
| Sulfabromomethazine | 10 | 8 (96) |
| Sulfadimethoxine | 7 | 5 (60) |
| Sulfamethazine | 10 | 8 (96) |
| Sulfisoxasole | 10 | 8 (96) |
| Thiabendazole | 3 | 8 (96) |

## DAIRY—CALF DRUG LIST

| Active ingredients | Withdrawal (days) |
|---|---|
| **INJECTABLES** | |
| Ampicillin trihydrate | 9 |
| Dihydrostreptomycin | 30 |
| Erythromycin | 14 |
| Levamisole | 7 |
| Oxytetracycline | 15 - 22 |
| Procaine penicillin G | 5 |
| Procaine penicillin G and dihydrostreptomycin sulfate | 30 |
| Sodium sulfachlorpyridazine | 5 |
| Sulfamethazine | 10 |
| Sulfadimethoxine | 7 |
| Tylosin | 8 |
| **ORAL USE** | |
| Ampicillin trihydrate | 7 |
| Amprolium | 1 |
| Chlorhexidine dihydrochloride and dihydrostreptomycin sulfate | 3 |
| Chlortetracycline hydrochloride | 1 - 3 |
| Chlortetracycline hydrochloride and chlortetracycline bisulfate (water) | 3 |
| Chlortetracycline and sulfamethazine (feed) | 7 |
| Chlortetracycline and vitamin B | 3 |
| Chlortetracycline and neomycin | 1 |
| Dihydrostreptomycin | 10 |
| Famphur (feed) | 4 |
| Haloxon | 7 |
| Levamisole | 2 |
| Ronnel | 10 |
| Streptomycin | 30 |
| Sulfabromomethazine | 10 |
| Sulfachlorpyridazine | 7 |
| Sulfadimethoxine | 7 |
| Sulfamethazine | 10 |
| Sulfamethazine, streptomycin and phthalysulfathiazole | 10 |
| Tetracycline hydrochloride (water) | 5 |
| Thiabendazole | 3 |
| **TOPICALS** | |
| Famphur and xylene | 35 |
| Fenthion | 35 - 45 |
| | (add 45 days if retreated |

## SWINE DRUG LIST

| Active ingredients | Withdrawal (days) |
| --- | --- |

**INJECTABLES**

| | |
| --- | --- |
| Dihydrostreptomycin | 30 |
| Erythromycin | 7 |
| Lincomycin | 2 |
| Oxytetracycline | 20 - 26 |
| Procaine penicillin G | 5 |
| Procaine penicillin G and dihydrostreptomycin | 30 |
| Sulfamerazine and sodium sulfathiazole | 10 |
| Sulfamethazine | 15 |
| Sulfathiazole and sulfapyridine | 10 |
| Tylosin | 4 |

**Oral Use**

| | |
| --- | --- |
| Ampicillin trihydrate | 1 |
| Arsanilic acid | 5 |
| Carbadox | 70 (10 weeks) |
| Chlortetracycline (feed or water) | 1 - 5 |
| Chlortetracycline bisulfate (water) | 3 |
| Chlortetracycline bisulfate and sulfamethazine (feed) | 15 |
| Chlortetracycline, sulfamethazine and procaine penicillin (feed) | 15 |
| Chlortetracycline, sulfathiazole and procaine penicillin (feed) | 7 |
| Furazolidone | 5 |
| Hygromycin B | 2 |
| Levamisole (feed or water) | 3 |
| Lincomycin (feed) | 6 |
| Nitrofurazone | 5 |
| Procaine penicillin G and streptomycin sulfate (water) | 2 |
| Pyrantel tartrate | 1 |
| Roxarsone | 5 |
| Sodium arsanilate | 5 |
| Sodium sulfachlorpyridazine | 4 |
| Sodium sulfathiazole | 10 |
| Sulfamethazine | 15 |
| Sulfaquinoxaline | 10 |
| Tetracycline hydrochloride (water) | 4 |
| Tylosin (with vitamins) | 2 |
| Tylosin and sulfamethazine | 5 |

## BABY—PIG DRUG LIST

| Active ingredients | Withdrawal (days) |
|---|---|
| **INJECTABLES** | |
| Iron dextrin complex and neomycin sulfate | 42 |
| Lincomycin | 2 |
| **ORAL USE** | |
| Chlortetracycline hydrochloride and chlortetracycline bisulfate (water) | 1 |
| Spectinomycin dihydrochloride pentahydrate | 21 |
| Thiabendazole paste | 30 |

## SHEEP AND GOAT DRUG LIST

| Active ingredients | Withdrawal (days) | Milk discard Milkings (hours) |
|---|---|---|
| **INJECTABLES** | | |
| Dihydrostreptomycin | 30 | --- |
| Erthromycin | 3 | 6 (72) |
| Procaine penicillin G | 5 | 6 (72) |
| Procaine penicillin G and dihydrostreptomycin | 30 | 4 (48) |
| Sulfamethazine (sheep only) | 10 | --- |
| **ORAL USE** | | |
| Diethylstilbestrol (sheep only) | 14 | --- |
| Haloxon | 7 | --- |
| Levamisole (sheep only) | 3 | --- |
| Crufomate | 7 | --- |
| Sulfamethazine | 10 | --- |
| Sulfaquinoxaline | 10 | --- |
| Sulfasoxasole | 10 | --- |
| Thiabendazole | 30 | 8 (96) |
| **IMPLANTS** | | |
| Diethylstilbestrol (lambs only) | 120 | --- |
| Zeranol (feedlot lambs only) | 40 | --- |
| **TOPICALS** | | |
| Flurgestron acetate | 30 | --- |

**Intramammary Infusion Mastitis Products Approved by FDA**
**(as of August, 1977)**

| Active Ingredient(s) | Representative Trade Names | Lactating or Dry Cow | OTC or Rx | Milk Discard Times | Pre-Slaughter Withdrawal Times |
|---|---|---|---|---|---|
| 400 mg Novobiocin | Biodry | Dry | OTC | (a) | 30 days |
| procaine penicillin G 100,000 units | Aqua-Pen & Four-Pen | L | OTC | 84 hours | 4 days |
| procaine penicillin G 100,000 units | Hanford's Penicillin | L | OTC | 60 hours | 3 days |
| procaine penicillin G 100,000 units | Formula A-34 | L | OTC | 60 hours | 3 days |
| potassium hetacillin equiv. to 62.5 mg ampicillin | Hetacin-K | L | Rx | 72 hours | 10 days |
| 1,000,000 U penicillin & 1 g dihydro-streptomycin | Quartermaster | Dry | Rx | 6 wks post-treat & 96 hr post-partum | 60 days post-treat & 96 hr post-partum |
| benzathine cloxacillin 500 mg | Orbenin-DC | Dry | Rx | (a) | 30 days |
| benzathine cloxacillin 500 mg | Dry-Clox | Dry | Rx | (a) | 30 days |
| benzathine cloxacillin 500 mg | Boviclox | Dry | Rx | (a) (b) | (c) |
| penicillin 100,000 U & novobiocin 150 mg | Albacillin & Special Formual 17900 Forte | L | OTC | 72 hours | 15 days |
| sodium cephapirin 200 mg/dose | Cefa-Lak & To-Day | L | OTC | 96 hours | 4 days |
| 426 mg oxytetra-cycline HCL | Liquamast | L & D | OTC | 72 hours | None established |
| 300 mg erythromycin | Gallimycin 36 Sol'n | L & D | OTC | 36 hours | None established |
| 500 mg furaltadone | Valsyn Gel | L & D | OTC | 96 hours | None established |
| 60 mg nitrofurazone | Furacin Sol'n | Dry | OTC | 72 hours | None established |

(a) Not to be used within 30 days of calving.
(b) Milk taken from treated cows prior to 72 hours after calving must not be used for food.
(c) Not to be slaughtered for food from time of infusion until 72 hours after calving.

# Types of Toxic or Adverse
# Drug Reactions

A. **ALLERGIC HYPERSENSITIVITY**

1. **A manifestation of the immune response**

   A) Many drugs or their metabolites may act as antigens.

   B) Many drugs (hapten) conjugate with a body protein to form an antigen.

      1) Upon the animal's first exposure to the drug (antigen), the antigen stimulates the body to produce antibodies that are specific for the drug.

      2) Upon the animal's second exposure to the drug:

         a) The antigen (drug) and specific antibodies combine to produce a reaction.

         b) This reaction releases toxic substances in certain tissues (histamine, serotonin, heparin, acetylcholine). These substances cause the allergic response.

      3) Release of histamine and its effects on physiological functions will be discussed in the section on antihistamines.

2. **Three general types of allergic reactions:**

   A) *Atopic* — incomplete partial antibodies are formed which have special affinities for the skin, nose, and lung. Examples:

      1) *Urticaria* — a vascular reaction in skin, causing pale or red mild-to-severe patches. The resulting hyperemia and fluid leakage produce welts and edematous areas.

      2) *Hay fever type* — rhinitis, conjunctivitis, etc.

      3) *Asthma-like* — causes bronchiolar constriction and difficult breathing.

   B) *Anaphylactic*

      1) Rapid onset—usually within a few minutes, due to the production of mature, bivalent antibodies. Large numbers of these antibodies are present.

      2) The antibodies attach to tissue cells around vessels and/or bronchioles.

      3) The antigen/antibody reaction takes place in the cells mentioned above. This produces vascular collapse and respiratory collapse, leading to *shock*.

   C) *Delayed or contact dermatitis*

      1) Incomplete antibodies are produced and are still inside the cell.

      2) Antigen enters the cell; then allergic reaction occurs.

      3) Reactions usually occur within two to three days, rarely longer.

B. **PHOTOSENSITIVITY** — requires exposure to both sunlight and drugs. Energy of sunlight causes changes in the drug molecule. A drug thus changed can lead to toxic reactions by two mechanisms:

1. **Phototoxic** — a direct effect
    A) Energy is transferred from light to the drug. Drug molecule changes and may yield free radicals, peroxides and heat.

    Cellular alteration occurs in membranes, cytoplasm and/or nucleus , resulting in tissue damage .

    ↓

    B) Exaggerated sunburn-type reaction
    C) Nonimmunologic, no incubation period
    D) Occurs with first exposure to light
    E) Infrequent cross reactions occur between structurally related compounds.

2. **Photoallergic** — involves the allergic response
    A) Transfer of energy causes changes in the drug molecule and forms a new compound (hapten). Hapten is conjugated and forms an antigen. Antigen stimulates production of antibodies (cellular or humoral). Antigen/antibody reaction, upon reexposure of animal to drug and light, causes cell damage.
    B) Incubation period is necessary.
    C) Must be genetically susceptible; a small percentage of animals may be involved.
    D) Triggered by smaller amounts of drug.
    E) Urticaria type is most common.

3. **Schematic summary of photosensitization**

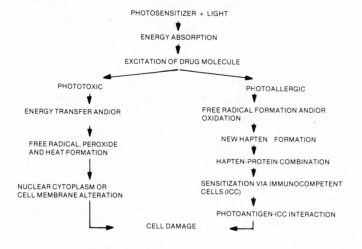

C.  **DRUG-INDUCED ORGAN INJURY** — caused by a direct injurious action of a drug upon cells, tissues and organs. Drugs can induce many different types of insults to tissues. These will be discussed by organ systems.

1.  **Blood Dyscrasias**

    A) *Aplastic anemia* — toxic effect is upon bone marrow. Blood cell-forming tissue is altered. May proceed to myeloblastic leukemia, which is usually fatal.

        1) *Signs*
            a) Weakness
            b) Pallor
            c) Hemorrhages
            d) Lessened resistance to infections

    B) *Agranulocytosis* (severe neutropenia)

        1) *Signs:* Explosive onset of severe infection characterized by necrosis and no pus.

        2) *Mechanisms:*
            a) An antibody-reaction mechanism has been proposed.
            b) The antibodies agglutinate leukocytes in the presence of the drug.
            c) Other possible mechanisms are not known.

    C) *Hemolytic anemia* — occurs when the drug increases destruction of RBCs. May be acute or chronic.

        1) *Signs:* Reduced concentration of hemoglobin after the drug is administered, with return to normal after the drug is withdrawn.

        2) *Mechanisms:*
            a) Animal may have a deficiency of a red-cell enzyme (glucose-6-phosphate dehydrogenase). This deficiency causes red blood cells to become more fragile, which increases their susceptibility to hemolysis by drugs.
            b) An antigen/antibody reaction could lead to disruption of cells.
            c) High levels of drug may directly disrupt cells by insulting the cell membrane.

    D) *Thrombocytopenia* (reduced number of platelets) — results in inhibition of the blood coagulation mechanism.

        1) *Signs:*
            a) Serious blood loss
            b) Brain hemorrhage
            c) Purpura

        2) *Mechanisms:*
            a) An antigen/antibody reaction occurs which damages the platelets and inhibits their function. It may also

result in an increase in the rate at which platelets are destroyed.
   b) Depression of production. *May be irreversible.*
   c) Drugs may be directly toxic to platelets and thus inhibit their function.

2. **Liver**
   A) *Disturbances of pigment metabolism* — may be caused by drugs. In all instances, the bilirubin is not properly excreted; therefore, it accumulates in the blood and body tissues.
      1) Pigment overload due to hemolytic reactions.
         a) Some directly produced; *e.g.*, drugs rupture RBCs.
         b) Some result from the antigen-antibody reaction which in turn increases the breakdown of RBCs.
      2) Decrease in hepatic uptake of bilirubin into liver cell
      3) Inhibition of bilirubin conjugation within liver cell
      4) Drug and bilirubin compete for biliary excretion.
   B) *Hepatic injury* — the drug directly injures the cell. The general pattern is as follows:
      1) Hepatocellular damage is the main effect, but the clinical disorder may be manifested in other organ systems. An example is impaired production of blood-clotting factors.
      2) Injury occurs in all individuals if the administered dose of drug is great enough. Can be consistently reproduced in experimental animals.
      3) Brief, uniform latent period
      4) Degree of injury is predictable
      5) Degree of injury is dose-related
   C) *Inflammatory reaction* — manifested by an acute hepatic necrosis and has a longer latent period. It is difficult to pinpoint a cause-and-effect relationship as exists with hepatitis.
      1) Pre-existing liver damage may be a prerequisite.
      2) Many drugs may lead, either directly or indirectly, to hypoxia. The liver is sensitive to a shortage of oxygen and the hypoxia causes the liver cells to function abnormally. Affected cells are more susceptible to an inflammatory-like insult by certain drugs.
   D) *Hypersensitivity* — a form of allergic reaction. It usually produces cholestasis (a plugging-up or backing-up of bile in the duct system of the liver).
      1) General pattern
         a) Variable histological changes
         b) Injury not restricted to liver; may also include skin rashes, fever, etc.
         c) No consistent dose relationship

       d) No consistent latent period

       e) Sporadic occurrence

       f) Unpredictable

       g) Cannot consistently be reproduced in experimental animals

    E) *Simple cholestasis* — Drug interferes with excretion of bile. With the aid of the electron microscope, changes in microvilli of bile canaliculi are seen. All individuals show some degree of cholestasis, depending upon degree of drug exposure.

3. **Kidney**

    A) *Direct toxic effect*

       1) Identifiable morphological or functional changes occur because of a direct toxic effect of the drug.

       2) Acute tubular necrosis may result.

       3) Chronic nephrotoxicity may last months or years.

    B) *Hypersensitivity* (allergic reaction)

       1) May affect the kidney cells.

       2) May affect the blood vessels of the kidney.

    C) Drug may induce a decrease in flow of blood and an oxygen to the kidney, resulting in:

       1) Inhibition of transport schemes; thus the result may be severe metabolic changes in the body. Example: loss of bicarbonate ($HCO_3$).

       2) Necrosis and inhibition of metabolism of kidney cells.

       3) Large doses of pressor agents (epinephrine and norepinephrine) in shock therapy can readily shut down blood flow to nephrons.

    D) *Predisposing disease.* A drug may simply aggrevate a pre-existing renal disease.

4. **Nervous system** — may be readily affected by many drugs. Generally, types of adverse effects of drugs on the nervous system include:

    A) Direct effect upon morphology of nervous tissue

    B) Disturbance of a physiological control system, because an organ-system response is manifested in other organs. Example: inhibition of the respiratory or vasomotor control areas.

    C) CNS may be depressed, resulting in coma and death.

    D) CNS may be stimulated, which can lead to convulsions, coma, and death.

    E) Impairment of special senses

       1) Deafness

       2) Vestibular disturbances (balance problems)

       3) Impaired or blurred vision

       4) Retinopathy, glaucoma and/or cataracts

5. **Heart and blood vessels**
   A) Impaired circulation due to changes in vessels or an inhibitory effect directly upon the heart.
   B) Some drugs may cause arrhythmias, even fibrillate the heart. Epinephrine, for example, given IV in too great a dose or for long periods may cause ventricular fibrillation.

6. **Lungs** — the mechanisms for drug-induced injury or decreased function are as follows:
   A) May irritate the secretory cells and cause excessive secretion and build-up of fluids in lungs.
   B) May constrict bronchioles and restrict air passage.
   C) May damage the membranes of gaseous exchange areas in alveoli.

7. **Gastrointestinal tract** — general types of drug-induced adverse reactions include:
   A) Irritation and corrosion of mucosae. Causes diarrhea and/or vomiting with loss of fluids, electrolytes and nutrients.
   B) May cause the formation of ulcers. Mechanisms include:
      1) Irritation
      2) Stimulation of excessive secretion of HCl
      3) Excessive production of digestive enzymes
      4) Depression of the rate at which the normal desquamated epithelium of the tract is replaced. This is an adverse action, an anti-inflammatory response. It may be brought about by an anti-inflammatory drug such as aspirin.

8. **Endocrine system**
   A) Direct toxic effect upon gland, causing a reduction of its function and decreased hormone output.
   B) Disturbance (excessive stimulation or inhibition) of control systems. Induced by influencing the feedback-scheme in the pituitary gland, and normal control of hormone levels.
   C) End-responses are seen in the organ systems, which are controlled by hormones. For example, extensive, prolonged corticosteroid therapy will shut down the adrenal cortex.

9. **Reproduction** — drugs may influence the reproductive process in many ways.
   A) *Impaired Fertility*
      1) Female
         a) Improper cycling and ovulation
         b) Improper implantation
         c) May contribute to uterine changes that lead to early embryonic death
      2) Male: Poor semen quality

B) May bring about *mutagenesis*
   1) Acts upon parent. Drug acts on the egg or the sperm.
   2) Deleterious effect on genes. Action precedes conception.
   3) May bring about lethal and sublethal gene action.
   4) May bring about teratogenesis via altered gene action that controls organogenesis.

C) May bring about *teratogenesis*
   1) Drug is given to pregnant animal. (*See* B above for exception.)
   2) Malformations of the fetus are induced.
   3) Deleterious effect is upon organogenesis. Cells are disrupted when they are differentiating to become a specific tissue.
   4) Exposure to drug must occur between implantation and the time of organogenesis.
   5) ★ **First trimester is critical time in most cases.**
   6) Stage of embryonic development is critical.
      a) Rapidly proliferating cells are unusually sensitive. This occurs in the first trimester.
      b) During organogenesis, injury or destruction of cells will lead to derangements in form or function.
   7) Mechanisms by which the embryo is affected:
      a) Directly, drug action is injurious to cells of embryo.
      b) Altered maternal environment, such as reduction of oxygen or nutrients to the embryonic cells
   8) When given at higher doses, drugs that produce teratogenic disturbances are likely to cause death and resorption of the fetus.

10. **Disturbances in body defense mechanisms**
   A) Depression of resistance to infection by:
      1) Inhibition of immune response and decreased production of antibodies; decreased production of interferon.
      2) Inhibition of the functional ability of phagocytic cells
   B) Depression of tissue repair and healing, most generally by an inhibition of protein synthesis

11. **Alteration of physiological schemes**
   A) Impaired absorption of nutrients from the GI tract. Example: Dilantin® decreases absorption of folic acid and/or vitamin $B_{12}$, thus reducing ability to manufacture red blood cells.
   B) Sterile gut — microflora are inhibited by antibiotics or sulfonamides given orally for an extended period of time. The reduction in microflora leads to altered digestion and vitamin synthesis. May lead to an abnormal increase in populations of resistant bacteria or fungi.

C) Alteration of endocrine feedback schemes.
  1) *Chemical castration* — extended use of testosterone inhibits the testicle by inhibiting the output of pituitary gonadotropins.
  2) *Steroid adrenalectomy* — same mechanism will cause the adrenal cortex to become dormant if steroids are given for several days.
D) Alteration of acid-base balance, water balance, and electrolyte balance
E) Change in binding or storage of endogenous substances
F) Interference with the process by which blood coagulates
G) Inhibition of the ability of hemoglobin to transport oxygen

12. **Carcinogenesis** — the cancer-producing ability of chemicals. Cancer is the excessive and uncontrolled proliferation of cells brought about by disruption in the biochemical make-up or control of DNA and RNA.
A) The effects of carcinogens are dose-dependent.
B) The effects of carcinogens are additive.
C) The effects of carcinogens are irreversible.
D) Carcinogenesis requires time.
E) Cellular changes that bring about carcinogenesis are transmitted to daughter cells.
F) Carcinogenesis can be influenced by factors that are not truly carcinogenic.
G) Carcinogenesis requires rapid proliferation of cells. Slow-dividing cells are not as susceptible.
H) May be long delays; *i.e.,* months or years may be involved before uncontrolled proliferation starts.
I) Importance in veterinary medicine
  1) Safety of our patients — does the drug cause cancer when given to the animal?
  2) Role of residues in food-producing animals and their potential to induce cancer in man

**REPORT ADVERSE DRUG REACTIONS**

The Bureau of Veterinary Medicine of the FDA wants veterinarians to continue reporting adverse drug reactions encountered in practice. The Bureau wants reports of (1) all unexpected reactions, particularly those that are serious, life threatening, or fatal; (2) increases in the number or severity of reaction(s); (3) problems concerning a product's effectiveness; and (4) possible association with congenital abnormalities or problems during pregnancy.

Veterinarians who need postpaid Adverse Drug Reaction Reporting Cards or information about the Adverse Reaction Reporting Program should write to:

Walter L. Graves, DVM
Director, Division of Surveilance, HFV-216
Bureau of Veterinary Medicine
Food and Drug Administration
5600 Fishers Lane
Rockville, MD  20857

An Adverse Drug Reaction Hot Line (301-443-4093) also can be used.

Single copies of the Annual Summary of the Adverse Reaction Reporting Program are available on request from the Industry Information Branch, HFV-226, at the above address.

CHAPTER

# 2

# Central Nervous System

## Physiological Principles

A. **FORM AND FUNCTION**
1. **The CNS is a complex organ system by which:**
    A) The animal is brought into functional reaction with its environment, *i.e.* the animal is able to adapt to changes.
    B) The animal's various parts and organ systems are controlled and coordinated.
    SUMMARY: *ADAPT and COMMUNICATE.*
2. **Two systems for communication between the animal's body parts:**
    A) *Nervous system* — messages are sent as impulses over a nerve-tract network. These impulses are electrical in nature and can be measured. Examples are nerve-action potentials or brain waves (EEG).
    B) *Endocrine system* — messages are sent as chemicals (hormones) traveling via the blood stream from site of origin to target tissue(s). They may act locally.

    These two systems function to bring about a response (effect) in a target tissue and hence influence organs and organ systems. The nervous system and the endocrine system are closely related structurally and functionally.

3. **Functional classification**
   A) *Central nervous system* (CNS)
      1) Brain
      2) Spinal cord
   B) *Peripheral nervous system*
      1) Cranial nerves
      2) Spinal nerves
      3) Autonomic nervous system (ANS)

   *Not a rigid classification; there is considerable overlap.*

**ORGANIZATION
OF THE NERVOUS SYSTEM**

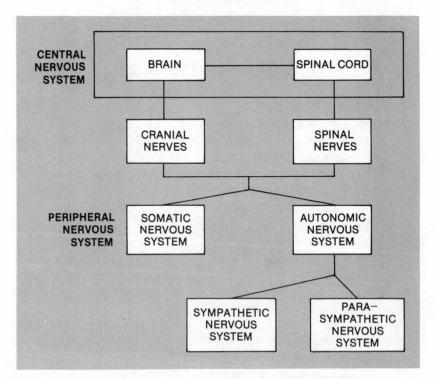

4. **Basic unit of the nervous system is the neuron** — a nerve cell that carries out the function of the nervous system.

## NEURON

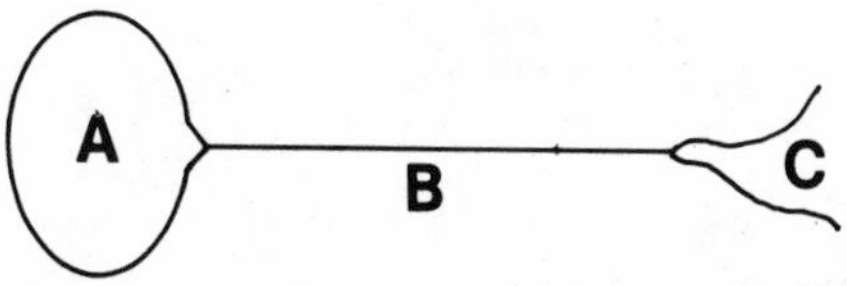

### A. DENDRITIC ZONE

Senses changes
Responds to a stimulus
Responds to neurotransmitters
Generates an impulse

### B. AXON

Conducts impulse from dendritic zone to nerve ending

### C. TELODENDRITIC ZONE (nerve ending)

Pass impulse to next structure, which is either:
  i.  another neuron, or
  ii.  an effector cell

Message carried via a chemical across the gap to the next structure. The chemical messenger is called a neurotransmitter.

5. **Basic functions of neurons:**
   A) *Generate* and *conduct* electrical impulses
   B) *Pass impulse* (message) to the next structure
   C) In order to reach the next structure, the impulse must cross a gap called a *junction* or *synapse.*
   D) Messages are carried across the junctions by chemicals called *neurotransmitters.*
   E) *Neurotransmitters* may be either *stimulatory* or *inhibitory.*
   F) *Neurotransmitters* may be either *mimicked* or *blocked* by closely related exogenous compounds (drugs). This is the mechanism by which many drugs act upon the CNS.

6. **Two types of junctions:**
   A) Synapse — the junction between two neurons
   B) Neuro-effector junction — the junction between a nerve ending and an effector cell. The effector cell carries out the instructions of the nervous system.

**SYNAPSE** — Junction between two neurons

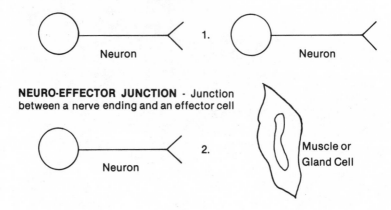

**NEURO-EFFECTOR JUNCTION** - Junction between a nerve ending and an effector cell

## SCHEMATIC
## OF A REFLEX ARC

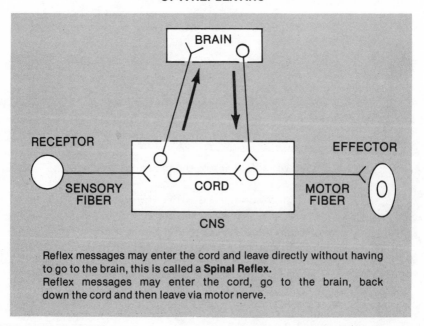

Reflex messages may enter the cord and leave directly without having to go to the brain, this is called a **Spinal Reflex.**
Reflex messages may enter the cord, go to the brain, back down the cord and then leave via motor nerve.

7. **The reflex arc** — carries out reflex actions. It is the basic functional unit of the nervous system. Utilizes several neurons. Five component parts of a reflex arc are:

   A) *Receptor* — senses changes and generates an impulse.
      1) *External* — receptors found in skin, ear, eye. Examples: hearing, sight, touch, pressure, pain, temperature.
      2) *Internal* — receptors found in the internal organs such as the brain, mouth, muscle and viscera. Examples: taste, hunger, thirst, fatigue, nausea, carbon dioxide and oxygen sensors, position and movement (stretch and contraction of muscles and tendons), blood pressure.

   B) *Sensory nerve fiber* — carries impulse to CNS.
   C) *Central nervous system* — integrates, modulates, and relays impulse to appropriate motor-output nerve fibers.
   D) *Motor-nerve fiber* — carries impulse from CNS to target cell.
   E) *Effector* cell — carries out or responds to the order brought by the impulse.

B. **FUNCTIONAL ANATOMY OF THE BRAIN**

   1. **Brain**
      A) *Cerebrum* — "higher centers" is the common term for the cerebral area.
      B) *Cerebellum*
      C) *Brainstem*
         1) Thalamus          4) Pons
         2) Hypothalamus      5) Medulla
         3) Midbrain          6) Reticular formation

   2. **Schematic of the brain** — illustrates the anatomic relationship of pharmacologically important areas.

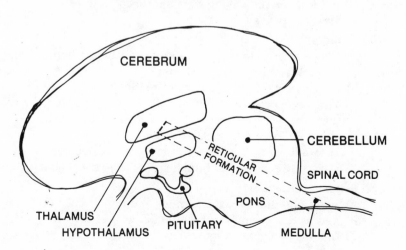

## C. FUNCTIONS OF THE CENTRAL NERVOUS SYSTEM

1. **Cerebrum** — motor and sensory. Association areas function to:
   A) *Regulate* muscular movement
   B) *Interpret* sensory input
   C) *Evaluate* and *integrate* stimuli, make decisions
   D) *Correlate* incoming sensory stimuli (listed below) with appropriate outgoing motor responses.

   | | |
   |---|---|
   | 1) Perception | 6) Reasoning |
   | 2) Emotion | 7) Sight |
   | 3) Sensation | 8) Sound |
   | 4) Memory | 9) Taste |
   | 5) Intelligence | 10) Hearing |

2. **Cerebellum** — synergizes motor movements relative to:
   A) Posture    B) Coordination    C) Balance

3. **Thalamus**
   A) *Relays* sensory input to cerebrum
   B) Is the area of crude *awareness* in the brain
   C) Enables recognition of *pain*

4. **Hypothalamus**
   A) *Controls* and *integrates* the autonomic nervous system; chief regulator of visceral activities
   B) *Receives* and *interprets* sensory input from the *viscera*
   C) Acts as principal *intermediary* between the nervous system and the endocrine system via the pituitary gland
   D) *Regulates* body temperature
   E) *Regulates* thirst and hunger
   F) *Regulates* water balance
   G) Helps *maintain* waking state and sleep patterns
   H) May be involved in *rage*

5. **Medulla**
   A) *Conduction pathway* for sensory and motor impulses between the brain and spinal cord
   B) *Respiratory center* — controls breathing
   C) *Vasomotor center* — control center for heart and blood pressure
   D) Other reflex centers located here:

   | | | |
   |---|---|---|
   | 1) Swallowing | 3) Vomiting | 5) Coughing |
   | 2) Sneezing | 4) Blinking | 6) Hiccoughing |

6. **Reticular formation**
   A) Sends impulses to higher centers and lower centers
   B) Acts as reinforcing or *background agent* of the CNS
   C) Inhibits exaggerated movements

D) Enables perception of *pain*

E) Regulates state of *wakefulness* and *sleep*
   1) Level of alertness
   2) Behavioral arousal

7. **Vital centers** (a functional term)
   A) Important physiological control centers which are vital to health
   B) Situated anatomically in the following areas of the brain:
      1) Thalamus          3) Medulla
      2) Hypothalamus      4) Brainstem
   C) May be affected by many drugs
      1) May be *stimulated* or *inhibited*
      2) May be affected for a therapeutic purpose. An example is Dopram® -V (A.H. Robins) or Metrazol® (Knoll) given to a deeply anesthetized animal to restore breathing.
      3) May suffer a serious side or toxic effect when a drug is used for another purpose. For example, anesthetics may depress the respiratory center.
      4) *Must use extreme care* — tampering with control centers can be serious and affect many organ systems. The key to successful use of CNS drugs, and specifically anesthetics, is: **pay attention to vital signs.**
   D) Vital control centers
      1) Respiratory    4) Water balance    7) Emetic
      2) Reflex         5) Cough            8) Body temperature
      3) Vasomotor      6) Urinary bladder  9) Emotion

      10) Hunger and thirst
      11) Sympathetic nervous system
      12) Parasympathetic nervous system
      13) Hypothalamic-pituitary axis; control of the endocrine system is centered here.

## D. INTERRELATIONSHIP OF NERVOUS AND ENDOCRINE SYSTEM

1. **Endocrine glands may be stimulated directly by nerve impulses;** *e.g.* motor fibers of the sympathetic nervous system stimulate the adrenal medulla to release epinephrine into the blood stream.

2. **Hormones may have a direct effect on the CNS.**
   A) *Estrogen* brings about behavioral estrus in the female.
   B) *Epinephrine* and *norepinephrine* increase aggressiveness.
   C) *Thyroxin* tends to stimulate the CNS.

  D) *Testosterone* creates sex drive in males.

  E) *Corticosteroids* may stimulate the CNS, producing euphoria.

  F) High levels of *progesterone* may inhibit the CNS.

3. **The nervous system plays a vital role in the control of endocrine glands** — influences the hypothalamus and the pituitary gland.

  A) Situational or environmental factors may influence the endocrine system through nervous-system input.

  B) Schematic of neuro-pituitary-endocrine relationships

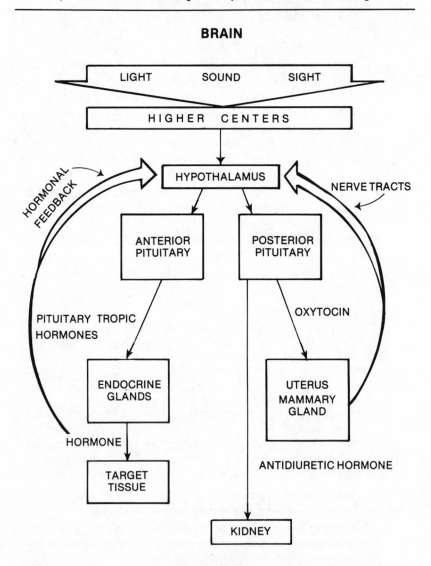

C) *Neurohormonal arc* — this physiological control scheme uses the basic concept of a reflex arc, except that the last part of the arc (the motor output) is carried out by a hormone, *oxytocin*. Three general schemes for this arc:

1) If a calf suckles or if the cow's udder and teats are washed with warm water, receptors in the skin generate an impulse which travels via nerves to the hypothalamus. The hypothalamus signals the posterior pituitary to release oxytocin into the blood. The oxytocin travels to the mammary gland and stimulates milk let-down.

2) The higher centers may also be stimulated by sights and sounds associated with milking (clanging milk buckets, milking machines, etc.) and signal the hypothalamus to initiate the release of oxytocin.

3) Nervous system receptors in the uterus, cervix and vagina also can initiate an impulse which is sent to the hypothalamus to release oxytocin as a part of parturition.

4. **Hormonal feedback control system** — the nervous system is sensitive to circulating levels of certain hormones via a scheme called *the feedback control mechanism.*

A) Activity of an endocrine gland is controlled by the circulating plasma level of the hormone produced by that gland. A check-and-balance system exists.

B) Feedback may be either positive or negative.

1) *Negative feedback scheme:*

a) High plasma levels of a hormone are sensed by the hypothalamus. The hypothalamus decreases the releasing factor (RF). The RF provides the mechanism by which the hypothalamus stimulates the anterior pituitary. The RFs are released from hypothalamic cells and travel via the blood from the hypothalamus to the anterior pituitary.

b) Reduced level of RF *decreases* the release of anterior pituitary hormones.

c) Reduced level of pituitary tropic hormones brings about *decreased activity* of target endocrine gland(s). The endocrine gland then becomes "dormant."

2) *Positive feedback scheme:*

a) Low plasma levels of a hormone are sensed by the hypothalamus. The hypothalamus increases levels of RF.

b) An increased level of RF *stimulates* the *pituitary* to release increased amounts of pituitary hormones.

c) An increased level of pituitary hormones brings about *increased activity* of target endocrine glands.

3) The hypothalamus may also be sensitive to and controlled
by drugs that are closely related to natural hormones.
   a) Estrogens, androgens and progestins are effective in
      the male or female. This is the basic mechanism for
      control and synchronization of estrus.
   b) Hydrocortisone and new synthetic anti-inflammatory
      steriods are all sensed by the hypothalamus, which
      cannot differentiate between natural hydrocortisone
      and synthetic relatives.

C) Schematic of hypothalamic-pituitary functional relationship:

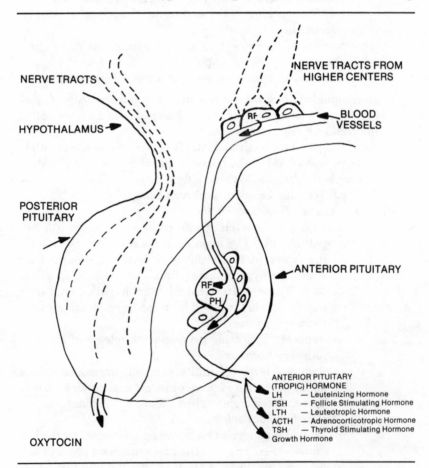

NERVE TRACTS

NERVE TRACTS FROM HIGHER CENTERS

HYPOTHALAMUS

BLOOD VESSELS

RF

POSTERIOR PITUITARY

ANTERIOR PITUITARY

RF
PH

ANTERIOR PITUITARY
(TROPIC) HORMONE
LH — Leuteinizing Hormone
FSH — Follicle Stimulating Hormone
LTH — Leuteotropic Hormone
ACTH — Adrenocorticotropic Hormone
TSH — Thyroid Stimulating Hormone
Growth Hormone

OXYTOCIN

5. **The nervous system plays a vital role in the animal's ability to react to stress and life-threatening situations** — the CNS provides the ability to return to and/or maintain the internal environment in normal homeostasis.

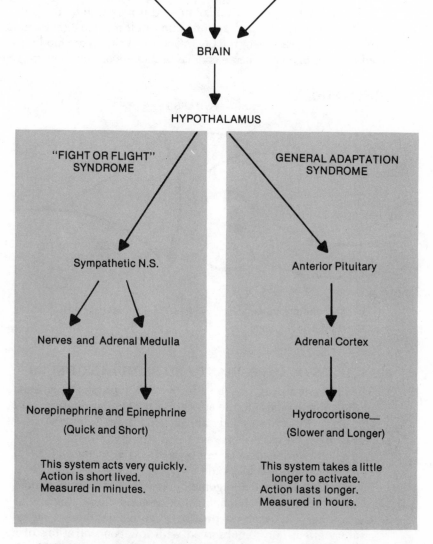

6. **Drugs may influence control systems** — depending on how they influence the CNS. They may be utilized as a therapeutic tool or may cause a side effect that should be kept in mind.

# Drug Actions on
# Central Nervous System

A. **MAY STIMULATE OR DEPRESS NEURONS**

B. **DRUGS INFLUENCE CENTRAL NERVOUS SYSTEM BY:**

1. **Acting directly on nerve cells**

2. **Influencing synaptic transmission** — this may well be the principal mechanism of drug action. The result may be either stimulation or depression of the CNS. Central synapses are modulated by both inhibitory nerve endings and excitatory nerve endings.

**SCHEMATIC:**

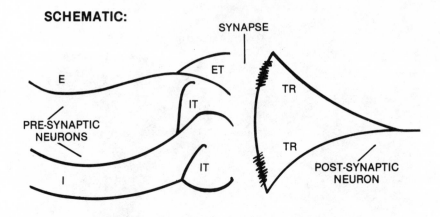

ET = Excitatory transmitter    TR = Transmitter receptor
IT  = Inhibitory transmitter

C. **PRINCIPLES OF DEPRESSANT AND STIMULANT DRUGS**

1. **The effect of a drug may be additive to the physiological state of the animal** — also to the effect of other similar depressant or stimulant drugs in the body at the same time.

2. **Antagonism between depressant and stimulant drugs**
   A) Called *physiological* or *opposite-effects antagonism*
   B) It is *not* receptor blockade
   C) An example is the antagonizing action of Metrazol® (Knoll) or Dopram-V® (A.H. Robins) on general anesthetics.

3. **Central nervous system depressants depress neurons** — an excitatory effect may be observed with low concentrations of a depressant drug due to depression of inhibitor neurons. This allows the excitatory neurons to dominate. The excitement that may be seen during induction of anesthesia is a typical example.

4. **Drugs that stimulate the central nervous system stimulate the neurons** — a depressant effect of a stimulant may also be observed when stimulation of inhibitor neurons causes the inhibitor to dominate. Example: amphetamine and Ritalin® (Ciba) have been used to treat hyperkinetic dogs and children.
5. **Acute, excessive stimulation of the central nervous system** is normally followed by depression.
6. **Acute depression** is not usually followed by stimulation.
7. **Chronic drug-induced depression** may be followed by hyperexcitability.

## D. DRUG INFLUENCE

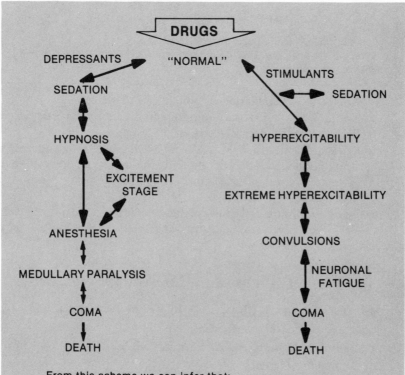

From this scheme we can infer that:
1. Excitement may occur with drugs that depress the CNS.
2. Sedation may occur with drugs that stimulate the CNS.
3. Both excitement and sedation may be by-passed.
4. Overdosage of either a CNS stimulant or CNS depressant may cause coma and death.
5. Usually, animals recover (return to normal) from CNS depression or stimulation by means of reverse flow of this same scheme.

E.  **DEPRESSANT DRUGS** (response terms)

 1. **Sedation** — slight depression. Patient is awake.
 2. **Hypnosis** — greater depression. Patient is asleep but can be awakened.
 3. **Narcosis** — patient asleep, can be awakened, will return to sleep. Implies very good analgesia.
 4. **Anesthesia** — without sensation. Patient asleep and cannot be awakened. Amnesia and loss of reflexes are present.

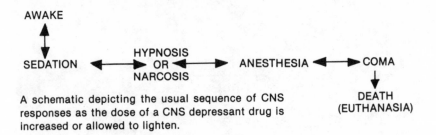

A schematic depicting the usual sequence of CNS responses as the dose of a CNS depressant drug is increased or allowed to lighten.

 5. **Analgesia** — alleviation of pain. Patient is alert.
 6. **Tranquilizer** — some sedation and hypnosis. Mainly alters behavior and the animal's reaction to its environment.
 7. **Cataleptic anesthesia or dissociative anesthesia** — superficial sleep, good analgesia and amnesia. Animal is not responsive to external stimuli. Rigid limbs, delirium characteristics and many reflexes present.
 8. **Basal anesthesia** — light anesthesia is induced with one agent, the basal anesthetic. Surgical anesthesia is maintained with another agent.

# Principles of Anesthesia

A.  **GENERAL ANESTHESIA** — attributes that characterize the patient under general anesthesia:

 1. **Failure of brain to receive impulses initiated by sensory stimuli — without feeling.**
 2. **Failure of arriving sensory impulses to pass into memory storage — amnesia.**
 3. **Failure of arriving sensory impulses to evoke an effect** — no response is shown.

B.  **CLINICAL CHARACTERISTICS OF GENERAL ANESTHESIA**

 1. **Animal will not respond to external stimuli.**
 2. **Animal is immobile.**
 3. **Varying degrees of muscular relaxation exist.**

4. **Certain reflexes are abolished.**
5. **Analgesia should be complete.**
6. **Amnesia exists.**

C. **CLASSIC STAGES OF ANESTHESIA** (based on effects of ether in man)

1. **Stage I** — Excitation
2. **Stage II** — Delirium
3. **Stage III** —Surgical anesthesia
Planes 1, 2, 3, and 4
Most surgery is done in planes 2 and 3
4. **Stage IV** —Medullary paralysis. Precedes death.

D. **EXCITATION AND DEPRESSION.** (**Multidirectional scheme adapted from Winter**)

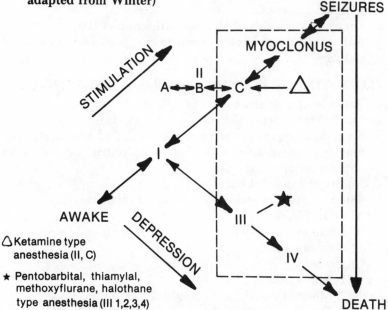

1. Uses the classical stages from above.
2. In Stage II, delirium, the letters A, B and C are used to denote increasing depth of depression within the delerium state, C being the most depressed.
3. An animal in any of the states within the dotted line box area is considered to be under anesthesia.
4. Some drugs such as ketamine and phencyclidine produce this state through an effect that is actually excitatory.
5. Anesthesia as a state, may in reality then, vary a great deal when produced by different single drugs.
6. This difference in the drug mechanisms to produce anesthesia is the basis for the use of drug combinations such as xylazine (a depressant type) plus ketamine (a stimulant type) to produce a desirable CNS state for general anesthesia.

E. **BASIC COMPONENTS OF BALANCED ANESTHESIA** — the fundamental pharmacological objectives are:
   1. **Sensory block** — analgesia
   2. **Mental block** — hypnosis
   3. **Motor block** — relaxation
   4. **Blocking of reflexes** — hyporeflexia

   Most drugs are weak in one or more of the above actions. Truly balanced anesthesia requires the use of more than one drug.

F. **SURGEON'S CRITERIA FOR IDEAL ANESTHESIA** — brought about by a drug or mixtures of drugs with any premedicants deemed necessary.
   1. **Patient should undergo surgery safely and pleasantly** — minimal anxiety and struggling are desired.
   2. **Surgeon's work should be made efficient and fast.**
   3. **Animal should promptly return to preoperative physiological status.**

G. **PROPERTIES OF AN IDEAL GENERAL ANESTHETIC:**
   1. **Rapid induction and emergence phases**
   2. **Not irritating to the patient**
   3. **No serious organ-system responses** — should accomplish the four fundamental pharmacological objectives of anesthesia without cellular toxic effects.
   4. **No fire or explosion hazards**
   5. **Suitability for general use** — the agent should be:
      A) *Inexpensive*
      B) *Easily handled and transported* — compressed gases have a disadvantage.
      C) *Stable*
         1) Nonexplosive
         2) Minimal deterioration in storage and use
         3) No decomposition to harmful substances
         4) Not affected by the alkali in carbon dioxide absorbers
      D) *Physically controllable* — without complex systems
      E) *Compatible with adjuvant drugs* — such as muscle relaxants, narcotics, tranquilizers
      F) *Compatible with other drugs* — such as antibiotics, sulfonamides, antispasmodics, digitalis
      G) *Pleasant and nonirritating* — to subject and operating room personnel
      H) Should not produce adverse effects in operating room staff
      I) *Noncorrosive* — especially to valves, meters, tubing, fittings and other equipment

6. **Ideal veterinary requirements:**
   A) *Useful* in a broad range of species
   B) *Easily administered and maintained* — minimal equipment, assistance and attention needed.
   C) *Adaptable* to current methods of administration
   D) *Adaptable* to equipment currently in use

# Barbiturates

A. **CHEMISTRY**
   1. **Derivatives of barbituric acid** (nonhypnotic)

   Urea + malonic acid→barbituric acid

   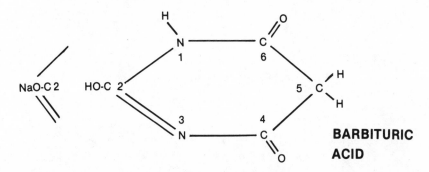

   A) White, odorless, bitter crystals or powder
   B) Stable in air, slightly soluble in water
   C) Weak acids
   D) Form salt by adding Na + on C#2. Salt forms are water-soluble and make highly alkaline (up to pH 11) solutions.

   2. **When both H's on C#5 are substituted, the compound is a potent hypnotic** capable of anesthesia.
      A) *Phenobarbital sodium* — long acting
      B) *Pentobarbital sodium* — short acting — Nembutal® (Abbott) and others.
      C) *Secobarbital sodium* — short acting — Seconal® (Lilly) and others.
      D) *Hexobarbital sodium* — ultra-short acting — (various manufacturers)
      E) *Methohexital sodium* — ultra-short acting — Brevane® (Squibb)

   3. **Sulfur analogues of the 5.5-substituted derivatives are formed**

by substituting S for the 0 at C#2. These are the thiobarbitu-
rates.
A) *Thiopental sodium* — ultra-short acting — Pentothal® (Ab-
bott), Dipentol® (Diamond)
B) *Thiamylal sodium* — ultra-short acting — Surital® (Parke-
Davis), Bio-tal® (Bio-Ceutic)
C) *Thialbarbitone sodium* — ultra-short acting — Kemithal®

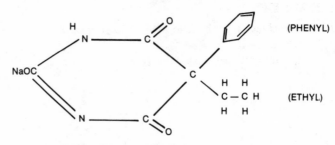

**PHENOBARBITAL SODIUM**

**PENTOBARBITAL SODIUM**

**THIOPENTAL SODIUM**

**SECOBARBITAL SODIUM**

**THIAMYLAL SODIUM**

B.  **PRINCIPAL RESPONSE TO BARBITURATES**
1.  **Central nervous system depression**
    A)  Clinical degree of CNS depression is dose-dependent. Ranges from:
        1)  Sedation
        2)  Hypnosis
        3)  Basal anesthesia
        4)  General anesthesia
        5)  Euthanasia
    B)  Other CNS responses
        1)  Some barbiturates (phenobarbital) selectively depress the motor cortex, thus giving an *anticonvulsant* effect.
        2)  *Poor analgesia* is provided in all stages short of general anesthesia. When low doses of barbiturates are given, the reaction to pain may be increased.
        3)  The threshold of *spinal reflexes* is raised.
        4)  The parasympathetic nervous system is slightly stimulated. This is especially true with reference to the thiobarbiturates.
    C)  Site of action is not well known, but does include the cerebral cortex, thalamus, and reticular-activating system.
    D)  Mechanism of action is not completely known.
        1)  An inhibitory effect on cellular respiration occurs.
        2)  Hypnotic and anesthetic ability is probably manifested by an effect on *synaptic transmission*.
    E)  Produces local anesthetic action when the drug is applied directly to the peripheral nerve.

C.  **OTHER RESPONSES OF ORGAN SYSTEMS TO BARBITURATES**
1.  **Respiratory system**
    A)  Sedative doses have little effect.
    B)  Hypnotic and anesthetic doses cause a progressive depression of the respiratory center. Respiration becomes progressively (and sometimes very abruptly) slower, and more shallow. Then, shallow abdominal respiration occurs.
    C)  Death from an excessive dose of barbiturates is caused by cessation of respiration.
    D)  Laryngeal reflex is reported to become hyperactive after administration of intravenous barbiturates. This leads to the risk of *laryngeal spasm*.

2.  **Cardiovascular system**
    A)  Sedative doses have little affect.
    B)  Hypnotic and anesthetic doses cause a progressive tendency

toward *hypotension* and a compensatory increase in heart rate. This is the result of:
1) Vasomotor-center depression
2) Peripheral vasodilation
3) High concentrations producing a negative effect on the strength of heart-muscle contractions (negative inotropic effect).

C) Thiobarbiturates may bring about *ventricular arrhythmia*
   1) Arrhythmias seen:
      a) Bigeminal rhythm
      b) Ectopic electrical waves of excitation for which there is no ventricular contraction and no corresponding pulse curve. The following is a typical ECG recording.

### SURITAL-INDUCED ARRHYTHMIAS

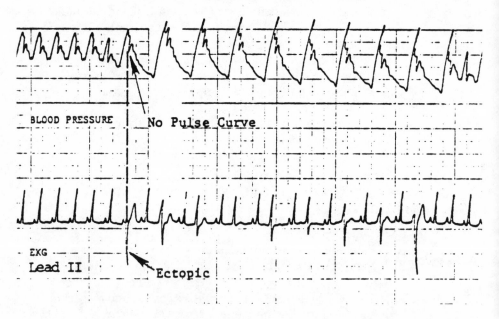

2) Clinical significance of arrhythmia:
   a) *All* anesthetics are associated with some hazard.
   b) Most arrhythmias are transient.
   c) 5% solutions of barbiturates are more likely to initiate arrhythmias than are 2.5% solutions. Thiamylal is reported more likely to induce arrhythmia than is thiopental.

d) Dogs are most susceptible, but arrhythmia may occur in cats.

e) Increases in epinephrine, either endogenously released or injected, exaggerate the situation.

f) Lidocaine, without epinephrine, given IV at a dose of 2-4 mg/lb, will reverse ventricular arrhythmias.

g) There probably is little increased risk in a dog or cat with a clinically normal cardiovascular system. An overdose will embarrass the respiratory system, and *hypoxia* will certainly render the heart more susceptible to arrhythmia. Arrhythmias, such as fibrillation, can quickly become serious.

h) Great care should be exercised when an animal with cardiovascular problems is anesthetized.

i) The thiobarbiturates are valuable agents for certain types of basal and general anesthesia and have been proven safe when used properly.

3. **Gastrointestinal system**
   A) Generally inhibitory
   B) May be followed by an increase in *smooth muscle* tone
4. **Skeletal muscle**
   A) Have some acetylcholine-blocking ability at the myoneural junction. Not observable clinically.
   B) Depress motor output centrally, act on motor area of the cerebral cortex.
   C) Muscular relaxation during surgical anesthesia is not quite as good as that produced by *inhalant anesthetics.*
5. **Renal system.** Impaired flow of urine, caused by reduced blood flow to kidney, and barbiturate-induced release of *antidiuretic hormone* from the posterior pituitary gland.
6. **Body temperature**
   A) Hypnotic and anesthetic doses cause a progressive drop in body temperature as a result of:
      1) *Peripheral vasodilation*, which increases heat loss
      2) Less skeletal muscle contraction, plus a decrease in the metabolic rate—a decrease in heat production
      3) Inhibition of temperature control center in the hypothalamus that makes the animal less capable of conserving body heat

D. **ABSORPTION**
   1. **Barbiturates are readily absorbed by all routes.**
   2. **They are very irritating if injected subcutaneously and they may produce tissue necrosis and sloughing of skin.**

E. DISTRIBUTION
   1. Occurs throughout body — highest in skeletal muscle, liver and kidney.
   2. Thiobarbiturates selectively distribute to skeletal muscle and fat. This redistribution stops their action.
   3. Readily cross the placenta into fetal blood — depress the fetal CNS, including respiration.
   4. Pass into milk — concentrations will not affect the nursling.

F. FATE
   1. Some barbiturates are excreted, largely unchanged, by the kidney — phenobarbital is an example.
   2. Most are biotransformed by the liver to inactive metabolites — a decrease in body temperature reduces rate of biotransformation. If body temperature is allowed to drop, the duration of pentobarbital anesthesia may be prolonged.
   3. Anesthetic action is stopped by various means.
      A) *Renal excretion* in the case of phenobarbital.
      B) *Biotransformation* to inactive metabolites occurs in the case of pentobarbital and secobarbital.
      C) *Redistribution to fat and muscle* occurs in the case of thiobarbiturates such as Surital®, Bio-tal®, Pentothal®, Dipentol® and Kemithal®. Intravenous anesthetics distribute very quickly, first to the brain, because of the large volume of blood per unit of time. As the blood continually passes through fat and muscle, thiobarbiturate is removed. As more and more thiobarbiturate is sequestered in fat and muscle, the drug level in the brain is reduced and the animal awakens. See schematic on following page.

G. BARBITURATE TOLERANCE
   1. Produces psychic and physical dependence in man
   2. Withdrawal symptoms will follow sudden abstinence after chronic use.

H. TOXICITY
   1. Barbiturates are relatively nontoxic to organs.
   2. Overdoses produce death by depression of the respiratory center and resultant respiratory failure.

I. INTERACTION OF BARBITURATES WITH OTHER DRUGS
   1. Summation occurs between barbiturates and other CNS depressants — additive effect.
   2. Hepatic microsomal enzyme inducers decrease the duration of action of pentobarbital. Phenobarbital, Phenergan® (Wyeth), phenylbutazone, etc. are enzyme inducers.

## DISTRIBUTION · ULTRA-SHORT BARBITURATES

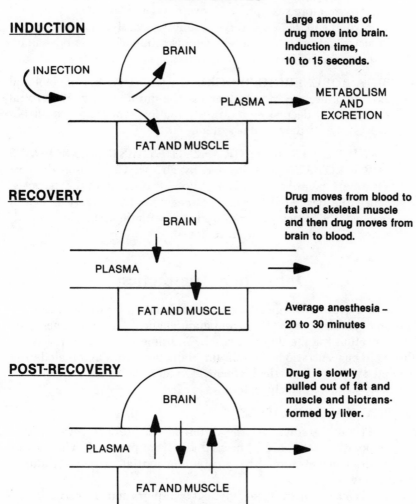

**INDUCTION**

INJECTION

BRAIN

PLASMA ⟶ METABOLISM AND EXCRETION

FAT AND MUSCLE

Large amounts of drug move into brain. Induction time, 10 to 15 seconds.

**RECOVERY**

BRAIN

PLASMA

FAT AND MUSCLE

Drug moves from blood to fat and skeletal muscle and then drug moves from brain to blood.

Average anesthesia – 20 to 30 minutes

**POST-RECOVERY**

BRAIN

PLASMA

FAT AND MUSCLE

Drug is slowly pulled out of fat and muscle and biotransformed by liver.

3. Chloramphenicol, a microsomal enzyme inhibitor, will prolong the sleeping time produced by pentobarbital — dogs, 120%; cats, 260%; monkeys, 165%; rats and mice, up to 3,500%.

J. **SPECIES DIFFERENCES TO BARBITURATE EFFECTS**

1. **Cats tend to sleep longer** — especially under pentobarbital. Repeated doses in cats tend to cause a *reverse tolerance*. Repeated doses produce great depth and a tendency toward respiratory embarrassment and a longer recovery period.

2. **Sight hounds are reported to be more sensitive to barbiturates and possibly all CNS depressants** — these dogs may sleep longer and are more susceptible to overdosage.
3. **Atropine (0.044 mg/kg) given subcutaneously, may prolong the sleeping time of dogs** after administration of thiopental—an increase of 205% has been reported.

K. **BETA ADRENERGIC BLOCKING AGENTS** — propanolol and alprenolol are reported to increase the duration of pentobarbital anesthesia by decreasing biotransformation. They can also further depress the cardiovascular system.

L. **A UNIQUE METHOD FOR ANESTHETIZING LARGE BOARS FOR CASTRATION** (suggested by Dr. M. C. Chesson of Ivor, Virginia): pentobarbital is injected directly into the testicles. When the desired depth of anesthesia for the surgery has been reached, the testicles are removed, and with them the source of additional anesthesia has been removed.

# Inhalation Anesthetics

Onset and depth of surgical anesthesia depend on a threshold concentration of the drug in the brain and maintenance of a proper anesthetic concentration for the depth desired. The time required to reach the threshold concentration in the brain (induction) with an inhaled drug is related to certain physical, chemical and physiological principles. A summary of these principles follows.

A. **PHYSICAL PRINCIPLES**
   1. **Pressure gradient** — the difference in pressure between two points of reference (expressed as partial pressure). The greater the concentration, the greater the partial pressure (**Dalton's Law**).
   2. **Mass movement** — the physical transportation of a certain mass of anesthetic into and within the body.
   3. **Diffusion** — gas exchange in the body occurs by diffusion. The velocity of diffusion is inversely proportional to molecular weight. The larger the molecular weight, the slower the diffusion velocity. The lower the density, the greater the diffusion rate (**Graham's Law**). Diffusion rate of inhalant anesthetics across membranes may be altered by:
      A) *Partial pressure* — an increased partial pressure brings about an increased diffusion rate.
      B) *Solubility of drug in membrane* — the greater the lipid solubility, the greater the rate of diffusion.

        C) *Pressure gradient* — the greater the gradient, the faster the diffusion.

        D) *Surface area* and *thickness* of membrane — the greater the surface area and thickness of the membrane, the less the diffusion rate.

        E) *Density of gas or vapor* — an important variable in the comparison of anesthetics.

   4. **Solution** — the weight of gas dissolved in the solvent (blood) is proportional to the partial pressure of the gas (**Henry's Law of Distribution**). The drug is passed in the direction of greater solubility and down a concentration gradient.

## B. PHYSIOLOGICAL PRINCIPLES

   1. **Ventilation** — the movement of air into or out of the lungs. Tidal volume x respiratory rate = respiratory minute volume.

   2. **Gas exchange** — occurs across alveolar membrane and brain cell membrane by diffusion (passive transport).

   3. **Uptake of drug by the brain follows physical principles** — the rate depends on:

        A) Solubility of gas in blood

        B) Solubility of gas in brain relative to other tissues; *i.e.*, the preference of the drug to enter brain tissue as opposed to other body tissues. The more soluble the drug in other tissues, the longer the time required to induce anesthesia. Must reach a steady state.

        C) *Perfusion* of blood through the brain. The brain receives 8 to 10% of the cardiac output.

   4. **Excretion of gas and termination of action is via the lungs**

        A) Drugs are expired unchanged. Very little biotransformation occurs.

        B) The more soluble the drug in other tissues, the slower the elimination and the longer the recovery time. The drug remaining in other tissues acts as a reservoir that feeds back into the blood and into the brain.

## C. SUMMARY

   1. **Concentration of anesthetic within the brain** is proportional to the concentration in arterial blood.

   2. **Concentration in arterial blood** is proportional to the concentration in alveolar air.

   3. **Concentration in alveolar air** is proportional to the amount of anesthetic vapors inhaled.

4. **Anesthetic vapors in inhaled air** can be regulated very discretely, thus controlling the depth of anesthesia and changing the depth quickly and precisely.

## SCHEMATIC OF MOVEMENT OF INHALATION ANESTHETICS

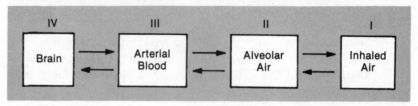

5. **Quickly alters the depth of anesthesia** — an advantage of inhalation anesthesia.
6. **Overdoses** may be reached just as rapidly with inhalation anesthetics.

D. **DEPTH OF ANESTHESIA** (factors influencing anesthesia)
   1. **Inhaled air** — concentration depends on:
      A) Volatility of anesthetic and *vaporization rate*
      B) Proficiency of vapor conduction to the patient. Loss or dilution may occur.
   2. **Alveolar air** — airway restrictions may have an important influence. Respiratory volume is an important variable in animals.
   3. **Blood** — pulmonary circulation and cardiac output control the blood flow through the lungs and hence the rate of gaseous exchange across alveolar membranes.
   4. **Brain** — circulation or rate of blood flow to the brain influences the depth of anesthesia. The lipid content of brain tissue is high.

E. **HYPOXIA** (oxygen shortage in tissues)
   1. **Must be alert to the possibility when any anesthetic is used**—depression of the respiratory center is a common cause of hypoxia.
   2. **Critical with inhalants because:**
      A) Of nature of administration. May inhibit ventilation.
      B) Inhaled vapors contain a certain percentage of anesthetic gas and that much less oxygen.
      C) A 100% potent anesthetic is an inhalant anesthetic that can induce deep surgical anesthesia (III-4) without causing hypoxia.
   3. **Heart, liver and brain cells are especially susceptible to insult by hypoxia** — they quickly show a decrease in function. For ex-

ample, hypoxia renders the heart prone to *arrythmias*.

4. **Hypoxia of brain tissue increases the permeability of membranes** — this increases the delivery rate of anesthetic drugs to the brain and may initiate a vicious circle.

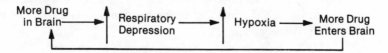

# Ether

A. **CHEMISTRY**

H $\overset{\displaystyle H}{\underset{\displaystyle H}{\overset{|}{\underset{|}{C}}}}$ — $\overset{\displaystyle H}{\underset{\displaystyle H}{\overset{|}{\underset{|}{C}}}}$ — O — $\overset{\displaystyle H}{\underset{\displaystyle H}{\overset{|}{\underset{|}{C}}}}$ — $\overset{\displaystyle H}{\underset{\displaystyle H}{\overset{|}{\underset{|}{C}}}}$ H    Ethyl ether or diethyl ether

1. **Volatile liquid**
2. **Use only Ether for Anesthesia U.S.P.** — up to 3% ethyl alcohol and/or water.
3. **Keep seal tight and protect from light and air** — exposure to light and air leads to formation of peroxides which:
   A) Are toxic
   B) Irritate the respiratory tract
   C) Lower the ignition temperature of the compound
4. **Highly flammable and explosive**

B. **PRINCIPAL RESPONSE**
   1. **Central nervous system depression**
      A) 100% potent
      B) All reflexes can be abolished
      C) Moderate analgesia in light planes of anesthesia and during the recovery period

C. **OTHER ORGAN RESPONSES**
   1. **Respiratory system**
      A) Respiration is *reflexly stimulated* in the early stages of induction by the irritating effect of ether on the mucous membranes of the respiratory tract.
      B) Progressively depresses the respiratory center. May totally inhibit the respiratory center and stop respiration.
      C) Irritation of mucous membranes stimulates the secretion of fluids in the lungs.

D) May initially induce breath-holding.

E) Surgical anesthesia can be maintained with little respiratory depression in a properly pre-medicated animal.

2. **Cardiovascular system**

A) May moderately stimulate the cardiovascular system during induction. Sympathetic tone is increased as a result of fright and struggling.

B) As CNS depression deepens, there is a tendency toward *hypotension* because the vasomotor center is depressed.

3. **Gastrointestinal tract**

A) May stimulate vomiting if induction is hurried

B) Vomiting may occur after anesthesia.

C) Inhibitory to tract during Stage III anesthesia

4. **Skeletal muscle**

A) Relaxation is good in Stage III, planes 3 and 4.

B) Mechanisms of skeletal muscle relaxation:

1) Potent curare-like action at myoneural junction. Blocks acetylcholine from post-junctional receptors.

2) Depresses motor output centrally. Less motor stimuli to muscles reduces tone.

5. **Cellular metabolism depressed** — blood glucose may rise as a result of:

A) Decreased utilization of glucose by cells

B) Mobilization from glycogen due to release of epinephrine during induction

6. **Body temperature tends to drop.**

D. **FATE**—excreted unchanged through the lungs. Small amounts are excreted through the kidneys.

E. **TOXICITY**—nontoxic. Among the safest general anesthetics for animals. Overdoses cause death by respiratory failure.

F. **INTERACTIONS WITH OTHER DRUGS**

1. **Additive with other CNS depressants**

2. **Summation with drugs that block myoneural junctions of skeletal muscle**—require extreme care when used together. (The muscles of respiration are skeletal.)

3. **Summation with antibiotics that paralyze skeletal muscle.**

# Halothane & Methoxyflurane

## A. CHEMISTRY

```
      F    Br                          Cl   F        H
      |    |                           |    |        |
F  -  C  - C  - Cl            H -  C  - C  - O- C  - H
      |    |                           |    |        |
      F    H                           Cl   F        H
```

Halothane                    Methoxyflurane

(Fluothane® — Ayerst)        (Metofane™ — Pitman-Moore)

1. Volatile liquid           1. Volatile liquid
2. Nonflammable,             2. Nonflammable,
   nonexplosive                 nonexplosive
3. Colorless                 3. Colorless
4. Sweetish odor             4. Fruit-like odor
5. Not stable when exposed   5. Stable
   to light
                             6. More soluble in plasma
6. More volatile than           (HOH)
   methoxyflurane
7. More lipid-soluble than
   methoxyflurane

## B. PRINCIPAL RESPONSE

1. Central nervous system depression
    A) 100% potency. Both drugs are more potent than ether. Halothane has four times the potency of ether. Methoxyflurane has eight times the potency of ether.
    B) Excellent analgesia in light planes of anesthesia and during recovery. Methoxyflurane is a better analgetic in light planes of anesthesia.
    C) Methoxyflurane acts slower. Induction takes longer because methoxyflurane is less volatile and lipid-soluble.
    D) Induction and recovery are rapid with halothane. Need trained help and greater care because halothane is more volatile and more soluble.

## C. SKELETAL MUSCLE RELAXATION — Good with both drugs

D. **FATE**

    1. Excreted unchanged, primarily through the lungs

    2. Small amounts are biotransformed by liver — particularly methoxyflurane.

E. **BLOOD PRESSURE**

    1. Produce a progressive fall in blood pressure caused by vasodilation and dependent on time and plasma concentration.

    2. Decrease in cardiac output — hypotensive

F. **RESPIRATION**

    1. Both produce a progressive dose-related inhibition.

    2. Surgical anesthesia can be maintained with little respiratory depression.

G. **TOXICITY**

    1. Low toxicity

       A) Hepatotoxicity is debatable. The role of hypoxia is thought to be a key: *no hypoxia, no hepatotoxicity.*

       B) Capable of sensitizing the myocardium to epinephrine. They induce *ventricular arrhythmias* and possibly *ventricular fibrillation.* The risk with methoxyflurane is reported to be less. Phenothiazine-derivative tranquilizers will protect against these arrhythmias.

       C) Nonirritating to the respiratory tract

       D) Death from overdosage results from respiratory paralysis.

H. **USED IN VARIETY OF SPECIES** including exotics and birds.

I. **INTERACTIONS WITH OTHER DRUGS**

    1. Summation with other CNS depressants—also with drugs, including some antibiotics, that paralyze skeletal muscle.

## Chloroform

$$Cl-\underset{\displaystyle Cl}{\overset{\displaystyle H}{\underset{|}{\overset{|}{C}}}}-Cl \quad \xrightarrow[\text{light}]{\text{air}} \quad \underset{\displaystyle Cl}{\overset{\displaystyle Cl}{\underset{|}{\overset{|}{C}}}}=O \quad \text{Phosgene \textbf{TOXIC}}$$

A. **NOT USED EXTENSIVELY IN VETERINARY ANESTHESIA**

B. **TOXICITY**

    1. More toxic than other agents

2. Very hepatotoxic
3. Sensitizes the myocardium to epinephrine—induced *ventricular arrhythmias* and fibrillation
4. Nausea and vomiting occur frequently.

# Nitrous Oxide (Laughing Gas, $N_2O$)

A. CHEMISTRY
   1. Colorless
   2. Odorless
   3. Nonflammable — however, high concentrations ($> 80\%$) combined with methoxyflurane are flammable.
   4. Nonexplosive

B. PRINCIPAL RESPONSES
   1. Not 100% potent when used alone
   2. Maximum depression without hypoxia in Stage III, plane l
   3. Pleasant induction in man
   4. Nontoxic, nonirritating to tissues of the respiratory tract
   5. Rapid induction and recovery
   6. Used with other inhalant anesthetics — such as with halothane or methoxyflurane for anesthesia in small animals
   7. Produces excellent analgesia — even in early stages of induction of anesthesia.
   8. Analgesia has been shown to be reversible by Nalline® (Merck, Sharp & Dohme) or naloxone, indicating that the analgesia is induced by an action on the opiate receptors.

# Cyclopropane

A. CHEMISTRY
   1. Colorless, odorless gas
   2. Flammable
   2. Explosive
   4. 100% potent

B. NOT COMMONLY USED IN VETERINARY MEDICINE

# Opiate Narcotics

A pharmacological term derived from narcosis. It means sedation *plus* hypnosis *plus* analgesia.

A. **CHEMICAL GROUPS**
 1. **Opium contains the following alkaloids:**
  A) Morphine — 10%
  B) Codeine, methyl morphine — 0.5%
  C) Papaverine — non-narcotic, smooth-muscle relaxant
  D) Noscapine — non-narcotic, smooth-muscle relaxant
 2. **Synthetic opium alkaloids** — prepared from a natural alkaloid
  A) Morphine derivatives
   1) *Heroin* (diacetylmorphine) — analgesia 2.5 times greater than that of morphine
   2) *Apomorphine* — potent emetic
   3) *Oxymorphone* (Numorphan® - Endo) — analgesia 10 times greater than that of morphine
  B) Codeine derivatives
   1) *Hydrocodone* — Hycodan® (Endo)
   2) *Oxycodone* — Percodan® (Endo)
   3) *Hydromorphone* — Dilaudid® (Knoll)
 3. **Synthetic compounds**
  A) *Meperidine* — Demerol® (Winthrop)
  B) *Methadone* — Dolophine® (Lilly)
  C) *Fentanyl* — Sublimaze® (McNeil)—one of the compounds in Innovar-Vet™ (Pitman-Moore)
  D) *Diphenoxylate* — Lomotil® (Searle)
  E) *Propoxyphene* — Darvon® (Lilly)
  F) *Pentazocine* — Talwin-V® (Winthrop)
 4. **Antagonists**
  A) *Nalorphine* — Nalline® (Merck, Sharp & Dohme) — morphine derivative
  B) *Levallorphan* — Lorfan® (Roche) — synthetic
  C) *Naloxone* — Narcan® (Endo) — synthetic
B. **OPIUM**
 1. **One of the oldest drugs used by man** (since 4,000 B.C.)
 2. **Opium** — derived from Greek, meaning *poppy juice*
  The coagulated, air-dried juice of the incised, unripe seed capsule of the opium poppy (*Papaver somniferum*).
 3. **Opium preparations** — contain all the alkaloids of opium
  A) *Laudanum* — tincture of opium
  B) *Paregoric* — camphorated tincture of opium

## C. MORPHINE

1. **Principal response:**
   A) CNS depression. Includes:
      1) Sedation, hypnosis, and mental clouding
      2) Analgesia. Mechanisms of morphine analgesia are:
         a) Threshold to pain is increased; patient is less able to perceive pain. Opiates act upon the same receptors as the brain's naturally released pain-relieving substances called endorphins.
         b) Reaction to pain changes; response to sensation (anxiety, fear, panic) is diminished.
         c) Of greatest value for pain from viscera or trauma; less valuable for pain of arthritis or from skin.
         d) Analgesia is greater if the patient is not disturbed.
      3) Euphoria (human responses)
         a) "Cloud nine"
         b) A feeling of total well-being
         c) The patient feels good

2. **Comparative actions of morphine and anesthetics**
   A) Anesthetics:
      1) Higher centers are depressed first, producing analgesia and hypnosis.
      2) The spinal cord is depressed next, producing muscular relaxation.
      3) Respiratory center and medulla are depressed last.
   B) Morphine
      1) The first area depressed is the respiratory center.
      2) The higher centers are affected next, resulting in analgesia and hypnosis.
      3) The spinal cord is stimulated last.

3. **Effects of morphine on central nervous system**
   A) Depresses the:
      1) Cerebral cortex, causing analgesia and hypnosis
      2) Hypothalamus and brainstem, causing sedation
      3) Medulla, which controls the respiratory center
      4) Cough center, thus raising the cough threshold, which in turn inhibits the cough reflex
      5) Vomiting center, causing *late* depression
   B) Stimulates the:
      1) Spinal cord, with a resultant strychnine-like effect
      2) Vomiting center, causing *early* stimulation
      3) Nucleus of 10th cranial nerve, the vagus nerve
      4) Nucleus of 3rd cranial nerve, which is the oculomotor

nerve, the apparent stimulus that produces a pin-point
pupil in man

4. **Other organ responses to morphine**
   A) Respiratory system
      1) Progressive depression of respiration is pronounced in
         both rate and depth.
      2) Response to carbon dioxide and hypoxia is diminished.
      3) Large doses will constrict bronchioles.
      4) Reflexes of the ANS are inhibited; respiration may be
         stimulated.
   B) Cardiovascular system
      1) Usual therapeutic doses have little effect.
      2) Large doses will stimulate vagal bradycardia (atropine
         will block).
      3) Vasomotor center is depressed, causing vasodilation and
         fall in blood pressure.
   C) Gastrointestinal system
      1) Vomiting center is first stimulated, then inhibited.
         a) Direct action on CNS. After primary emesis the center
            is blocked.
         b) Action is through the *chemoreceptor trigger zone*
            (CRTZ) situated next to the emetic center.
      2) Intestinal tract
         a) Stimulated first, with defecation usually resulting.
         b) Chronic administration causes constipation because of
            a state of *spastic tonus* (no motility).
   D) Cough center
      1) Inhibited
      2) Cough reflex blocked centrally
      3) Low doses are effective
   E) Urinary tract
      1) Reduces volume of urine voided
      2) Antidiuretic action was used in pre-insulin days to treat
         diabetes mellitus
      3) Urine retention in bladder
      4) Stimulates release of ADH (antidiuretic hormone) from
         posterior pituitary, which causes the kidney tubules to re-
         sorb more water and produce less urine.
   F) Pupil of the eye
      1) Contracts in man, rabbit, and dog
      2) Dilates in other domestic animals
      3) Birds are not affected
   G) Skin. Morphine stimulates the release of histamine, which
      may initiate itching.

H) Metabolic effects
  1) Reduces metabolic rate
  2) Mobilizes glycogen, resulting in *hyperglycemia*

5. **Absorption and distribution of morphine**
  A) It is rapidly absorbed from all sites.
  B) Uniformly distributed to all tissues. Small amounts reach the brain (very potent).
  C) Passes readily through the placenta into fetal circulation.
  D) Small amounts pass into the milk.

6. **Fate**
  A) Biotransformed principally by conjugation with glucuronic acid. Cats have poor ability to biotransform morphine.
  B) Conjugates are excreted principally in the urine.
  C) Small amounts of free drug and metabolites are excreted in bile, saliva, tears, and expired air.

7. **Tissues and organs**
  A) Not affected
  B) Death results from depression of the respiratory center.

8. **Contraindications**
  A) *Shock* — may add to circulatory and respiratory embarrassment already present.
  B) *Liver disease* — disrupted rate of morphine conjugation causes greater potential for toxicity.
  C) *Hypoxic states* — those occurring with chest wounds, pneumothorax, pulmonary edema.
  D) *Asthma* — may constrict bronchioles even further.
  E) *Strychnine toxicity* — both drugs stimulate the spinal cord. The effect would be additive.
  F) *Chronic lung disease*
  G) *Head injuries* — may mask symptoms. Respiratory center may already be depressed. Tendency toward convulsions.
  H) *Low metabolic rate* — hypothyroid animals would be very sensitive.
  I) *Old animals*
  J) *Young animals* — very susceptible. Morphine enters brain more readily.

9. **Species responses to morphine**
  A) *Canine* — CNS depression resembles response in man.
  B) *Feline* — Very low doses (0.1 mg/lb) cause analgesia. Higher doses cause CNS excitement and even mania.
  C) *Equine* — CNS is stimulated. Heroin and morphine have been used to "hop" race horses.
  D) *Other domestic animals* — show little or no response, but a

tendency toward CNS stimulation is sometimes detected.

10. **Pattern of central nervous system stimulation**
    A) Excitement
    B) Delirium
    C) Convulsions

D. **APOMORPHINE**
    1. **Chemistry**
       A) Morphine treated with hydrochloric acid yields *apomorphine.*
       B) Very unstable in solution. Turns green.

    2. **Centrally acting emetic**
       A) Acts directly on CRTZ
       B) Potent in dogs and is very reliable
       C) Poor response in cats

    3. **Little narcosis** — may be additive with other CNS depressants such as morphine.

    4. **Administer intravenously, subcutaneously, intramuscularly.**

    5. **Can produce excitement in large doses** — may lead to convulsions and death.

E. **CODEINE**
    1. **Synthetically prepared from morphine**

    2. **Central nervous system responses** (compared to morphine)
       A) Less potent analgetic
       B) Less CNS depression and less euphoria
       C) Less depression of respiratory center
       D) Less risk of addiction
       E) Little affect on emetic center
       F) Comparable inhibition of cough center

F. **MEPERIDINE** (Demerol® - Winthrop)
    1. **Synthetically prepared**

    2. **Central nervous system responses** (compared to morphine)
       A) Less potent analgetic, thus requires a larger dose
       B) Less potent CNS depressant
       C) Less respiratory depression
       D) Less risk of addiction

    3. **Biotransformed in liver** — quickly biotransformed by cats

    4. **Slower onset and shorter duration**

    5. **May be used in cats and horses**

G. **METHADONE** (Dolophine® - Lilly)
    1. **Synthetically prepared**

2. **Central nervous system responses** (compared to morphine)
   A) Similar analgesia
   B) Less sedation
   C) Less respiratory depression
   D) Less risk of addiction
   E) Less severe withdrawal syndrome. It is used in human medicine to treat morphine and heroin addiction.

3. **Onset of action** is slower than that of morphine but the action is more prolonged.

H. **FENTANYL** (Sublimaze® - McNeil)
   1. **Synthetically prepared**
   2. **One of the two ingredients in Innovar-Vet®** (Pitman-Moore)
   3. **An excellent analgetic** — fifty times more potent than morphine.
   4. **Short duration of action** — up to 30 minutes
   5. **Can be used intravenously** — rapid injection.

I. **PENTAZOCINE** (Talwin® and Talwin-V® - Winthrop)
   1. **Synthetically prepared**
      A) Less potent analgetic than morphine. Comparable to meperidine.
      B) Less respiratory depression
      C) Slight risk of addiction, not a controlled drug.
   2. **Fast onset of action, but short duration** — less than 1 hour.

J. **OXYMORPHONE** (Numorphan® - Endo)
   1. **A chemical derivative of morphine**
   2. **Central nervous system responses**
      A) Analgesic action 10 times greater than that of morphine
      B) Less sedation as compared to morphine
      C) Has good synergistic action with phenothiazine-derivative tranquilizers. Produces good neuroleptanalgesia.
   3. **Duration of action similar to that of morphine**
   4. **Has been used in dogs, cats and horses**

K. **ANTAGONISTS** (Nalline® - Merck, Sharp & Dohme; Lorfan® - Roche; Naloxone®, Narcan® - Endo)
   1. **Competitive antagonists at receptor sites**
      A) Nalline® and Lorfan® are *partial antagonists.*
      B) Naloxone® is almost a *pure antagonist.*
   2. **Reverses all central nervous system responses** — especially respiratory depression of morphine, Meperidine®, methadone, and fentanyl. Will also reverse M-99®.

3. **Use intravenously** — act quickly, usually in 10-60 seconds.

L. **CLINICAL USES AND NOTES**
1. **Analgesia**
   A) *Dog* — all drugs may be used.
   B) *Cat* — Demerol®, morphine may be used in very small dose. Oxymorphone and Darvon® may also be used.
   C) *Horse* — Demerol®, Talwin® and Numorphan® may be used.
   D) *Sheep* — Demerol® may be used.
2. **Preanesthetic medication** — aids in handling the patient. Smoother induction of anesthesia, less anesthetic needed, and good analgesia follows anesthesia.
3. **Decrease motility of gastrointestinal tract**
4. **Use atropine with this group of drugs.**
5. **Tolerance will develop to all drugs in this group except:**
   A) *Codeine* — cough center
   B) *Apomorphine* — emetic center

# Tranquilizers

A. **TERMINOLOGY RELATED TO PSYCHOPHARMACOLOGIC AGENTS**

1. **Psychotropic** — any substance that alters mental processes or behavior.
2. **Psycholeptic, neuroleptic** — exerts a depressing or inhibiting action; example: sedative, tranquilizer.
3. **Psychoanaleptic** — has a stimulating or enhancing action; anti-depressive action.
4. **Tranquilizer** — difficult to define. The following are patient responses:
   A) Allay fear, anxiety and nervous tension without impairing conscousness.
   B) Reduce emotional tension.
   C) *Ataractic* — from the Greek meaning *undisturbed*. Small doses of hypnotics may also produce tranquilizing effect.
   D) Tranquilizers in large doses do not produce anesthesia.
   E) Restraint is accomplished with less stress and irritation to the animal.
   F) Enables animals to adapt to threatening environments.
   G) *Phenothiazine*-derivative tranquilizers are most commonly used in veterinary medicine.

5. **Antipsychotic drug** — major tranquilizer.  ⎰Terms from
6. **Antianxiety drug** — minor tranquilizer.    ⎱human use
7. **Phenothiazine-derivative tranquilizers** — major tranquilizers.

B. **CHEMICAL GROUPS OF TRANQUILIZERS**
   1. **Phenothiazine derivatives:**
      A) *Chlorpromazine* — Thorazine® (Norden)
      B) *Promazine* — Sparine® (Wyeth)
      C) *Isobutrazine* — Diquel® (Jen-Sal)
      D) *Propiopromazine* — Tranvet® (Diamond)
      E) *Piperacetazine* — Psymod® (Pitman-Moore)
      F) *Acetylpromazine* — Acepromazine® (Ayerst)
      G) *Triflupromazine* — Vetame® (Squibb)
      H) *Trifluomeprazine* — Nortran® (Norden)
      I) *Promethazine* — Phenergan®, Temaril-P® (Norden)
      J) *Trimeprazine* — Temaril® (Norden)

   2. **Rauwolfia alkaloid:** *Reserpine* — Serpasil® (Ciba)

   3. **Butyrophenones**
      A) *Droperidol* — Inapsine® (Critikon). The tranquilizer in In-
         novar-Vet® (Pitman-Moore)
      B) *Lenperone* — Elanone-V® (Robins)

   4. **Propanediol and butanediol derivatives** (alkyl diols)
      A) *Meprobamate* — Equanil® (Wyeth) or Miltown® (Wallace).
         Central muscle relaxant tranquilizers.

   5. **Minor tranquilizer**
      A) *Diazepam* — Valium® (Roche). Used in veterinary medicine
         as an anticonvulsant.

C. **PHENOTHIAZINE-DERIVATIVE TRANQUILIZERS**
   1. **Mechanism and site of action**
      A) Affect the central nervous system
         1) Mechanism not well understood
         2) Thought to act by blocking dopamine, one of the stimula-
            tory neurotransmitters in the brain. Dopamine is a cate-
            cholamine, a chemical relative of epinephrine and nor-
            epinephrine.
         3) Act on many different parts of the brain
         4) Depression of hypothalamic function, which may alter
            the function of the pituitary gland.

   2. **Principal response**
      A) Central nervous system depression
         1) Animal's behavior is altered; patient becomes more docile.
         2) Conditioned reflexes are inhibited. Example:

a) Animals are conditioned, on an auditory cue, to avoid a punishing shock by climbing a pole.

b) After receiving chlorpromazine, animals ignored the warning signal but could still escape by climbing the pole when shocked.

c) After receiving barbiturates, animals ignored the warning signal; their escape was inhibited.

3) Hostility is decreased.

4) Spontaneous motor activity is reduced.

5) Sedative and hypnotic effects; drug may be used for pre-anesthesia medication.

6) The CRTZ is blocked or inhibited, thus vomiting is suppressed.

7) Indifference or slowing of responses to external stimuli occurs. Alarming environmental conditions are less stressful.

### The LD$_{50}$ of Amphetamine (IP)
Example:

a) Isolated mice............................. 111 mg/kg

b) Crowded mice, 3 mice/small cage........ 15 mg/kg

c) Crowded mice + phenobarbital.......... 110 mg/kg

d) Crowded mice + chlorpromazine........ 110 mg/kg

e) Both phenobarbital and chlorpromazine reduce the damaging influence of crowding. More amphetamine was needed to produce death in 50% of the test animals.

f) Phenobarbital was needed at anesthetic levels.

g) Chlorpromazine caused no loss of consciousness.

8) Emotional quieting occurs.

9) Threshold for convulsions may be lowered (most likely in animals with a history of, or a predisposition to seizures). Also important if the animal is concurrently receiving other drugs that tend to increase susceptibility to seizures.

10) Phenothiazine-derivatives will not produce analgesia; they only change reaction to pain.

11) Occasionally causes excitation, (has occurred in all species) particularly if given intravenously. Horses seem to be especially vulnerable.

12) Alpha adrenergic blocking agents (ANS) are affected by phenothiazine-derivatives.

a) Block epinephrine and norepinephrine from alpha adrenergic receptors.

b) Can reverse action of epinephrine. Epinephrine in this case causes a drop in blood pressure.

c) Protect against epinephrine-induced ventricular arrhythmias and fibrillation.

3. **Other organ system responses to phenothiazines derivatives**
   A) Respiration
      1) Little effect at usual doses
      2) Initially stimulated
      3) Large doses progressively inhibit
      4) Little depression of fetal respiration
   B) Cardiovascular
      1) A tendency toward hypotension
         Inhibition of vasomotor area
         Adrenergic blockade.
         Negative inotropic effect on heart; *i.e.*, decrease contractility
         Vasodilation
   C) Kidney — slight diuretic affect
   D) Endocrine
      1) Affect the hypothalamus. Phenothiazine inhibits output of releasing factors which normally stimulates the anterior pituitary.
         a) Decrease release of ACTH from the anterior pituitary
         b) Decrease release of gonadotropins from the anterior pituitary. Block ovulation, thus suppressing the estrous cycle.
         c) Decrease release of growth hormone from the anterior pituitary
      2) May inhibit release of oxytocin
      3) Slight skeletal muscle relaxation
4. **Toxicity**
   A) Relatively nontoxic
   B) Cholestatic jaundice in man
   C) Overdoses bring about cardiovascular and respiratory collapse, predominately through inhibition of control centers.
   D) Paralysis of penis in the horse after administration of Tranvet® (Diamond) and Acepromazine (Ayerst). Seen in stallions and geldings given testosterone.
5. **Interactions and clinical precautions**
   A) Summation (suggested potentiation) with other CNS depressants
   B) Use with care in debilitated animals.
   C) Use with care in animals with cardiac disease.
   D) Reverse the effect of epinephrine; blood pressure falls
   E) Do not use in conjunction with organophosphates; will potentiate their toxicity.
   F) May potentiate the toxicity of procaine
   G) May produce CNS stimulation, restlessness, disorientation,

excitement and even convulsions
   H) Accidental intracarotid injection in the horse may cause signs listed in G.
   I) Rapid intravenous injection may cause fall of blood pressure sufficient to cause cardiovascular collapse.
6. **Absorption** — well absorbed by all routes
7. **Fate**
   A) Biotransformed in the liver; many metabolites produced
      Glucuronic acid conjugation
      Oxidation to sulfoxides
8. **Clinical uses**
   A) Chemical restraint. Animals are easier to handle or confine.
   B) Preanesthesia prior to general anesthesia or local anesthesia.
   C) Antiemetic—prevents chemical-induced or motion-induced (car sickness) vomiting in dogs and cats.
   D) *Antipruritic* — primarily Phenergan® (Wyeth) and Temaril® (Norden).
   E) *Antitussive* — primarily Phenergan® (Wyeth) and Temaril® (Norden).
   F) Antistress effect when patient is exposed to high ambient temperatures; cattle and swine conditioning.
   G) Hyperexcitable sow in parturient hysteria
   H) Beneficial effect in long-standing shock. Cause increased blood flow to kidneys through alpha adrenergic blockade.

D. **DROPERIDOL** (Inapsine® - Critikon) — the tranquilizer in Innovar-Vet™ (Pitman-Moore)

E. **DIAZEPAM** (Valium® - Roche) — a mild sedative with anti-seizure activity, a muscle-relaxant effect

F. **TRANQUILIZER** (antihistamine group) — compounds that have attributes of both groups: Phenergan®, Temaril®, in Temaril-P® (Temaril® plus prednisolone)
   1. **Phenothiazine derivatives**
   2. **Responses of phenothiazine-derivative tranquilizers** — also have some antihistamine responses

G. **RESERPINE** (Serpasil® - Ciba)
   1. **Chemistry** — an alkaloid of botanical origin, from the shrub *Rauwolfia serpentina* (Indian snake root)
   2. **Mechanism of action** — proposed to be by depletion of neurotransmitters in synapses in the brain. Reserpine lowers brain levels of norepinephrine, dopamine and serotonin.
   3. **Very potent** — total dose for a horse is 2-5 mg.

4. **Used to calm unruly show and race horses** — not as predictable as is desirable.

5. **Onset after intravenous injection is 2 to 6 hours** — clinical response to one dose has persisted for 1 to 2 weeks.

6. **Adverse reactions**
   A) Drooping eyelids and tail
   B) Diarrhea, colic and pain possible
   C) Penile extension at larger doses

7. **Antidote** — methamphetamine (Desoxyn® - Abbott).

# Other Central Nervous System Depressants

A. **INNOVAR-VET®** — approved for use in dogs only, but it has been used in sows.

1. **Drug combination** — composed of a short-acting narcotic (Fentanyl® - Critikon) plus tranquilizer (Droperidol® -Critikon).

2. **Actions in central nervous system**
   A) A narcotic plus tranquilizer (action termed *neuroleptanalgesia*). Consciousness is not completely lost. Sedation,
   B) Hypnosis *plus* analgesia = *narcosis*.
   C) A stimulant action has been noted in cattle, sheep, cats, and horses.

3. **Other organ responses**
   A) Salivation
   B) Defecation, flatulence, but no emesis
   C) Bradycardia
   D) Respiratory depression or panting
   E) Adrenergic blockade; antagonizes the pressor response of epinephrine.

4. **Clinical uses and notes**
   A) Chemical restraint
   B) Minor surgical procedures
   C) Preanesthesia and postanesthesia
   D) Intravenous or intramuscular administration
   E) Should be preceded by atropine to block salivation and bradycardia
   F) Respiratory depression countered by narcotic antagonists, Nalline® (Merck, Sharp & Dohme) or naloxone.
   G) Good relief of pain

B.  **XYLAZINE** (Rompun® — Haver-Lockhart)

1.  **Best classified pharmacodynamically as a narcotic**

2.  **Central nervous system responses**
    A) Sedative *plus* analgesia = *narcosis*
    B) Centrally acting muscle relaxant
    C) Analgesia in legs of horses is of short duration (7 to 10 minutes).
    D) Sedation lasts longer than analgesia.

3.  **Other organ responses**
    A) Emesis occasionally occurs in dogs, especially if the drug is given subcutaneously or intramuscularly—rarely if given intravenously. Emetic action is blocked later. Cats are especially sensitive; 90% vomit within 5 minutes after administration.
    B) Bradycardia with partial A-V blocks sometimes occurs.
    C) Respiratory depression

4.  **Clinical uses and notes**
    A) Approved for dogs, cats and horses. Available in concentrations of 20 mg/ml and 100 mg/ml. Widely used in cattle, hogs, sheep and goats.
    B) Chemical restraint and immobilization of wild animals
    C) Minor surgical procedures
    D) Relief of pain
    E) Preanesthesia
    F) Major surgery. Used in conjunction with local anesthesia.
    G) Relatively safe for use in older animals
    H) Premedication with atropine may be needed.
    I) Use intravenously or subcutaneously. Some swelling produced in horses.
    J) *Do not use* in conjunction with tranquilizers.
    K) Increased dosage will increase the duration of activity but will not proportionally increase the depth.
    L) Contraindicated in the pregnant cat
    M) *Cattle* — may induce uterine contractions
    N) Injection into the carotid artery may cause seizure and collapse.
    O) Used in combination with ketamine
    P) Cattle dose (0.25 mg/kg) is approximately 1/10 that of the equine dose per kilogram. *Use extreme care!*
    Q) Overdoses may be antagonized by treating with:
       1) *Atropine* — for bradycardia and hypotension
       2) *Dopram-V®* (A.H. Robins) — for respiratory depression

C. **CHLORAL HYDRATE** — Chloral hydrate *plus* ethyl alcohol = a "Mickey Fin". One of the oldest sedative hypnotics.

  1. **Chemistry** — a derivative of ethyl alcohol.

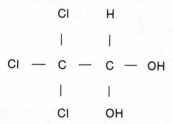

  2. **Central nervous system**
     A) Sedative, hypnotic, light anesthetic
     B) Poor margin of safety as an anesthetic
     C) Analgesia not achieved without anesthesia
     D) Respiratory center depressed by large doses

  3. **Clinical uses**
     A) Orally as a sedative
     B) An ingredient in combination solutions for intravenous anesthesia in large animals

D. **LARGE ANIMAL ANESTHESIA COMBINATIONS**

  1. **Chloral hydrate + pentobarbital + magnesium sulfate** — Equi-Thesin® (NA\*), LA-Thesia®, Chloropent® (Fort Dodge)

  2. **Chloral hydrate + magnesium sulfate** (Chloral-Thesia®)

  3. **Intravenous use only**

  4. **Used in cattle, horses, sheep**

E. **PHENCYCLIDINE** (Sernylan® —Bio-Ceutic)

  1. **Central nervous system responses**
     A) Cataleptic anesthesia
     B) Immobilizing agent for nonhuman primates when used alone
     C) In other species, may cause CNS stimulation associated with disorientation, erratic behavior, excitement and convulsions
     D) Known as PCP, Peace Pill, Angel Dust, or DOA (Dead On Arrival) by drug abusers

  2. **No longer legally available**

F. **KETAMINE** (Ketoset® - Bristol; Vetalar® - Parke-Davis)

  1. **Chemical relative of phencyclidine**

\* Not available

2. **Central nervous system responses**
   A) Cataleptic (dissociative) anesthesia. Stages I and II. Produces anesthesia through a stimulant action.
   B) Induces paralysis with some muscle rigidity
   C) Analgesia is good
   D) Many reflexes are maintained
      1) Swallowing
      2) Coughing
      3) Pedal
      4) Corneal
   E) Slight effect on medullary centers. Action appears to be primarily in the cerebral cortex.
   F) Eyes open, animal does not blink. Cornea is not lubricated by tears. Eye ointment should be used to protect cornea from drying out.
   G) Slight adrenergic effects
   H) Large doses may produce seizure-like activity in canine and other species.
   I) Hallucinogenic in man and apparently in animals

3. **Clinical uses and notes**
   A) Approved for use in cats and subhuman primates
   B) Used in subhuman primates, pigeons, parakeets, snakes. Used in combination with other drugs in horses, swine, cattle and dogs.
   C) Given intramuscularly to cats but may be administered intravenously
   D) Depression in cats depends on dose. Used for restraint, minor surgery, major surgery.
   E) The following premedications are recommended to minimize the side effects of ketamine:
      1) Atropine
      2) Rompun® (Haver-Lockhart)
      3) Acepromazine (Ayerst)
      4) Numorphan® (Endo) combined with Vetame® (Squibb)
      5) Opiate narcotics

4. **Excreted unchanged in urine and as metabolites in urine** — use with care in renal disease or obstruction.

5. **May be redistributed**

6. **Recovery may take up to 24 hours**

7. The following physiograms demonstrate the difference in the way the neurons of the brain respond to typical depressant-type anesthetics (pentobarbital and halothane) and a stimulant-type anesthetic (ketamine). Two points of special interest:

A) The EEG A (dog given pentobarbital) and the EEG B (dog given halothane) are of the deep-sleep pattern. An EEG for a patient given ketamine is of the stimulatory type.

B) If a patient is given an overdose of pentobarbital or halothane the EEG becomes quieter and quieter until it becomes isoelectric, denoting no neuronal activity.

### A and B: Classical EEG of general anesthesia or "deep sleep"

#### A. Pentobarbital

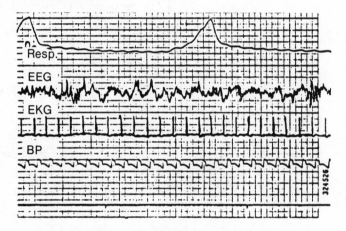

#### B. Surital and halothane (30%)

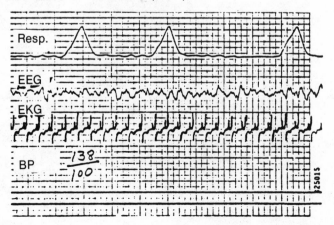

If a patient is given an overdose of ketamine the EEG becomes progressively indicative of heightened neuronal activity (as seen in recordings C, D, and E). Increased jerking and chomping movements are seen. In recording E notice the bursts of seizure-like activity (*arrow*).

C. 10 mg/lb ketamine

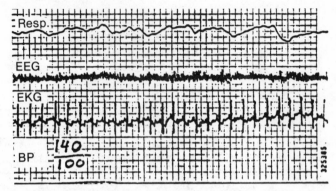

D. 20 mg/lb ketamine

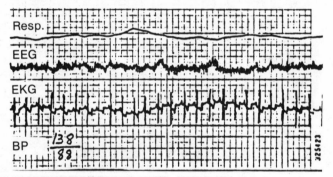

E. 30 mg/lb ketamine

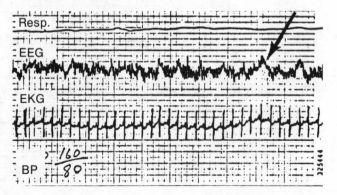

G. **KETASET-PLUS®** (Bristol)

1. **A combination product** — contains ketamine with promazine and aminopentamide

2. **Labeled for use in cats**

3. **Actions of ingredient drugs:**
   A) Ketamine — dissociative anesthesia
   B) Promazine (phenothiazine-derivative tranquilizer) — sedation, centrally mediated muscle relaxant
   C) Aminopentamide, Centrine® (Bristol) — cholinergic blocker, atropine-like, 12-hour duration

4. **Administer intramuscularly**

5. **With larger dose (20 mg/lb ketamine):**
   A) Surgical anesthesia lasts 30 to 45 minutes
   B) Recovery takes up to 24 hours

H. **EXPERIMENTAL GENERAL ANESTHESIA**

1. **Alpha-chloralose** — **a chemical combination of glucose and chloral**

2. **Urethane Ethyl carbamate**

3. **Used singly or in combination of 1 and 2**

4. **ANS reflexes are not inhibited as with other anesthetics.**

I. **ETHYL ALCOHOL** (included for general information)

$$\begin{array}{cc} H & H \\ H\,C & - & C - OH \\ H & H \end{array}$$ Ethanol, Grain Alcohol
Proof Spirit

1. **Central nervous system responses**
   A) Depressant — sedative, tranquilizer, hypnotic, anesthetic
   B) May produce excitement at low plasma levels. Suppresses inhibitors of central synapses.
   C) Plasma levels, CNS response, and the law:

| Percent | | Response |
|---------|---|----------|
| 0.05% | ( 50 mg/100 ml) | Relaxed |
| 0.1 % | (100 mg/100 ml) | Impaired faculties |
| 0.15% | (150 mg/100 ml) | Legally drunk (6 oz whiskey or 6 bottles of beer) |
| 0.3 % | (300 mg/100 ml) | Very drunk |
| 0.5 % | (500 mg/100 ml) | Average fatal level |

2. **Other organ responses**
   A) *Respiratory* — progressive depression
   B) *Cardiovascular* — vasodilator. Direct action on smooth muscle and depression of vasomotor center.
   C) *Urinary* — diuretic. Increases urine formation. Ultimate site of action is the cells of the kidney tubules.
      1) Decreases tubular reabsorption of water
      2) Inhibits release of ADH from the posterior pituitary. Less ADH results in resorption of less water by the tubules.
   D) *Gastrointestinal* — increases release of hydrochloric acid. A questionable aid in digestion.

3. **Metabolic activity** (man)
   A) A food carbohydrate. Each gram yields 7 calories. Can metabolize 6-8 g/hr or 1200 calories/day. Equal to: one-half bottle of 4% beer/hour or 0.5 oz 90-proof liquor/hour.
   B) Can alter intermediary metabolism and may produce a hyperlipemia

4. **Body temperature**
   A) Increases heat loss through cutaneous vasodilation
   B) Decreases heat production at levels that induce hynosis

5. **Other actions**
   A) Local
      1) Precipitation and dehydration of protoplasm
      2) Irritation of mucosae
      3) Irritation of skin
   B) Antibacterial activity. Bactericidal in 70% solution.

6. **Well absorbed from the gastrointestinal tract**

7. **Fate**
   A) Oxidized to carbon dioxide and water, yielding energy by alcohol dehydrogenase scheme
   B) Small amounts excreted unchanged in expired air and urine

# Anticonvulsant Drugs

A. **CANINE SEIZURES**
   1. **Idiopathic canine epilepsy**
      A) Basic pathogenesis unknown. Genetics play a major role.
      B) Usually generalized
      C) Commonly begins at 6 months to 5 years of age
      D) Convulsions are sometimes precipitated by flashing lights or sharp, abrupt stimuli.

2. **Altered function**
   A) Instability of neuronal cell membrane, resulting in excessive depolarization
   B) Sudden recurring neuronal discharge in the brain exceeding a seizure threshold
   C) Clinically described as a CNS dysfunction or a *seizure*

B. **DIPHENYLHYDANTOIN OR PHENYTOIN** — Dilantin® (Parke-Davis) is a sodium salt. Ekko® (Fleming) is the base drug prepared for timed release.

1. **Central nervous system responses**
   A) Selective depression of motor discharge from cortex
   B) Action appears to be at the synapse. Stabilizes excitable neuronal membrane. No action on normal neuronal membrane.
   C) Not a hypnotic

2. **Gastrointestinal**
   A) Absorbed slowly
   B) Used orally. An injectable form is available for use in man.
   C) Requires 7-10 days to reach essential level when given orally
   D) Label dosage has been shown to be inadequate to provide proper blood levels of $10\,\mu g/ml$. Authors suggest dosage of 35 mg/kg, t.i.d.

3. **Fate**
   A) Biotransformed by liver
   B) Excreted in bile
   C) Resorbed and excreted in urine
   D) Plasma t½ is three hours in the dog.
   E) Concurrent treatment with phenobarbital speeds up disappearance from plasma by increasing hepatic biotransformation. One study shows a reduction of blood levels to one-third of blood levels substained with phenytoin alone.
   F) Concurrent treatment with chloramphenicol inhibits biotransformation, thus causing an increase in plasma levels; may become toxic.

4. **Toxicity**
   A) Relatively nontoxic
   B) Overdose leads to cardiovascular collapse
   C) Tolerance does not develop
   D) May inhibit absorption of folic acid, which can predispose animal to anemia
   E) Salicylates and phenylbutazone may displace diphenylhydantoin from plasma binding sites. The plasma levels of free (active) phenytoin are increased.

C. **PHENOBARBITAL**
1. **Central nervous system**
   A) Affects all areas of CNS
   B) Brainstem and spinal cord are very sensitive
   C) Inhibits synaptic function
   D) Inhibits excessive motor discharge with little effect on sensory areas at required dosage levels. Sedative action is slight.

2. **Gastrointestinal**
   A) Well absorbed when given orally
   B) May be used intravenously, but it is the slowest acting of the commonly used barbiturates. May require 15 to 40 minutes to achieve maximum activity.
   C) Threshold levels are achieved 15 hours after oral dose.

3. **Fate**
   A) Excreted unchanged in urine. Small amounts are biotransformed.
   B) Tolerance to sedative effect will develop, causing physical dependence.
   C) Development of little tolerance to antiseizure effect

D. **MEPHOBARBITAL** (Mebaral® — Winthrop)
1. **Chemistry** — close chemical relative of phenobarbital

2. **Fate**
   A) Biotransformed to phenobarbital
   B) Conversion is 100% when given intravenously, but only 50% when given orally.

E. **MEBROIN-V®** (Winthrop)
1. **Combination of Mebaral® (Winthrop) and diphenylhydantoin — fixed-dose combination does not allow flexibility.**

2. **Potentiation is claimed.**

3. **Do not use in cats.**

F. **PRIMIDONE®** (Ayerst)
1. **Mylepsin® (Fort Dodge), Anadone® ( Bio-Ceutic)**

2. **Central nervous system actions**
   A) Similar to phenobarbital
   B) Structurally related to phenobarbital
   C) Approximately 25% is biotransformed to phenobarbital in the body. Drug and metabolite are both active.
   D) Not recommended for use in cats even though it has been used successfully in cats at a lower dosage. The dose given to dogs may produce neurotoxicity in cats.

2. **Toxicity** — ataxia, anorexia, tachycardia and hyperventilation have occurred with a dosage of 150 mg/kg/day in a dog

G. **DIAZEPAM** — Valium® (Roche)

  1. **A tranquilizer and skeletal-muscle relaxing agent**

  2. **An effective antiseizure agent**
    A) Can be used intravenously for initial dose and/or by intravenous drip
    B) Rapid onset. Effective in treating *status epilepticus*.

H. **DRUGS FOR HUMAN USE** (have been used to control seizures)

  1. **Carbamazepine** — Tegretol® (Geigy)

  2. **Paramethadione** — Paradione® (Abbott)

I. **CLINICAL USES AND NOTES**

  1. **Indications**
    A) Idiopathic epilepsy
    B) Epileptiform convulsions
    C) Aid in controlling neurologic disorders such as the aftermath of virus encephalitis, distemper, and hard pad disease

  2. **During acute seizure or status epilepticus use intravenous pentobarbital, phenobarbital or Valium®** — give slowly to effect.

  3. **Phenytoin requires 7 to 10 days to reach an effective level** — dogs may be started on phenobarbital and phenytoin, then phenobarbital should be withdrawn after two weeks.

  4. **Inconsistent, intermittent medication is a common cause of treatment failure** — owners should be impressed with the importance of following directions.
    A) Use minimal but adequate daily doses.
    B) Therapy should be individualized and periodically reviewed.

  5. **Contraindications** — the following drugs are contraindicated for use in canine epilepsy, in acute seizures, or in animals with a history of seizures.
    A) Chloramphenicol and penicillin
    B) Phenothiazine-derivative tranquilizers
    C) Central nervous system stimulants
    D) Large doses of local anesthetics; *e.g.* procaine, lidocaine

## Central Nervous System
## Stimulants
## Classified According to Therapeutic Activity

**Cerebral or psychic** (psychoanaleptics)
   **Xanthines:**
      caffeine, caffeine sodium benzoate
   **Adrenergics:** (group related to epinephrine
   and norepinephrine)
      amphetamine — Benzedrine® (SmithKline & French)
      dexedrine
      methamphetamine — Desoxyn® (Abbott)
      ephedrine
      cocaine
   **Diphenylmethane derivatives:** methylphenidate
   hydrochloride — Ritalin® (Ciba)
      dibenzazepine (stimulant in depressed individuals)
      Imipramine
      psychotomimetic (hallucinogenics)
      cocaine
      lysergic acid (diethylamide — LSD)
      marijuana (Indian hemp, hashish)
      mescaline (peyote)
      amphetamine, Dexedrine® (SmithKline & French)
      and methamphetamine
      atropine, hyoscayamine and scopolamine
      phencyclidine and ketamine

**Brainstem:** (selective medullary-area stimulants)
      nikethamide — Coramine® (Ciba)
      pentylenetetrazol — Metrazol® (Knoll)
      picrotoxin
      bemegride — Mikedimide® (Parlam)
      doxapram — Dopram-V® (Robins)
      camphor and menthol

**Spinal cord:**
      strychnine

**Medullary reflex:**
      nicotine, lobeline
      cyanide
      veratrum
      apomorphine
      aromatic spirits of ammonia

# Central Nervous System
# Stimulants

A.  **CEREBRAL GROUP** — Site of action is the higher centers.

1.  **Caffeine**
    A) Chemistry — *Methyl xanthine* is the same as theophylline and theobromine.
    B) Central nervous system
        1) Stimulates sensory cortex
        2) Increases wakefulness (the daily lift from coffee)
        3) Combats drowsiness
    C) Diuretic and cardiovascular stimulant action

2.  **Amphetamine** — Benzedrine® (SmithKline & French)
    A) Chemically related to epinephrine
    B) Actions on the central nervous system
        1) Potent cerebral stimulant
        2) May produce convulsions
        3) Psychic stimulation
            a) Brighter spirits
            b) Euphoria
            c) Increased mental alertness
            d) Combats drowsiness
        4) Inhibits awareness of fatigue
        5) Stimulates medullary area and is a respiratory stimulant
    C) Is a potent adrenergic with action on the autonomic nervous system. It increases heart rate and blood pressure.

3.  **Dextroamphetamine** — Dexedrine® (SmithKline & French)
    A) More potent cerebral stimulant than amphetamines
    B) Less potent adrenergic than amphetamines

4.  **Ephedrine**
    A) Potent cerebral stimulant
    B) Potent medullary stimulant
    C) Potent adrenergic

B.  **MEDULLARY GROUP** (brainstem, midbrain group) — respiratory analeptics

1.  **Central nervous system actions**
    A) Tend to have a specific affinity for respiratory center
    B) Large doses can produce convulsions.
    C) If respiratory center is depressed by a hypnotic, this group causes increased respiratory rate and depth (*mostly depth*).
    D) Physiological antagonism (opposite effects) of anesthetic overdoses

2. **Doxapram** — Dopram-V® (A.H. Robins)
   A) Indirectly stimulates the cardiovascular system. Stimulates the vasomotor center in the brainstem. Effect is through stimulation of sympathetic nerves and increased action of epinephrine and norepinephrine.
   B) Stimulates pituitary adrenal system, resulting in an increased corticosteroid release
   C) Increases the secretion of hydrochloric acid and the excretion of saliva
   D) Raises body temperature
   E) Increases urine flow
   F) Excessively high doses will produce a marked respiratory stimulation and concurrent increase in arterial pH of 0.2 to 0.3 units.
   G) Has the best safety margin between respiratory analeptic dose and convulsant dose
   H) Used intravenously in dogs, cats, cattle, and horses. May be given sublingually (topical) or injected into the umbilical vein of the newborn.

3. **Pentylenetetrazol** — M'Zol® (Summit Hill)
   A) Used intravenously for respiratory analeptic action
   B) Used orally in geriatric medicine
      1) Stimulates respiration and increases oxygen flow to the tissues
      2) Circulatory stimulant
      3) Overall pick-up. Patients eat and drink better.
   C) Has more stimulatory effect on cerebrum than Dopram®
   (*See* facing page)

Note the return of EEG brain waves a few seconds after intravenous injection of Metrazol. Onset of spontaneous breathing followed shortly thereafter.

## Physiogram of a dog given an overdose of pentobarbital

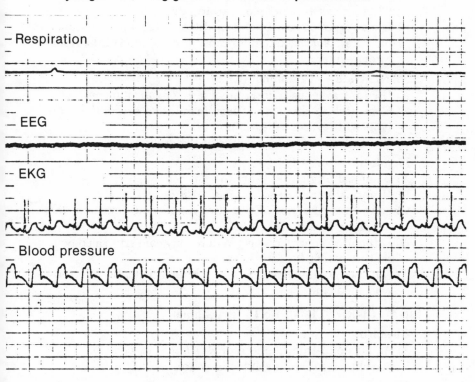

## Physiogram of the same dog after it was given Metrazol®

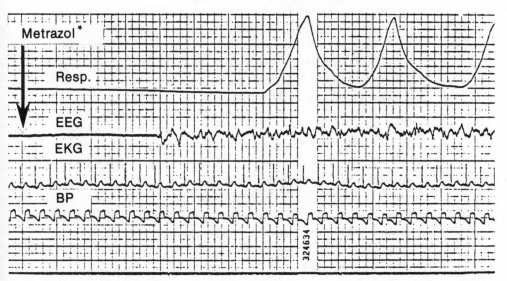

* Tradename now M'Zol®.

4. **Bemegride** — Mikedimide® (Parlam)
   A) Close chemical relative of barbiturates
   B) Once suggested as a true competitive antagonist to the barbiturates. *Not so!* Action is simply a stimulation of the respiratory center.

5. **Nikethamide** — Coramine® (Ciba)
   A) Used intravenously, intramuscularly or subcutaneously
   B) Converted in the body to nicotinamide, a *B-complex vitamin*; will reverse pellegra in dogs.
   C) Weakest respiratory analeptic of the group

6. **Picrotoxin**
   A) Botanical origin. Seeds are the source.
   B) Historically used to poison fish. *Fish berries.*
   C) Slow onset of action. Even after intravenous injection, the lag phase is several minutes.
   D) Difficult to control dosage. Will readily convert to a convulsant. A potent CNS stimulant.
   E) Not used to any extent as a respiratory analeptic in veterinary medicine

C. **SPINAL CORD STIMULANTS** (strychnine)

1. **Chemistry**
   A) An alkaloid, from the seed of *strychnos nux vomica.*
   B) Strychnine sulfate is soluble in water.

2. **Central nervous system**
   A) *Postsynaptic block* of inhibitory synapses in the spinal cord is the mechanism of strychnine action.
   B) The cord is stimulated *indirectly.* The slightest stimulus becomes exaggerated and will lead to convulsions.
   C) Tonic convulsions. Produces *tonic extensor rigidity. Opisthotonos* (legs extended, arched neck and back) is produced.
   D) Experiment to illustrate indirect action:
      1) Frog *plus* strychnine produces convulsions.
      2) No convulsions when the frog is given a cocaine bath and strychnine. Peripheral stimuli are eliminated by local anesthetic action of cocaine. *No stimuli, no convulsions.*

3. **Therapeutic value in veterinary medicine as a tonic for the gastrointestinal tract is questionable** — it will possibly increase thirst and appetite when given orally.

4. **Important to veterinary medicine because of its malicious use** — to poison animals, especially dogs.

5. **Toxicity**
   A) Animal dies of anoxia. Respiratory muscles are in spasm and

there is no ventilation. This is a mechanical interference with respiration.

B) Treatment
  1) Early: Empty stomach and/or precipitate the alkaloid with tannic acid, or oxidize with potassium permanganate.
  2) Late: *If convulsions are evident,* induce light anesthesia. Give pentobarbital intravenously to effect. Robaxin® (A.H. Robins) may be used. Works well for follow-up therapy.

C) *Degree of susceptibility* — dog > cat > man > cow > horse.

## D. MEDULLARY REFLEX GROUP

1. **Not used therapeutically** — adverse affects are too severe.
2. **Reflexly stimulates respiratory center in medulla** — through the carotid sinus.

CHAPTER

# 3

# Autonomic Nervous System

## General Principles

The autonomic nervous system (ANS) controls and integrates the action of the visceral-organ systems. It maintains the animal with a stable, relatively constant and proper internal environment (homeostasis). It allows the animal to adjust to internal and external changes such as sleep *versus* wakefulness, rest *versus* exercise, blood loss, changes of blood pH, and the influence of disease.

A. **REFLEX ARC** — the basic functional unit of the autonomic nervous system. Basic components of the reflex arc are:

1. **Receptors** — sense change and generate impulse
2. **Afferent leg** — sensory impulse carried to CNS
3. **Central nervous system** — impulses integrated and directed
4. **Efferent leg** — motor impulses carried to effector cell
5. **Effector cells** — give response

### A.N.S. REFLEX ARC

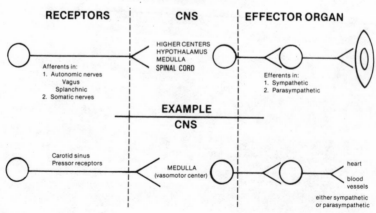

B. **MOTOR OUTPUT** — the ANS is divided into the *sympathetic* and *parasympathetic* divisions.

1. **Most organs receive a motor supply from both divisions.**
2. **Effects of the divisions are usually in opposition,** providing a check-and-balance system.
3. **Motor impulses may be stimulatory or inhibitory to the recipient organ.**
   A) *Sympathetic* — stimulates the heart and inhibits the gastrointestinal tract.
   B) *Parasympathetic* — stimulates the gastrointestinal tract and inhibits the heart.
4. **The two divisions also are suited to different types of controls and responses.**
   A) *Sympathetic* — has widespread distribution. Pooled postganglionic neurons are capable of rapid, mass discharge, and diffuse responses. *Fight or flight* response and the *emergency* response are typical.
   B) *Parasympathetic* — is not as widely distributed. Preganglionic to postganglionic fiber ratio is 1:1. Responses are more discrete and organ-specific.

**Schematic Showing the Motor Output
of the Automatic Nervous System**

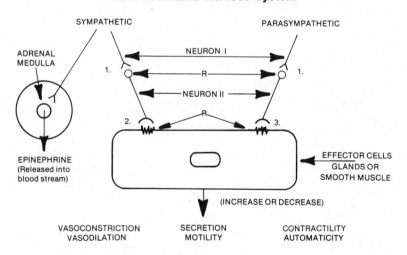

Receptor substances (R):
   Ganglionic site (1). Acetylcholine—natural transmitter substance.
   Adrenergic site (2). Norepinephrine—natural transmitter substance.
   Cholinergic site (3). Acetylcholine—natural transmitter substance.

C. **JUNCTIONAL TRANSMISSION** — the phenomenon by which an impulse is carried across a junction. The two types of junctions or gaps in the ANS efferents are:

1. **Synapse** — neuron I to neuron II.

2. **Neuroeffector junction** — neuron II to effector cell. An impulse is conducted along a nerve fiber and transmitted across a junction by a chemical substance called a neurotransmitter, neurohormone, or mediator.

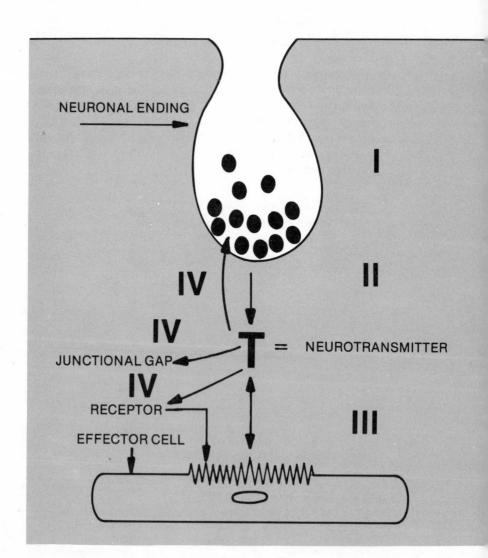

D. **AUTONOMIC DRUGS** — influence or modify one or more steps or events in junctional transmission. Examples of the mode of action of selected autonomic drugs:

1. **Is the actual transmitter** (epinephrine) **or mimics the transmitter** — excites the postjunctional receptors
2. **Blocks interaction of the transmitter and the postjunctional receptors** — causes competitive antagonism (atropine or curare)

## SEQUENCE OF EVENTS IN
## JUNCTIONAL TRANSMISSION

1. **Biosynthesis** of the transmitter and its **storage** in vesicles (secretory granules). The transmitter is *potentially* active (I).
2. An impulse to the neuronal ending causes the **release** of quantal amounts of the transmitter into the junctional gap (II).
3. The transmitter **meshes** with the post junctional membrane or receptor(s) and this brings about *depolarization* or excitation and this gives action (III).
4. **Removal** of the transmitter from the gap *terminates the action*
   Transmitter removal may be by: (IV)
   a. *Diffusion* out of the gap
   b. *Re-entry* into the neuronal ending
   c. *Destruction* by specific enzymes in the gap
5. The post-junctional membrane is now free to *repolarize* and is then ready to be excited by the next transmitter release and meshing.

3. **Interferes with transmitter release** — *e.g.* botulinus toxin, bretylium

4. **Interferes with storage or binding** — brings about depletion of the stored form by:
   A) Releasing stored form (ephedrine)
   B) Preventing re-entry of the transmitter into the neuronal ending (reserpine)

5. **Interferes with the enzymatic destruction of the transmitter** — *e.g.* neostigmine and organophosphates

6. **Inhibits transmitter biosynthesis**

7. **Postpones repolarization by continued presence of a depolarizer** — *e.g.* succinylcholine

E. **TERMS USED TO DESCRIBE DRUG ACTION ON THE ANS**

1. **Parasympathomimetic** — denotes action similar to stimulation of parasympathetic nerves.

2. **Sympathomimetic** — denotes action similar to stimulation of sympathetic nerves.

3. **Adrenergic** — an action (or site) mediated by epinephrine or norepinephrine.

4. **Cholinergic** — an action (or site) mediated by acetylcholine.

5. **Ganglionic** — a site, between neuron I and neuron II, mediated by acetylcholine.

6. **The cells of the adrenal medulla have the same embryologic origin and innervation as a sympathetic ganglion** — may be considered a unique sympathetic ganglion.

7. **Nicotinic and muscarinic are specific terms that:**
   A) Apply only to cholinergic sites or actions
   B) Are based historically upon the observed actions of the two alkaloids, nicotine and muscarine
      1) *Nicotinic* — refers to actions at sympathetic and parasympathetic ganglia, the junction at the adrenal medulla and the myoneural junction of skeletal muscle.
      2) *Muscarinic* — refers to actions at neuroeffector junctions at autonomic nerve endings where acetylcholine is the mediator.

F. **ANATOMICAL SUMMARY OF CHOLINERGIC AND ADRENERGIC FIBERS**

1. **Cholinergic fibers** — acetylcholine is the mediator.
   A) Autonomic preganglionic nerve endings
   B) Parasympathetic postganglionic nerve endings

      C) Sympathetic postganglionic nerve endings in:
        1) Sweat glands in man, dog, cat (most species except horse and sheep)
        2) Some vasodilator fibers
      D) Sympathetic fibers (preganglionic) to *adrenal medulla*
      E) Somatic motor-nerve endings (myoneural junction)

  2. **Adrenergic fibers**
      A) Norepinephrine is the principal mediator.
      B) Epinephrine is also a mediator.
      C) Sympathetic postganglionic nerve endings except certain sweat glands and blood vessels (for exceptions see C above).

G. **STIMULATION OF THE AUTONOMIC NERVOUS SYSTEM —** may be accomplished by:

  1. **Electrical stimulation of nerve fibers (experimental).**

  2. **Physiologically** — creates a need for compensatory action. This initiates the normal scheme of endogenous-transmitter release. If blood pressure falls, the sympathetic system is stimulated and heart rate and blood pressure increase.

  3. **Pharmacologically** — giving a drug that influences gap transmission. It may either *mimic* or *block* the neurotransmitters.

**Schematic of the Autonomous Nervous System**

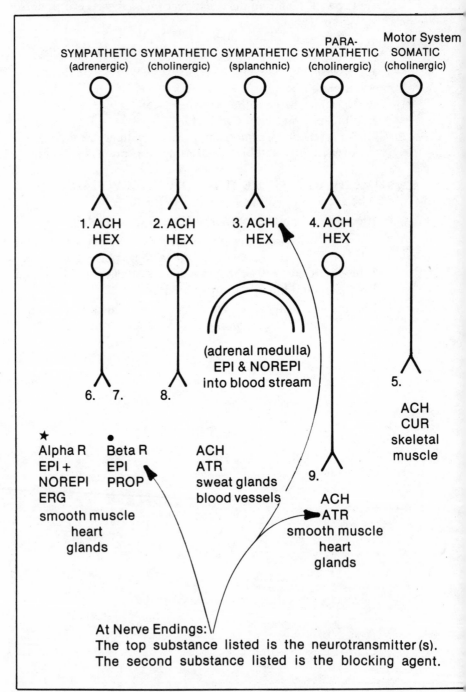

**LEGEND FOR SCHEMATIC**

The action of acetylcholine (ACH) at sites 1, 2, 3, 4, 5 is referred to as **nicotinic.**

The action of acetylcholine (ACH) at sites 8 and 9 is referred to as **muscarinic.**

Hexamethonium (HEX) blocks the nicotinic action of acetylcholine at sites 1, 2, 3, 4. It does **not** block the **nicotinic action** of acetylcholine at 5.

D - tubocurarine (CUR) blocks the **nicotinic action** of acetylcholine at site 5, but does **not** block the nicotinic action of acetylcholine at sites 1, 2, 3, and 4.

Note that neither HEX nor CUR block the **muscarinic action** of acetylcholine at sites 8 and 9.

Atropine (ATR) blocks the **muscarinic action** of acetylcholine at sites 8 and 9, but does **not** block the **nicotinic action** of acetylcholine at sites 1, 2, 3, 4, 5.

Ergotamine (ERG) blocks the **alpha adrenergic action** of epinephrine (EPI) at site 7.

Propanolol (PROP) blocks the **beta adrenergic action** of epinephrine (EPI) at site 7.

Sympathetic affector cells may have alpha or beta receptors or both. Cells of a sympathetically innervated organ generally have a preponderance of one type.

**● BETA RECEPTORS (R)**

**Heart rate increase**
 contractility increase
**Vessels**
 skeletal muscle — dilate
 viscera — dilate
**Bronchiole smooth muscle** – dilate

**★ ALPHA RECEPTORS (R)**

**Vessels**
 skeletal muscle — contract
 viscera — contract
 skin — contract

**Epinephrine** — stimulates both alpha and beta.

**Norepinephrine** — stimulates both alpha and beta, but is predominately an alpha stimulator.

**Isoproterenol** — stimulates predominately beta.

# PHYSIOLOGICAL SUMMARY:
## ACTIONS OF THE AUTONOMIC NERVOUS SYSTEM

| Organ or Structure | Cholinergic Parasympathetic | Adrenergic Sympathetic "Fight or Flight" |
|---|---|---|
| **Heart** | Slows | Accelerates |
| | Weaker contractions | Stronger contractions |
| | Slower and weaker conduction | More rapid conduction |
| | Shortens refractory period | Increases irritability |
| **Smooth Muscle** | | |
| A. Eye | | |
| 1. Radial m. of iris | — — — — | Contraction |
| 2. Sphincter m. of iris | Contraction | — — — — |
| 3. Ciliary m. | Contraction | ? Relaxation |
| B. Bronchioles | Constriction | Dilation |
| C. Gastrointestinal System | | |
| 1. Motility and tone | Increased | Inhibitory |
| 2. Sphincters | Inhibitory | Increases tone |
| D. Blood Vessels | | |
| 1. General | Dilatation | Constriction |
| 2. Skin | Dilatation | Constriction |
| 3. Kidney | — — — — | Constriction |
| 4. Uterus | — — — — | Constriction |
| 5. Skeletal | Dilatation | Dilatation |
| 6. Coronary | Constriction or ? Dilatation | Dilatation |
| E. Urinary Bladder | | |
| 1. Detrusor | Contraction | Relaxation |
| 2. Sphincters & Trigone | Relaxation | Contraction |
| F. Ureters | Increase tone and motility | Relaxation |
| G. Pilomotor Muscles | — — — — | Contraction |
| H. Miscellaneous | | |
| 1. Liver | — — — — | Glycogenolysis |
| 2. Salivary glands | Copius serous secretion | Scanty mucus secretion |
| 3. Spleen capsule | — — — — | Constricts |
| 4. Mucous glands (respiratory tract) | Secretion | — — — — |

The responses listed under *adrenergic* are those required to provide for the needs of an animal during severe exercise. The *cholinergic* responses are just the opposite.

## SUMMARY DRUG LIST

## AUTONOMIC NERVOUS SYSTEM
## AND MYONEURAL JUNCTION

**Cholinergic Drugs**
    A. Receptor Activators (Direct)
       Alkaloids: Pilocarpine, arecholine, muscarine

       Synthetic Drugs: Acetylcholine, methacholine (Mecholyl® —J.T. Baker),
          carbamylcholine (carbachol, Lentin® , Caride®), carbamylmethylcholine
          (Urecholine® —Merck, Sharp & Dohme)

    B. Cholinesterase Inhibitors (Indirect)
       Reversible: physostigmine (Eserine® , neostigmine (Prostigmin® —Roche,
          Stiglyn™—Pitman-Moore)

       Irreversible: alkylphosphates, organophosphates, parathion, malathion,
          DDVP

    C. Cholinesterase Reactivators
       2-pyridine aldoxime methiodide (2-PAM) (Protopam® —Ayerst)

**Cholinergic Blocking Agents**
    A. Parasympatholytic (Muscarinic Block): atropine, scopolamine, meth-
       scopolamine, atropine methylnitrate, homatropine methylbromide,
       glycopyrrolate (Robinul-V® —A.H. Robins), aminopentamide
       Centrine® —Bristol)

    B. Ganglionic Blocking Agents: tetraethylammonium, hexamethonium

    C. Neuromuscular Blocking Agents: (to be discussed under *Muscle Relaxants*)
       Stabilizers: d-tubocurarine, gallamine (flaxedil)

       Depolarizers: succinylcholine, decamethonium

**Adrenergic Drugs**
    A. Alpha and Beta: epinephrine (Adrenalin® —Parke, Davis)

    B. Alpha: norepinephrine (Arterenol® , Levophed® , Levarterenol®),
       ephedrine, phenylephrine (Neo-Synephrine® —Winthrop)

    C. (CNS) Alpha: amphetamine, dexedrine, methamphetamine

    D. Beta: isoproterenol (Isuprel® —Winthrop, Iprenol® —Vitarine),
       dopamine (Intropin® —Arnar-Stone)

**Adrenergic Blocking Agents**
    A. Alpha
       Ergot alkaloids: ergotamine

       Dibenamine, Dibenzyline®

       Phenothiazine-derivative tranquilizers

    B. Beta: propanolol (Inderal® —Ayerst)

# Cholinergics

There are two general mechanisms of action: *direct* action of the drug on the receptors of effector cells, and *indirect* action by inhibition on the cholinesterase enzymes.

A. **DIRECT-RECEPTOR ACTIVATORS ON EFFECTOR CELLS** — acetylcholine is a good prototype for a study, but is not used clinically. It is quaternary ammonium compound chemically, biosynthesized from choline and active acetate via the enzyme, choline acetylase.

1. **Actions** — mimic vagal stimulation (PG 1)
    A) *Cardiovascular effects*
       1) Heart is inhibited. Chronotropic (rate) and inotropic (strength) are both decreased; *i.e.* negative chronotropic and inotropic effects.
       2) Decreased peripheral resistance. Vasodilation occurs via relaxation of arteriolar smooth muscle.
       3) Together, these two effects produce a sharp drop in blood pressure. (PG 2, *facing page*)
    B) *Gastrointestinal tract effects*
       1) Increased motility
       2) Increased salivation (profuse and watery)
       3) Increased flow of pancreatic juice
       4) Increased secretion of intestinal mucus
       5) Slight increase in bile flow (has been questioned)
    C) *Eye effects*
       1) Pupil contracts (miosis) if drug is given systemically
       2) Reduces intraocular pressure
       3) Increases outflow of aqueous humor
    D) *Respiratory system effects*
       1) Early stimulation caused by a compensatory reaction to the drop in blood pressure
       2) Later inhibition due to:
          a) Direct inhibition of respiratory center
          b) Constriction of bronchioles
          c) Increased mucous secretions of respiratory tract
          d) Combination of actions creating poor gaseous exchange
    E) *Urinary system effects*
       1) Reduced blood pressure. If drastic, output of urine may be decreased because of a drop in *effective filtration pressure* at the glomerulus. Decreased renal blood flow and glomerular filtration rate.
       2) Increased tone of bladder wall and relaxation of bladder

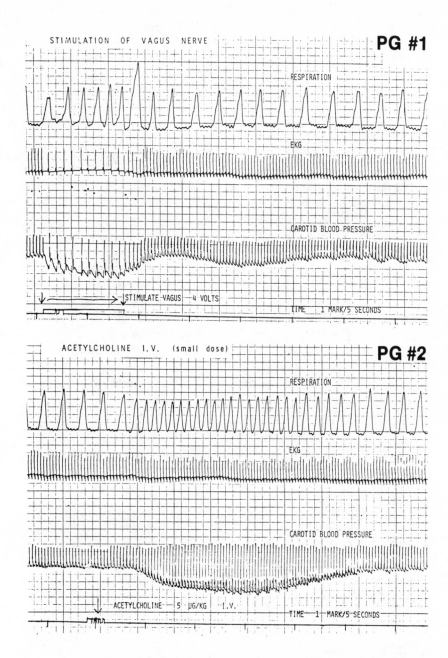

sphincter cause urinary incontinence.

    F) *Skeletal-muscle effects:* stimulates contraction only in exaggerated dosages

2. **As a neurotransmitter, plays an important role in CNS function—** injected acetylcholine is not important in this respect because it

is destroyed too rapidly and enters the CNS poorly.

3. **Mechanism of action**
   A) Acetylcholine meshes with cholinergic receptor sites.
   B) Rapidly biotransformed by specific acetylcholinesterase in tissue sites and non-specific esterases of plasma and liver. Acetylcholine is split (hydrolysis) into acetate and choline. This is a very, very fast reaction.
   C) Acetylcholine has a very short duration of action (30 to 60 seconds) after intravenous injection.
   D) Acetylcholine is not used clinically because of its extremely short duration of action.

4. **Other cholinester cholinergics**
   A) *Carbachol* (Lentin®, Caride®)
      1) Carbamylcholine chloride
      2) Usually given subcutaneously. Potent; use carefully.
      3) Has both nicotinic and muscarinic actions
      4) A potent stimulator of uterine smooth muscles; potency increases in direct relation to the duration of pregnancy. This is postulated to be due to estrogen potentiation.
      5) Rapid onset. Duration of action is 10 to 30 minutes. (PG 3, *below*)
      6) Available as a parenteral solution (1 mg/ml) and in combinations

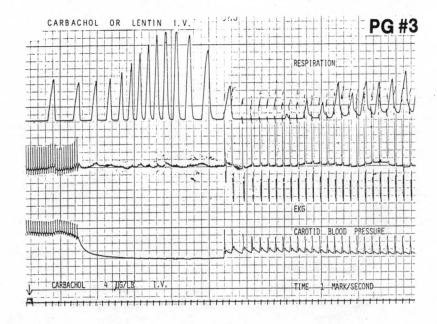

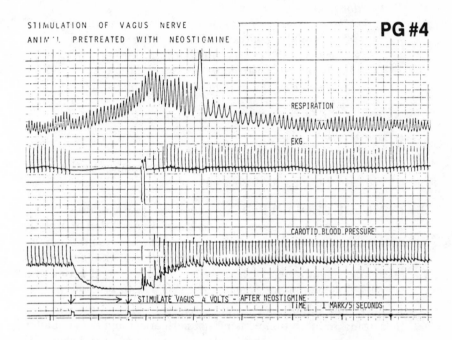

STIMULATION OF VAGUS NERVE
ANIMAL PRETREATED WITH NEOSTIGMINE

PG #4

RESPIRATION

EKG

CAROTID BLOOD PRESSURE

STIMULATE VAGUS 4 VOLTS - AFTER NEOSTIGMINE
TIME 1 MARK/5 SECONDS

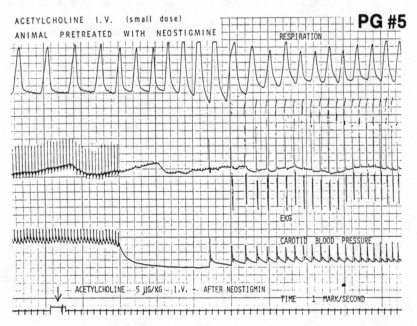

ACETYLCHOLINE I.V. (small dose)
ANIMAL PRETREATED WITH NEOSTIGMINE

PG #5

RESPIRATION

EKG

CAROTID BLOOD PRESSURE

ACETYLCHOLINE 5 μG/KG I.V. AFTER NEOSTIGMIN
TIME 1 MARK/SECOND

B) *Bethanechol chloride* (Myotonachol® —Glenwood; Urecho-
line® — Merck Sharp & Dohme; carbamylmethylcholine)

5. **Alkaloid cholinergics of botanical origin**
   A) *Pilocarpine*
      1) Eye response follows systemic or local administration.
         a) Stimulates contraction of the sphincter muscle of the
            iris and the ciliary muscle of the lens
         b) Pupillary constriction lasts 12 to 24 hours
         c) Loss of accomodation lasts 2 to 3 hours
         d) Onset of activity takes 10 to 15 minutes
      2) Available for oral, parenteral or ophthalmic use
   B) *Arecoline*
      1) Has been used as a teniacide
      2) Stimulates rather violent peristaltic action in the intes-
         tinal tract and washes out the worms

B. **INDIRECT CHOLINERGICS** — cholinesterase inhibitors.
   Tie up the cholinesterase enzymes and inhibit the hydrolytic
   destruction of acetylcholine. The increased concentrations of acetylcholine that result bring about increased action at cholinergic sites
   of glands, smooth muscle, and skeletal muscle. Vagal action and
   acetylcholine action are exaggerated. (PG 4 & 5, *previous page*)

   1. **Reversible inhibitors of cholinesterase** — bind to the enzyme,
      causing an inhibition which is not permanent and does not alter
      the enzyme. When the inhibitor is removed, the enzyme is
      functional again.
      A) *Physostigmine* (Eserine® — O'Neil, Jones & Feldman)
         1) Alkaloid of botanical origin
         2) Eye responses are pupillary constriction and spasm of ac-
            commodation. When drug is applied locally, the onset is
            within 5 to 60 minutes and duration is 12 to 24 hours.
         3) Stimulates skeletal muscle
            a) Esterase is inhibited, leading to increased concentra-
               tion of acetylcholine at the myoneural junction.
            b) Direct stimulatory action on muscle cells
      B) *Neostigmine* (Prostigmin® — Roche;
         Stiglyn™ — Pitman-Moore)
         1) Synthetic compound
         2) Actions similar to physostigmine

   2. **Irreversible inhibitors of cholinesterase** — *i.e.* organophos-
      phates and alkylphosphates (insecticides and anthelmintics).
      Gives a more nearly permanent binding to the enzyme, causing
      permanant inhibition. Irreversibility relates to:
      A) The particular compound, which varies among the group

B) The duration of the binding (aging increases the irreversibility)

C) Toxicity to mammals (indirect cholinergic potency) relates directly to degree of binding or irreversibility. Some cholinesterase inhibitors can be used to treat animals; others are too toxic. Responses related to toxicity are manifested as excessive action of acetylcholine on the CNS and the ANS.

# Cholinergic Blocking Agents

A.  **CHOLINERGIC BLOCKING AGENTS** — drugs that block the action of acetylcholine at smooth-muscle and glandular sites (muscarinic). The prototype is the belladonna alkaloids of botanical origin. They belong to the group of deadly nightshade plants.

1. **Atropine and scopolamine** — mechanism of action is one of competitive antagonism for muscarinic receptors. Receptors are blocked. Atropine exhibits a quantitative difference in affinity for the various receptor sites. Its strongest action occurs at the muscarinic sites, the basic sites of action for its clinical use.

2. **Responses**
   A) *Central nervous system*
      1) At the usual therapeutic doses, response is slight. A slight depression is seen initially.
      2) At higher doses, the cerebral cortex is stimulated. As plasma levels increase, the excitement increases; convulsions, coma, and death can ensue.
      3) Scopolamine has more-pronounced CNS effects than atropine and may be used as a hypnotic.
   B) *Cardiovascular*
      1) Block the vagal influence to the heart, causing an increase in heart rate (PG 6, *following page*)
      2) Block the peripheral vasodilator action of acetylcholine (PG 7, *following page*)
      3) May bring about a drop in diastolic blood pressure by a direct relaxation effect upon arteriolar smooth muscle.
      4) At therapeutic levels, there is little change in heart rate or blood pressure. Depends upon ANS tone to cardiovascular system at time of atropine action. Initially, there is bradycardia followed by tachycardia.
      5) Increase the automaticity of heart muscle. May increase the incidence of cardiac arrhythmias after induction of anesthesia, particularly with thiamylal.
   C) *Respiratory*
      1) Small doses may slightly stimulate

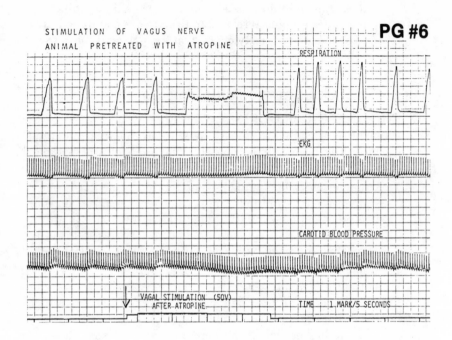

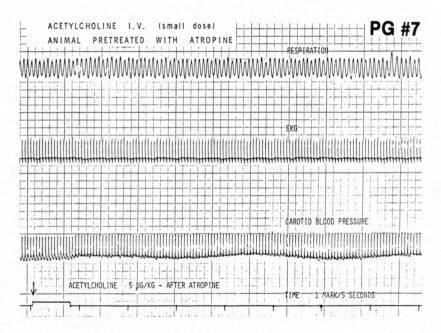

      2) Toxic doses severely inhibit respiration

      3) Decrease mucous secretions

      4) Dilate bronchioles

   D) *Gastrointestinal tract*

      1) Decrease intestinal motility and tone

      2) Decrease gastric secretions

      3) Slight to no decrease in flow of pancreatic and intestinal juices

      4) Decrease salivary secretions

      5) Relax bile duct

   E) *Eye*

      1) Pupil dilates (mydriasis) because sphincter muscle and ciliary muscles are relaxed

      2) Cycloplegia (lens suited for distant vision)

      3) May increase intraocular pressure

   F) *Urinary system*

      1) Relax ureters and bladder wall

      2) Tend to increase tone of sphincter

      3) Overall tendency is toward retention of urine

   G) *Miscellaneous responses*

      1) Inhibit sweating (not in horse), which may result in an increase in body temperature

      2) Inhibit sensory receptors of skin and cornea when applied locally. Similar to a topical anesthetic.

3. **Atropine may be given orally or parenterally.**

   A) Biotransformed by esterases of plasma and liver

   B) Enzyme levels and distribution vary considerably between species and individuals

   C) Excreted by the kidney, partly unchanged and partly as metabolites

   D) Duration of action in most species is 4 to 6 hours

4. **Other muscarinic blockers**

   A) *Methscopolamine* — a quaternary nitrogen compound

      1) Responses similar to those of atropine, but does not penetrate CNS as readily; hence, fewer CNS effects.

      2) Available for oral use

   B) *Methyl atropine nitrate* — Metropine® (Ciba), a quaternary nitrogen compound that produces less CNS activity

   C) *Glycopyrrolate* — Robinul-V® (A. H. Robins)

      1) Labeled for use in dogs

      2) Quarternary nitrogen compound

      3) Poor penetration of the CNS

      4) Reported to be especially effective in reducing the volume and free acidity of gastric juice.

      5) Usual doses have little effect on respiration, blood pressure, or heart rate.

      6) Peak effect is reached in 30 to 45 minutes after intramuscular or subcutaneous injection.

      7) Duration of the action is up to 7 hours

   D) *Aminopentamide* — Centrine® (Bristol)

      1) Labeled for use in dogs

      2) Inhibits motility; secretions of the gastrointestinal tract are more pronounced than with atropine.

      3) Mydriatic effect and inhibition of salivary secretions are less pronounced than with atropine.

   E) Banthine® (Searle) and Pro-Banthine® (Searle) — labelled for human use.

B. **RESPONSE OF ATROPINIZED DOG TO ACETYLCHOLINE GIVEN INTRAVENOUSLY**

1. **Small dose** (5 μg/kg) — causes no change in heart rate, blood pressure, respiration, or secretions. At this low dose level, acetylcholine would normally act only at muscarinic sites, and these sites are blocked (PG 7)

2. **Larger dose** (150 μg/kg) — sufficient to act at both muscarinic and nicotinic sites and will bring about:

   A) Increased respiration rate and amplitude

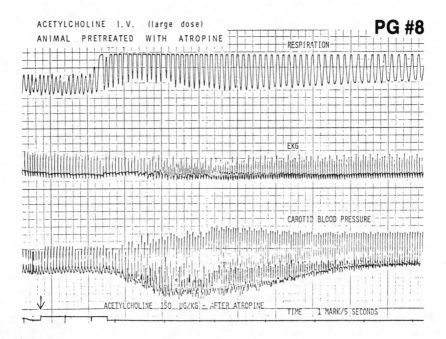

ACETYLCHOLINE I.V. (large dose)         **PG #8**
ANIMAL PRETREATED WITH ATROPINE    RESPIRATION

EKG

CAROTID BLOOD PRESSURE

ACETYLCHOLINE 150 μG/KG - AFTER ATROPINE
TIME    1 MARK/5 SECONDS

B) Heart stimulation, increase in rate and force

C) Rise in blood pressure (PG 8, *facing page*)

3. **Mechanisms for the response of acetylcholine in a dog given atropine:**

A) In smaller doses, the acetylcholine is blocked at all muscarinic sites. The plasma level is not sufficient to stimulate ganglionic sites.

B) In larger doses, the acetylcholine is blocked at muscarinic sites, but:

   1) Ganglionic sites of both divisions are stimulated.

   2) Postganglionic fibers of both divisions are stimulated and transmitters are released at the neuroeffector junction.

   3) Parasympathetic (muscarinic) sites are blocked by atropine, hence no action occur at these sites.

   4) Sympathetic (adrenergic) sites are excited, releasing norepinephrine and giving action.

   5) Norepinephrine and epinephrine are also released from the adrenal medulla, circulating through the blood and giving action.

   6) The overall effect is *adrenergic*.

C. **CHOLINERGIC BLOCKAGE AT GANGLIONIC SITES** — results in a blockage of acetylcholine from the postjunctional membrane in ganglionic sites. This blockage is not utilized to any extent in veterinary medicine.

1. **The net response** is loss of tone to an organ system.

   A) The response of a specific organ depends on which division is primarily responsible for maintenance of tone.

   B) The cardiovascular response is tachycardia because the heart rate is under vagal control. Peripheral vasodilation results from the loss of adrenergic tone.

   C) The gastrointestinal tract is inhibited because vagal tone is lost.

2. **Nicotine and acetylcholine**

   A) Historically important

   B) Small doses stimulate; large doses block.

3. **Hexamethonium** — the classic prototype.

4. **Tetraethylammonium** (Etamon®)

# Adrenergics

Adrenergics use two main mechanisms to induce action at sites mediated by epinephrine and/or norepinephrine. These mechanisms are: 1) direct activation of the receptor as the transmitter or as a mimic of the transmitter, or 2) release of the transmitter into the junction.

A. **ADRENERGIC RECEPTORS**
    1. **Beta receptors** — recently subclassified, $B_1$ and $B_2$.
        A) The $B_1$ are the beta receptors of the heart which, when stimulated, produce an excitatory response. Both epinephrine and norepinephrine apparently stimulate these $B_1$ receptors.
        B) The remainder are classified at $beta_2$

B. **ADRENERGIC RECEPTORS AND ACTIONS**
    Alpha . . . . . . . . . . . . . Arteries & veins . . . . . Vasoconstriction
    $Beta_1$ . . . . . . . . . . . . . . Heart . . . . . . . . . . . . . Increase contractile
                                       force, increase rate,
                                       increase automaticity
    $Beta_2$ . . . . . . . . . . . . . Arteries . . . . . . . . . . . Vasodilation
    Dopaminergic . . . . . . Mesenteric & renal
                                 arteries . . . . . . . . . . . Vasodilation

C. **ADRENERGIC ACTION ON HEART MUSCLE**

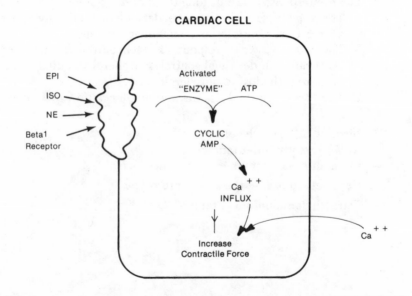

**CARDIAC CELL**

EPI
ISO
NE
Beta1
Receptor

Activated
"ENZYME"    ATP

CYCLIC
AMP

$Ca^{++}$
INFLUX

Increase
Contractile Force

$Ca^{++}$

D.  **ADRENERGIC RECEPTOR ACTIVATORS OR STIMULATORS**
1.  **Norepinephrine** — predominately alpha, some $B_1$.
2.  **Epinephrine** — alpha, $beta_1$, and $beta_2$.
3.  **Isoproterenol** — $beta_1$ and $beta_2$
4.  **Dopamine** — Low doses = $beta_1$ and $beta_2$
    High doses = alpha, $beta_1$, and $beta_2$
5.  **Ephedrine** — predominately alpha.
6.  **Phenylephrine** — predominately alpha.
7.  **Amphetamine** — predominately alpha.

E.  **EPINEPHRINE** (Adrenalin® — Parke-Davis)
1.  **Catecholamine** — chemically biosynthesized from the amino acid, tyrosine. The sequence is: from tyrosine to DOPA to dopamine to norepinephrine to epinephrine.
2.  **Actions**
    A)  *Heart* (beta receptors) $beta_1$
        1)  Increases rate of SA-node firing
        2)  Increased conduction through the AV node
        3)  Increases contractility and irritability of heart muscle; increases automaticity and the likelihood of arrhythmias.
    B)  *Blood vessels* — beta receptors are very sensitive.
        Examples:
        Skeletal muscle—alpha sites—constriction
        Skeletal muscle—$beta_2$ sites—dilation
        Skin—alpha sites—constriction
        Viscera—alpha sites—constriction
        Viscera—$beta_2$ sites—dilation
        Viscera—constriction dominates if both alpha and $beta_2$ are stimulated

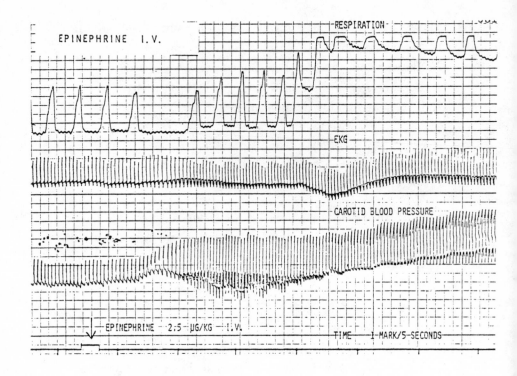

C) *Cardiovascular summary (see* above)
1) Increased systolic pressure
2) Decreased diastolic pressure
3) Mean pressure is unchanged or increased. As dose is increased, pressure increases proportionately.
4) Increased heart rate
5) Decreased peripheral resistance
6) Increased cardiac output
7) If mean pressure rises sufficiently, the heart rate may be decreased by compensatory vagal action.
8) Excessive levels may be toxic to myocardium, thus producing ventricular arrhythmias and even fibrillation.
D) *Bronchial muscle*
1) Beta-dilation is pronounced.
E) *Respiration* — temporarily increased rate and depth; then decreased, including possibility of apnea.
F) *Gastrointestinal smooth muscle*
1) Alpha and beta stimulation produces decreased motility.
2) Gastrointestinal sphincters are alpha, which produces contraction.
3) Decreased secretions (questionable)

        4) Salivary glands are alpha. Secretion is thick and ropey.
   G) *Urinary*
        1) Bladder wall is beta, producing relaxation.
        2) The sphincter of the urinary bladder is alpha, producing contraction.
        3) Reduced formation of urine — the afferent arterioles into the glomerulus are constricted; thus the blood pressure in the glomerulus is reduced. Reduced blood pressure drops the effective filtration pressure; hence, urine formation decreases.
   H) *Eye*
        1) Radial muscle and iris are alpha, producing contraction (mydriasis).
        2) Ciliary muscle is beta, producing relaxation.
        3) Withdrawal of nictitating membrane occurs.
   I) *Pilomotor muscles* — alpha will produce contraction and raise hair.
   J) *Sweat glands* — stimulated in the horse.
   K) *Spleen capsule* — alpha produces contraction.
   L) *Metabolism*
        1) Beta and/or undifferentiated
        2) Increased oxygen consumption
        3) Increased blood glucose from glycogen (and protein)
        4) Increased mobilization of free fatty acids
   M) *Central nervous system*
        1) May be a stimulant with little or no effect at usual doses.
        2) May cause release of corticotropin-releasing-factor from the hypothalamus, which stimulates the anterior pituitary to release more ACTH.

3. **Gastrointestinal tract**
   A) Poorly absorbed from subcutaneous injection. Constricts the vessels locally and hence inhibits its own absorption.
   B) Well absorbed after intramuscular injection, giving a rapid response (2 to 5 minutes). *Inject intravenously with great caution* (response 2 to 5 seconds).

4. **Biotransformed rapidly by tissue enzymes**
   A) Monoamine oxidase and catechol-O-methyl transferase
   B) Action is stopped by re-entry into adrenergic nerve ending and/or biotransformation (re-entry may predominate).

5. **Parenteral aqueous solution of 1:1000**
   A) If exposed to air and sunlight will oxidize to pink, red, then brown. Discard if discolored.
   B) Has been used in oil vehicle for injection.

F.  **NOREPINEPHRINE** — arterenol, levarterenol bitartrate (Levophed® — Winthrop)

   1. **Actions**

      A) Mostly alpha stimulation

      B) *Cardiovascular* (a pressor agent)

         1) Slight increase in rate and force of heart

         2) Potent vasoconstrictor; is alpha in skeletal muscle, skin, and viscera

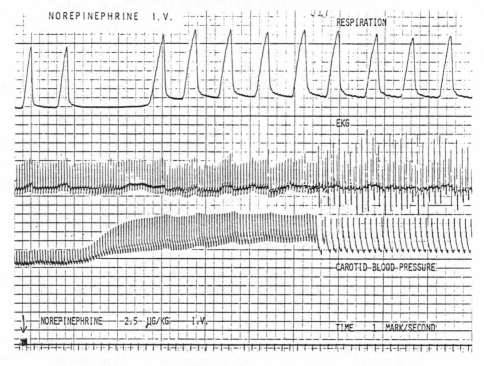

        a) *Cardiovascular summary* (*see* above)

           (1) Increased systolic pressure

           (2) Increased diastolic pressure

           (3) Increased mean pressure

           (4) Initial slight increase in heart rate, then rate slows because of the increased mean blood pressure. The rise of mean pressure causes decreased heart rate by compensatory vagal action.

           (5) Increased peripheral resistance

           (6) Decreased cardiac output because the heart has to pump against a high pressure.

      C) Less potent than epinephrine as a bronchodilator

      D) Little metabolic response

      E) Potent ability to suppress urine formation because afferent arterioles in the nephron are constricted

  2. **Usually given intravenously** — slow drip

  3. **Rapidly biotransformed** — similar to epinephrine. Action is terminated primarily by re-entry into nerve ending.

  4. **Available as levarterenol bitartrate (Levophed®** — Winthrop) — a solution for injection containing 0.1 mg/ml, supplied in 2-ml ampules.

G. **ISOPROTERENOL** (isopropylnorepinephrine) Isuprel® (Winthrop), Iprenol® (Vitarine)

  1. **Actions**

    A) *Purely beta stimulatory*

    B) *Heart*

      1) Stimulated to increase rate and force

      2) Marked vasodilation

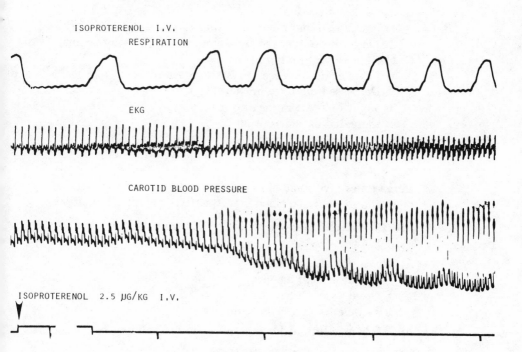

ISOPROTERENOL I.V.
RESPIRATION

EKG

CAROTID BLOOD PRESSURE

ISOPROTERENOL 2.5 μG/KG I.V.

    C) *Cardiovascular summary* (*see* above)

      1) Slightly increased systolic pressure

      2) Greatly decreased diastolic pressure

      3) Decreased mean pressure

      4) Greatly decreased peripheral resistance

   5) Increased heart rate
   6) Increased cardiac output
   7) May cause venous dilation, venous pooling, and decreased venous return, which may reduce cardiac output.
   C) *Potent bronchodilator* — ten times more potent than epinephrine
   D) *Resembles epinephrine* in metabolic response

2. **Available as Isuprel®** (Winthrop) — tablets for sublingual use. Also available: inhalation preparations, oral elixirs and injectable solutions containing 0.2 mg/ml in 1- and 5-ml ampules.

H. **DOPAMINE** Intropin® (Arnar-Stone)

1. **Actions**
   A) *Heart*
      1) Rate slightly increased
      2) Contractions stronger
      3) Automaticity increased
   B) Visceral vessels dilated
      1) Increased renal blood flow and formation of urine
      2) Action is not blocked by alpha or beta blocking agents.
   C) *Cardiovascular summary*
      1) Little or no increase in systolic pressure
      2) Decreased diastolic pressure
      3) Slight increase in mean pressure
      4) Increased cardiac output
      5) Less increase in myocardial consumption of oxygen, resulting in less tendency toward tachycardias and arrhythmias.

2. **Large doses** give some alpha action, increase peripheral resistance and reduce renal blood flow, thus reducing urine formation.

I. **PHENYLEPHRINE** Neosynephrine® (Winthrop)

1. **Actions**
   A) *Alpha stimulator*
      1) Potent pressor agent
      2) Nasal vasoconstrictor
      3) Little effect on myocardium

2. **Available as solutions for inhalation and injection**

J. **EPHEDRINE AND AMPHETAMINE**

1. **Actions**
   A) *Alpha stimulators*
   B) *Vasoconstrictors*
      1) Cause weak positive inotropic and chronotropic effects
      2) Combination of the two causes blood pressure to rise

   C) *Bronchodilator effect* — less than epinephrine, but more
      prolonged
   D) *Potent stimulators of* CNS

2. **Mechanism of action**
   A) *Adrenergic* — results from the release of the transmitter,
      norepinephrine, from nerve endings.
   B) *Direct stimulation of* CNS

3. **Slower onset of action** — longer duration of action than other
   alpha stimulators

4. **Available as oral tablets and injectable solutions**

5. **Antiphrine®** — an antihistamine and ephedrine combined.

# Adrenergic Blocking Agents

Drugs are used that will block either alpha sites or beta sites, but none that will block both. Activation of receptors is blocked by adrenergic compounds whether they are released naturally or given exogenously.

A. **ALPHA ADRENERGIC BLOCKERS** (*See* below)

 1. **Alpha adrenergic blockade** — competitive antagonism prevents the excitation of alpha receptors and prevents their specific response. This antagonism applies to compensatory responses as well as to responses from injected drugs and responses to sympathetic tone. If the specific alpha response is understood the action of the blocker can be predicted. Apparently some will block $B_1$ receptors also.

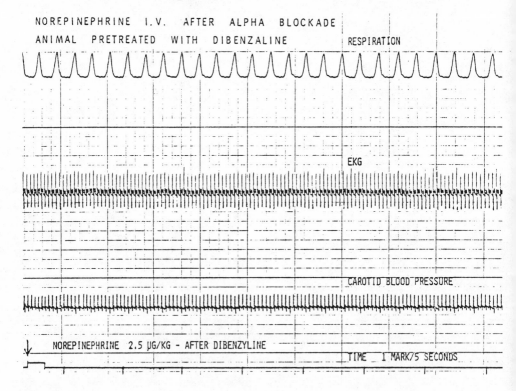

NOREPINEPHRINE I.V. AFTER ALPHA BLOCKADE
ANIMAL PRETREATED WITH DIBENZALINE     RESPIRATION

EKG

CAROTID BLOOD PRESSURE

NOREPINEPHRINE 2.5 µG/KG - AFTER DIBENZYLINE

TIME   1 MARK/5 SECONDS

 2. **Ergotamine** — an alkaloid from ergot (a fungus).
    A) Historically important. It was the first *alpha blocker.*
    B) Stimulates smooth-muscle contraction via a *direct* action on the smooth-muscle cells. This action is not related to the action of ergotamine as a blocker of alpha sites.

      1) Vasoconstriction occurs, causing a rise in blood pressure.

      2) Contraction of uterine smooth muscle (ergot alkaloids will be discussed with drugs that act on the uterus)

3. **Phenoxybenzamine** Dibenzyline® (SmithKline & French); alpha blockade is sometimes categorized as irreversible because of its long duration (weeks in man).

4. **Phenothiazine-derivative tranquilizers** (Acepromazine—Ayerst; Sparine® — Wyeth; Thorazine® — SmithKline & French)

   A) Central nervous system activity as tranquilizers

   B) Alpha blockade and beta$_1$ blocked

   C) Action is clinically important

B. **BETA ADRENERGIC BLOCKERS** propranolol (Inderal® — Ayerst)

1. **Inhibit the responses by competitive antagonism, which results from adrenergic stimulation of beta receptors.**

2. **Decrease excitability of the heart** — give a negative inotropic effect. May be used to prevent or treat arrhythmias.

C. **EPINEPHRINE-REVERSAL PHENOMENON** (*See* below)

1. **Response of a normal dog to an injection of epinephrine is a rise in systolic and mean blood pressure.**

2. **If the dog is pretreated with an alpha blocker in sufficient quantity, all alpha sites are blocked.**

3. **After the alpha sites are blocked, injection of epinephrine produces a drop in diastolic and mean blood pressure.**

EPINEPHRINE I.V. AFTER ALPHA BLOCKADE
ANIMAL PRETREATED WITH ACEPROMAZINE

4. **Mechanism of epinephrine reversal**
   A) Epinephrine excites both alpha and beta sites.
   B) The pressor effect is blocked. Alpha sites are vasoconstrictors and are blocked.
   C) Vasodilation is pronounced due to stimulation of the beta site.
   D) Overall peripheral resistance is reduced.
   E) Blood pressure falls.

# Therapeutic Applications of Autonomic Drugs

A. **ADRENERGICS**
   1. **Hypotension** — use norepinephrine and/or epinephrine for treatment of early hypovolemic or hypotensive shock.
   2. **Cardiac arrest** — inject epinephrine directly into the heart.
   3. **Anaphylactic shock** — inject one-third of the dose of epinephrine IV. Give the remainder IM.
   4. **Long-standing shock** — use isoproterenol or dopamine to enhance the heart action and improve renal, intestinal, and hepatic blood flow without causing vasoconstriction.
   5. **Allergic disorders** — use epinephrine or ephedrine.
   6. **Topical hemostasis** — use epinephrine, ephedrine, neosynephrine to produce vasoconstriction and hemostasis.
   7. **To reduce nasal vasodilation and resultant congestion** — use neosynephrine.
   8. **Addition of adrenergics to local anesthetic solutions** — reduces their absorption and prolongs their action. Use epinephrine and ephedrine.

B. **ADRENERGIC BLOCKERS**
   1. **Long standing shock** "irreversible" to correct extensive vasoconstriction of viscera and improve blood flow to viscera. Use alpha blocker (Dibenzyline® [SmithKline & French], phenothiazine derivative tranquilizers).
   2. **May possibly allow** administration of higher doses of digitalis without causing arrythmia.
   3. **Ventricular premature beats and certain atrial arrythmias.** Use beta blocker (propanolol [Inderal® —SmithKline & French]) for anti-arrhythmic effect.

4. **Phenothiazine derivative tranquilizers** have been shown to protect against (prevent) epinephrine induced cardiac arrythmias in an animal that has been given chloroform, halothane or methoxyflurane.

C. **CHOLINERGICS**

1. **Eye** — use as a miotic to reduce intraocular pressure in glaucoma.

2. **To treat urinary retention** of neurogenic origin, use neostigmine.

3. **To stimulate** motility and secretions of the GI tract, use neostigmine or carbachol.

4. **As an aid in parturition**, use carbachol.

D. **ANTICHOLINERGIC, CHOLINERGIC BLOCKERS**

1. **Use as preanesthetic medication** to inhibit secretions; appear to prevent cardiac arrest through vagal inhibition. Use to maintain patent airways, by dilating bronchioles and decreasing secretions. They inhibit peripheral vasodilation and reduce the tendency toward hypotension.

2. **Use to decrease motility or hyperperistalisis** in cases of diarrhea. In some concepts of diarrhea therapy, the value of this action is questioned.

3. **Slight anti-emetic effect;** applies also to use as preanesthetic medication.

4. **Eye** — dilate pupil for examination, prevent adhesions. Alternate with administration of a miotic agent.

5. **To treat for organophosphate toxicity.** Use higher than usual doses.

6. **For symptomatic relief** of difficult breathing or heaves.

7. **For relief of pain** from spasm of urinary tract (renal colic). Make use of antispasmodic property.

8. **To manage urinary incontinence** if it is caused by excessive cholinergic tone.

CHAPTER

# 4

# Analgesic, Antipyretic and Anti-inflammatory Drugs

## General Principles of Inflammation

A. **CIRCULATORY AND CELLULAR REACTION** — the body tissues react to injury or irritation.

B. **INJURIOUS AGENTS THAT MAY PRODUCE INFLAMMATION**

    1. **Bacteria and their toxins**
        A) Viruses        D) Chemical
        B) Rickettsia    E) Irradiation
        C) Fungi

    2. **Trauma**
        A) Mechanical    D) Protozoa
        B) Thermal       E) Internal and external parasites
        C) Electrical

    3. **Crush of tissues**

    4. **Death (necrosis) of tissue resulting from cell destruction**

    5. **Toxins released as a result of allergic reaction**

C. **TYPES OF INFLAMMATION**

    1. **Acute** — changes occur within a few minutes to a few days after exposure to injurious agents.

    2. **Chronic** — of long duration, sometimes months or years.

D. **OBJECTIVES OF INFLAMMATION**

    1. **Body defense mechanism against injury**
        A) Destroys, removes, neutralizes or walls off the action of in-

jurious agent(s)

B) Repairs the damage and restores the tissues to normal

E. **THE CARDINAL SIGNS OF INFLAMMATION**
1. **Redness**    3. **Swelling**
2. **Heat**       4. **Pain**        5. **Loss of function**

F. **RESULTS OF THE INFLAMMATORY REACTION** — is initially protective, but may proceed to be injurious to insulted tissue or even the whole animal.

1. **Changes in microcirculation** (in sequence):
   A) Dilation and increased flow of blood (hyperemia), which produces the redness and heat.
   B) Flow begins to slow.
   C) White cells migrate to and adhere to vessel walls.
   D) Red cells clump.
   E) Platelets may aggregate.
   F) Stasis or sludging of blood results.

2. **Increased permeability of vessel walls:**
   A) Results in increased loss of fluids and protein into tissues
   B) Results in swelling and edema
   C) May be induced by release of cell toxins such as histamine, kinins, and prostaglandins

3. **Emigration of white cells and phagocytosis occur.**
   A) Phagocytic cells are activated.
   B) Cells leave through the intact vessel wall and enter the surrounding tissue.
   C) Phagocytic white cells engulf the injurious agents, if present, and render them inactive.
   D) When infection is present, dead white cells and necrotic tissue form pus.

4. **Integrity of cell membranes is lost.**
   A) Lysis of cells may occur.
   B) Lysosomal digestive enzymes are released.

5. **Dead cells and injured cells release many cell toxins.**
   A) May cause further insult and may cause pain
   B) Time summary of cell toxins released:
      1) **Rapid** — takes just a few minutes
         a) Histamine and serotonin
      2) **Delayed** — ½ to 3 hours to begin the process
         a) Kinins                c) Prostaglandins
         b) Superoxide oxygen     d) Lysosomal enzymes

6. **Loss of function may be the ultimate result, due to:**
   A) Poor perfusion of tissues
   B) Lack of oxygen to cells
   C) Released cell toxins

## G.  HEALING

1. **Removal of inflammatory products and dead tissues — accomplished by liquefaction and absorption.**

2. **Repair or replacement of damaged or dead tissues occurs by:**
   A) Repair — the laying down of connective tissue or scar tissue and/or
   B) Regeneration — the replacement of destroyed cells with cells of the same kind

## H.  MECHANISM THAT MEDIATES INFLAMMATORY RESPONSE IN THE CELLS (*See* schematic on facing page)

1. **The injurious agent or insult alters the cell** — results in activation of cellular lipases and cell membrane phospholipases.

2. **Free arachidonic acid is made available.**

3. **Free arachidonic acid is converted by the enzyme cyclooxygenase** — forms many prostaglandins.

4. **Prostaglandins are not stored in the tissues** — they are present only when biosynthesized and released by injury or insult.

5. **The prostaglandins formed and released are the chemical mediators** — they bring about:
   A) Inflammation
   B) Platelet aggregation
   C) Lung-tissue responses of anaphylaxis
   D) Pain — locally at injured cells and also in the pain-perception areas of the brain.
   E) Fever — the prostaglandins are believed to act on the body-temperature control center in the hypothalamus.

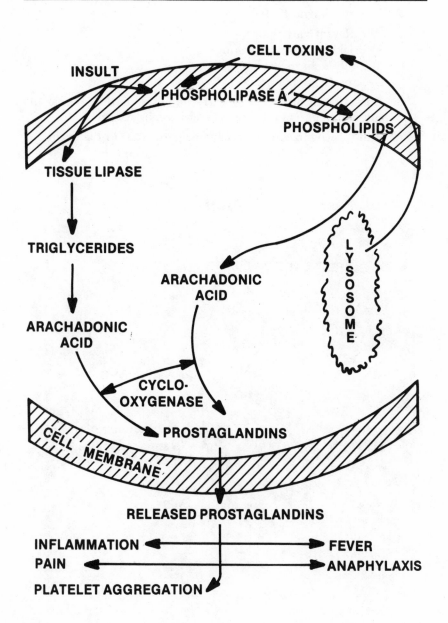

# General Principles of Pain

A. **PAIN**
   1. **A protective mechanism** — signals an injured area
   2. **A useful diagnostic tool**
   3. **Of different varieties**
      A) Pricking, burning, aching
      B) Dull or sharp
      C) Superficial or visceral
   4. **Pain afferent pathways** — carry impulses via the somatic and autonomic nerves into the central nervous system.
   5. **Pain is recognized (appreciated or perceived) in the brain.**

## PAIN

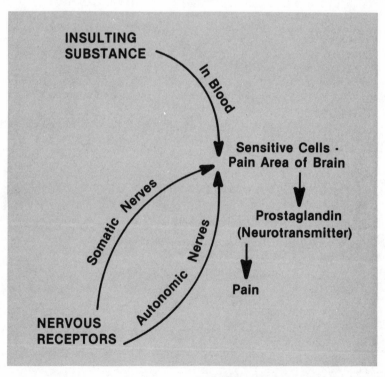

B.  **PHARMACOTHERAPEUTIC MECHANISMS FOR PRODUCING ANALGESIA**

1.  **Increases the threshold of pain in the pain areas of the brain** — there are two general mechanisms to accomplish this:
    A) Opiate drugs — act on the same receptors as the brain's own pain-relieving substances called *endorphins*. Included are:

    1) Morphine      3) Methadone      5) Pentazocine
    2) Meperidine     4) Oxymorphone     6) Fentanyl
                                        7) Codeine

    B) Interference with biosynthesis of specific prostaglandins — this takes place in certain areas of the brain. Included are: aspirin, flunixin, and phenylbutazone.

2.  **Anti-inflammatory drugs may produce analgesia by:**
    A) Blocking prostaglandin synthesis — reduces inflammation.
    B) Reducing tissue swelling and edema peripherally — reduces pressure on nerve endings. Fewer painful stimuli are initiated and there is less pain.

3.  **Inhibit input from sensory nerves by using local anesthetics**
    A) Blocks conduction along nerve fibers
    B) Infiltrates to block sensory receptors

4.  **General anesthesia**

# General Principles of Fever

A.  **FEVER** — an elevation of body temperature to above normal. It is an important and quick reflection of altered body function and hence a valuable clinical sign.

B.  **BODY TEMPERATURE** — brought about and controlled by means of a balance between heat production and heat loss.

1.  **Body heat is produced by:**
    A) Contraction of skeletal muscle
    B) Metabolic activity of glands, heart, liver, and brain

2.  **Body heat is lost via:**
    A) Radiation and conduction from body surfaces
    B) Evaporation of sweat

3.  **Body temperature** — is regulated in the hypothalamus where the thermostat is located.
    A) The thermostat is bathed in blood. It monitors the temperature of body organs via the temperature of circulating blood. (*See* schematic on following page.)

**Reaction of Body Temperature-Regulating
System to Disease**

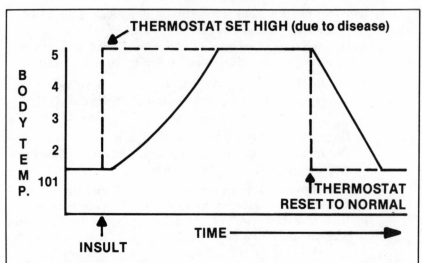

1.  **Normal setting is 101 F** — loss and production of body heat are balanced, resulting in a body temperature of 101 F.

2.  **At the point of insult, cellular products of a microorganism (pyrogen) circulate via the blood to the hypothalamus** — this brings about the formation of certain specific prostaglandin(s) which causes the thermostat cells to reset at a higher level.

3.  **Body temperature (101 F) is now below the thermostat setting,** *e.g.* 105 F — the body temperature control center now turns on the two schemes to raise body temperature.
    A)  Mechanisms for increasing heat production
        1)  Shivering
        2)  Sympathetic excitement caused by release of epinephrine and an increase in cellular metabolism
        3)  An increased output of thyroxine to increase cellular metabolism
    B)  Mechanisms for conserving body heat
        1)  Vasoconstriction in the skin
        2)  Decrease sweating
        3)  Piloerection to trap air for insulation

4.  **Body temperature reaches the new setting (105 F)** — the control center then will balance heat production and heat loss and maintain the body temperature at 105 F until the thermostat is reset to normal by:
    A)  The microorganisms (pyrogens)
    B)  Drug that can lower an elevated setting

5.  **When the thermostat is reset to normal (101 F),** — the body temperature (105 F) is now higher than the setting and the body-temperature control center now turns on the schemes to increase loss of body heat by causing:
    A)  Vasodilation in the skin
    B)  Increased sweating or panting-type respiration
    C)  Mobilization of water into blood

## C. MECHANISM FOR ANTIPYRETIC DRUG ACTION

1. **Lowers the setting of an elevated hypothalamic thermostat —** this only occurs in the presence of fever.

2. **Action is caused by blocking the production of and/or the release of certain prostaglandins —** the neurotransmitter that resets the normal thermostat to the fever level.

# Nonsteroidal
# Anti-Inflammatory Drugs

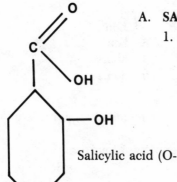

A. **SALICYLATES** (aspirin)
1. **Chemistry —** Salicylic acid derivatives
   A) Sodium salicylate
   B) Acetylsalicylic acid (aspirin)
   C) Methylsalicylate (oil of wintergreen)

Salicylic acid (O-hydroxy benzoic acid)

2. **Actions**
   A) Analgesia
      1) Effective against aches and pains of low intensity
      2) Effective against superficial pain, joint pain, and pain of the musculoskeletal system
   B) Antipyretic — reduces body temperature
   C) Anti-inflammatory action
   D) Other organ responses
      1) *Respiratory* — initial stimulation; depression ensues if the patient is overdosed.
      2) *Cardiovascular* — little effect at proper dose
      3) *Skin* — is local irritant (oil of wintergreen) with antibacterial and antifungal effects
      4) *Metabolic effects*
         a) Uncouples oxidative phosphorylation
         b) Decreases liver glycogen
         c) Generally increases metabolism

3. **Mechanism of action** — inhibits production of prostaglandins by inhibiting cyclo-oxygenase, the enzyme that biosynthesizes prostaglandin.

4. **Metabolism**
   A) Well absorbed after oral administration — absorption is rapid and begins in the stomach.
   B) Rapidly distributed to all tissues and fluids
   C) Tight binding with plasma proteins — results in an effective competition with other competitors (such as thyroxin, bilirubin, and penicillin) for relatively limited binding sites.
   D) Biotransformation
      1) Principally conjugated with a variety of substances
      2) Extreme species variation occurs — cats biotransform aspirin very poorly.

   | Plasma T½ | | |
   |---|---|---|
   | Man ... | 1.5 | hours |
   | Horse .. | 5 | hours |
   | Dog ... | 8 | hours |
   | Cat .... | 30 | hours |

   E) Fate
      1) Excreted by kidney
         a) Unchanged in free form, as metabolites and as conjugates
         b) Alkaline urine favors excretion of the free drug.

5. **Toxicity**
   A) Irritating to gastric mucosa
      1) Causes vomiting
      2) May produce hemorrhagic ulcers
      3) Buffering will reduce nausea
   B) Acid-base imbalances are produced with toxic doses.
      1) Initially causes respiratory alkalosis
      2) Later, a respiratory and metabolic acidosis may occur.
   C) Respiratory depression can occur late, which inhibits the respiratory center.
   D) Hepatotoxic
   E) Causes hypoprothrombinemia and depressed blood clotting.
   F) Toxic reactions vary among species. Toxicity is probably related to plasma concentration. Relative overdoses are possible. Cats are very susceptible. The dose for dogs is potentially lethal to cats and will kill a cat within 3 to 7 days. The maximum dose for cats is one-half a baby aspirin/day because of the drug's long half-life in that species.

6. **Aspirin has been reported to inhibit anaphylactic shock and anaphylactic bronchoconstriction and apnea in calves and ponies.** In experimental acute interstitial pneumonia of calves

caused by *Ascaris suum*, therapy with aspirin (100-250 mg/kg orally, b.i.d.) provided complete symptomatic control of the clinical signs, reducing or abolishing the characteristic setback. Treatment of the same condition with antihistamines and antiserotonin drugs caused no clinical improvement.

B.  **PHENYLBUTAZONE** (Butazolidin® — Jen-Sal, Tevcodyne® — Tevco, Equi Bute® — Fort Dodge, Bizolin® — Bio-Ceutic, Robizone-V® — A. H. Robins)

1.  **Chemistry** — a pyrazolone derivative

2.  **Actions**
    A)  Labeled for use in horses and dogs only
    B)  Anti-inflammatory
    C)  Analgesic and antipyretic properties are relatively weak. Used as an aid in relieving inflammation involving the musculoskeletal system.

3.  **Mechanism of action**
    A)  Inhibits the biosynthesis of prostaglandins by inhibiting the enzyme cyclo-oxygenase.
    B)  Prostaglandins are now said to be the principal mediators of the inflammatory response.

4.  **Metabolism**
    A)  Well absorbed when given orally
    B)  In the liver is biotransformed to the metabolite oxyphenbutazone, which is also active.
    C)  Phenylbutazone plasma half life:
        1)  Horse — 3.5 to 6 hours
        2)  Dog — 2.5 to 6 hours
        3)  Man — 72 hours.
    D)  Active metabolite, oxyphenbutazone, is found in horse urine for 48 hours.
    E)  Phenylbutazone is a hepatic microsomal enzyme inducer. When used chronically it will accelerate its own inactivation. Because its metabolite is also active, the decrease in activity is not great.

5.  **Relatively nontoxic at proper dosage in dogs and horses**
    A)  Fatal hemorrhagic syndrome, biliary stasis, and renal damage in dogs have been reported. Phenylbutazone given to cats (44 mg/kg b.i.d.) resulted in death. Signs of toxicity are: loss of appetite, loss of weight, CNS depression, dehydration, and vomiting. Medication should be discontinued when signs appear.
    B)  In horses, 2 g/day for 32 days produced a necrotizing

phlebitis of the portal veins.

C) Has produced blood dyscrasia in man. It is potentially very toxic to man. A 20-year-old professional jockey died from aplastic anemia which developed after he took phenyl-butazone about 20 times over a three-year period. Blood dyscrasias in man are thought to be dose-related.

D) Blood dyscrasia caused by phenylbutazone is not reported to be a problem in veterinary medicine, but care should be taken with its use.

1) Do not overdose.

2) Do not use any longer than needed and do not use in-discriminately or routinely.

3) Use appropriate dose and frequency of administration for each species.

D) Monitor hemogram if the drug is used for extended periods.

E) Intracarotid injection produces excessive stimulation and convulsions.

C. **OXYPHENBUTAZONE** (Tandearil® — Geigy)

1. **Metabolite of phenylbutazone**

2. **Used in human medicine**

3. **Not as widely used in veterinary medicine**

D. **DIPYRONE, METHAMPYRONE** (Myovin® , Analate® , Novin® )

1. **Chemistry** — a derivative of pyrazolon and aminopyrine

2. **Actions**
    A) Labeled for use in the horse, dog, cat
    B) Slight anti-inflammatory
    C) Analgesic and antipyretic
    D) Smooth-muscle relaxant, particularly of intestinal tract (antispasmodic)

3. **Mechanism of action**
    A) Not well understood
    B) Apparently has little action on normal spontaneous motility of the intestinal tract
    C) Inhibits kinin-induced intestinal spasms

4. **Toxicity**
    A) Agranulocytosis and leukopenia have been found when drugs have been used for extended periods.
    B) Overdoses may cause convulsions.
    C) Bleeding time tends to increase.
    D) Dipyrone and chlorpromazine used simultaneously can result in serious hypothermia.

E. **DIMETHYLSULFOXIDE** (DMSO) (Domoso® — Diamond)

1. **Chemistry**
   A) Water-white to straw-yellow (depending on purity) liquid
   B) Powerful solvent of inorganic and organic compounds
   C) Freely water-soluble
   D) Extremely hygroscopic

2. **History**
   A) Synthesized in Germany in 1867
   B) Economical method of production as a by-product of paper manufacturing was developed in 1950s. Used as a commercial solvent to synthesize certain synthetic fibers.
   C) In 1960 used in biological application as a preservative for various tissues and cells
   D) In 1964, first used as a medicinal compound. A broad range of potential uses was claimed. In veterinary medicine it was used to treat acute traumatic injuries.

3. **Responses**
   A) Anti-inflammatory; *i.e.*, it reduces acute swelling.
   B) Has been reported to inhibit the availability of arachidonic acid and its conversion to prostaglandin
   C) Enhances the percutaneous absorption of many substances, but not all
   D) May potentiate the activity of atropine, insulin, and endogenous steroids
   E) Some evidence that it is a cholinesterase inhibitor. Has been associated with:
      1) Lowering of vagal threshold
      2) Increased smooth-muscle tone in gastrointestinal tract
      3) Spontaneous skeletal-muscle fasciculations
   F) Evidence for a positive inotropic heart action

4. **Recommended for topical use in dogs and horses only** — available as a solution and a gel.

5. **Side effects**
   A) Transient and local erythema and burning or smarting
   B) Dry skin
   C) Breath odor
   D) Ocular changes
      1) Changes in refractive index; tendency toward myopia
      2) Dependent on dose and duration of treatment

6. **Precautions**
   A) Apply with rubber gloves.
   B) Use good judgment when appling with other drugs, especially those affecting the cardiovascular system and CNS.

C) Do not use simultaneously or within a few days before or after treatment with other cholinesterase inhibitors (organophosphates), cholinergics, or succinylcholine.
D) Bandaging may cause irritation.
E) Contraindicated in dogs and horses intended for breeding purposes. *May be teratogenic.*

F. **ENZYMES**

1. **Reduce inflammation, inflammatory barriers, and edema —** when associated with acute insult such as trauma.

2. **May act via their fibrinolytic action**

3. **No action on living cells**

4. **Chymotrypsin** (Kymar® — Burns-Biotec)
    A) Available for IM use
    B) Available as an ointment containing chymotrypsin, trypsin, neomycin and hydrocortisone

5. **Streptokinase** (Streptase® —Hoechst-Roussel) — Fibrinolytic

G. **METALLIC COMPOUNDS**

1. **Gold salts**
    A) Mechanism is not well understood
    B) Questionable value
    C) Gold sodium thiosulfate (various manufacturers)
    D) Myochrysine® (Merck, Sharp & Dohme) in a dosage of 1 mg/kg/week for several weeks, is reported to be beneficial as the sole treatment for rheumatoid arthritis in dogs.

2. **Orgotein** (Palosein® — Diagnostic Data); for horses and dogs
    A) Chemistry
        1) A group of soluble metalloprotein congeners
        2) Isolated from bovine liver
        3) Contains copper and zinc
        4) Includes hepato- and erythro-cuprein and the enzyme, superoxide dismutase
    B) Responses  ·
        1) Anti-inflammatory in soft tissue;˙associated with the musculoskeletal system of horses and dogs
        2) Wide safety margin
        3) Poorly immunogenic
        4) Not immunosuppressive
        5) Protects from shock reactions produced by antigenic challenge after prior sensitization; inhibits immediate hypersensitivity
        6) Preliminary data suggest an antiviral activity.

C) Summary for mechanism of the anti-inflammatory action of orgotein:

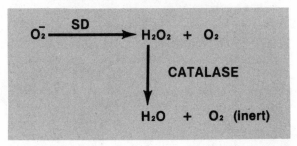

### Inactivation of Superoxide
### (Superoxide Dismutase)

$$O_2^- \xrightarrow{\text{SD}} H_2O_2 \; + \; O_2$$
$$\downarrow \text{CATALASE}$$
$$H_2O \; + \; O_2 \text{ (inert)}$$

   1) Inflammatory insult occurs which activates phagocytes. This causes an increase in cellular respiration and an aggregation of cells. The sharply increased cellular respiration results in excessive production of the superoxide radical, oxygen. Superoxide causes hyaluronic acid to depolymerize. The result is loss of function of hyaluronic acid in synovial fluid. The viscosity and lubricating property of the synovial fluid are thus reduced. The enzyme, superoxide dismutase (SD), in orgotein catalyzes the inactivation of the superoxide radical, reducing the amount of the offending agent.
   D) Should be given IM to horses, every other day. Give IM to dogs, daily for 6 days, then every other day.

H. **INDOMETHACIN** (Indocin® — Merck, Sharp & Dohme)
   1. **Has anti-inflammatory properties similar to aspirin.** Inhibits the biosynthesis of prostaglandins.
   2. **Relatively safe**
      A) May cause nausea or anorexia.
      B) May cause CNS effects such as vertigo or confusion.
      C) Use with care in patients with epilepsy.
      D) Side effects are usually dose-dependent.
   3. **Give orally**

I. **SELENIUM + TOCOPHEROL** (Seletoc® — Burns-Biotec)
   1. **Combination of sodium selenite and vitamin E** (*d*-alpha tocopheryl acetate)

*4-5mg/10# Body wt daily 7 days then once or twice weekly*

*50mg*

*100mg*

2. **Actions**

   A) Anti-inflammatory. It inhibits the formation of peroxides and highly reactive free radicals which can damage cellular materials.

   B) Serves as a catalyst or coenzyme in calcium and protein metabolism. It inhibits metastatic calcification and restores muscle tone.

   C) It plays a role in the maintenance of cellular, muscle and erythrocyte integrity.

3. **Indications**

   A) Arthritic and muscular disorders

   B) To improve muscle tone in hip dysplasia

   C) Certain skin conditions

4. **Side effects**

   A) Nausea and vomiting

   B) Irritation of gastrointestinal tract

5. **Selenium is potentially toxic. Do not overdose!**

   A) Anorexia

   B) Muscle weakness

   C) CNS stimulation, followed by depression

   D) Respiratory depression

   E) Chronic excessive doses cause pathological changes in heart, spleen, kidney and pancreas.

6. **Given orally, IM, or SC**

   A) Initially may be given daily, then every third day.

   B) If no response has been noted after 14 days, the diagnosis should be reevaluated.

   C) Maintenance therapy may be given, if beneficial.

J.  **MECLOFENAMIC ACID** (Arquel® — Parke-Davis)

1. **Chemistry** — an anthranilic acid derivative that is not related chemically to steroids, salicylates, indomethacine or phenylbutazone.

2. **Actions**

   A) Analgesic

   B) Antipyretic          C) Anti-inflammatory

3. **Mechanism of action**

   A) Acts centrally in the brain to raise the threshold to pain via inhibition of prostaglandin synthesis

   B) Acts at tissue sites

      1) Anti-inflammatory action on cells and blood vessels

      2) Inhibits the release of tissue prostaglandins by inhibiting cyclo-oxygenase

4. **Metabolism**
   A) Well absorbed when given orally
      1) Plasma levels reached in 30 minutes
      2) Peak plasma levels reached in 1 to 4 hours
   B) Metabolized by liver
   C) Eliminated by fecal and urinary excretion
   D) Appreciable concentrations are found in synovial fluid and articular cartilage after administration.

5. **Toxicity**
   A) Toxicity shown at four times the recommended dose
   B) Intolerance occurs, causing signs of:
      1) Colic, diarrhea and anorexia
      2) Occult blood in feces, followed by a lowered hematocrit
   C) Signs of chronic toxic dosage:
      1) CNS depression
      2) Ulcers in mouth
      3) Diarrhea
      4) Subcutaneous edema
      5) Tachycardia
      6) Loss of body weight

K. **NAPROXEN** (Equiproxen® — Diamond)
   1. **Not related chemically to the salicylates or steroids**
      A) Is a substituted naphthalene acetic acid compound
      B) Virtually insoluble in water
   2. **Approved for use in horses not intended for food**
   3. **Actions**
      A) Anti-inflammatory
         1) Inhibits the biosynthesis of prostaglandin
         2) Most effective against problems of soft-tissue origin; *i.e.* myostitis or the typing-up syndrome.
         3) Effective in reducing pain and inflammation associated with muscle damage
         4) Probably does not influence the actual rate at which tissue is repaired
      B) Analgesia is the result of the anti-inflammatory action.
      C) Antipyretic activity
      D) CNS depression has resulted from administration of large doses.
   4. **Metabolism**
      A) Well absorbed when given orally.
      B) 90% excreted via kidneys; almost totally eliminated in 48 hours
      C) Treat twice daily

5. **Toxicity**
   A) Three times the therapeutic dose caused no overt lesions in horses.
   B) Principal adverse effects shown experimentally were gastro-intestinal irritation and ulceration.
   C) After large doses, neuropathy was occasionally seen in rats, mice and rabbits, but not in monkeys or miniature pigs.

L. **FLUNIXIN MEGLUMINE** (Banamine® — Schering)
   1. **Chemistry** — a highly substituted nicotinic acid
   2. **Actions** — horse
      A) Anti-inflammatory
      B) Antipyretic
      C) Analgesic, colic pain especially.
   3. **Mechanism of action** — inhibits biosynthesis of prostaglandin
   4. **Action**
      A) Onset — 2 hours; peaks in 12 to 16 hours
      B) Duration — 24 to 36 hours
   5. **Can be given intramuscularly or intravenously**
   6. **Excreted in urine** — plasma T½ is 1.6 hours
   7. **No adverse reactions reported** — at doses up to five times daily dose for 5 days.

# Glucocorticosteroids
# Anti-Inflammatory Steroids

A. **HISTORY**

1855—Sir Thomas Addison described adrenal cortical insufficiency.
1856—Brown-Sequard showed that adrenalectomy was fatal to dogs.
1938—Reichstein synthesized deoxycorticosterone.
1948—Sarett synthesized cortisone.
1949—Hench and Kendall (Mayo Clinics) described and utilized the beneficial effects of cortisone in treating rheumatoid arthritis.
Mid to late 1950s—Ability to utilize the Mexican yam as a source for the basic steroid nucleus ushered in the era of the synthetic corticosteroids at a price that is feasible for widespread therapeutic use in human and veterinary medicine.

B. **PHYSIOLOGICAL ROLE**

Glucocorticosteroids maintain homeostasis in the face of the many and varied conditions to which an animal is exposed. The principal benefit is to enable the animal to react to stress. This phenomenon has been described by Dr. Hans Selye as the *general adaptation syndrome.*

C. **PRINCIPAL FUNCTIONS RELATIVE TO ADAPTATION ARE:**
   1. Regulation of volume and composition of body fluids
   2. Contribution to essential cellular metabolism

D. **PRIMARY PHYSIOLOGICAL ACTIVITY**
   1. **Glucocorticosteroids**
      A) Anti-inflammatory effect
      B) Influence carbohydrate and protein metabolism
      C) Principal natural steroid is *hydrocortisone* (cortisol)
   2. **Mineralocorticosteroids**
      A) Regulate the retention and excretion of sodium, potassium, and water; play an important role in water balance, electrolyte balance, and acid-base balance
      B) Essential for life
      C) The principal natural steroid is *aldosterone*

# Physiological Control

A. **SCHEME OF CONTROL** (*See* page 215)
   1. **The hypothalamus, the anterior portion of the pituitary gland and higher centers in the brain regulate the adrenal cortex —** they alter the blood level of glucocorticosteroids relative to the needs of the animal at a given time.
   2. **Physiological mechanism**
      A) Higher centers may send nervous signals to the hypothalamus.
      B) The hypothalamus sends a message by a special blood supply to the anterior pituitary via the *corticotropin releasing hormone* (CRF).
      C) CRF stimulates the anterior pituitary to release *adrenocorticotropic hormone* (ACTH).
      D) ACTH travels via the blood to the adrenal cortex where it causes the release of hydrocortisone into the animal's blood supply, thus distributing hydrocortisone it to all tissues of the body.

B.  **CONTROL SUMMARY** (*See* facing page)

1.  **Circulating plasma level of hydrocortisone (or chemical analogues)** — regulates release of hydrocortisone from the adrenal cortex by a feedback mechanism.

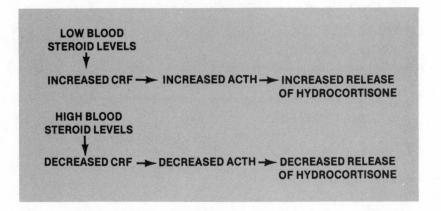

2.  **The nervous system is sensitive to changes in the animal's internal and external environment. The nervous system sends its messages to the hypothalamus, which in turn regulates release of hydrocortisone from the cortex.**

3.  **Many stimuli increase the release of ACTH and hydrocortisone** — this is called *stress*. The following are stressors:

    A) *External stressors* — environmental temperature (extreme heat or cold), noise, restraint, crowding, transporting, malnutrition, lack of water, lack of oxygen, debilitating disease, surgery, trauma, toxic reactions, allergic reactions, anaphylaxis.

    B) *Internal stressors* — pain, fear, anxiety, exercise, exhaustion, lactation, gestation, maximum production, tumors.

## Schematic of Physiological Control

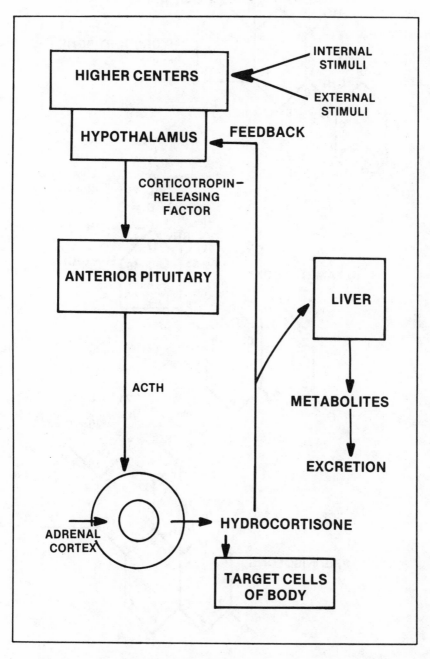

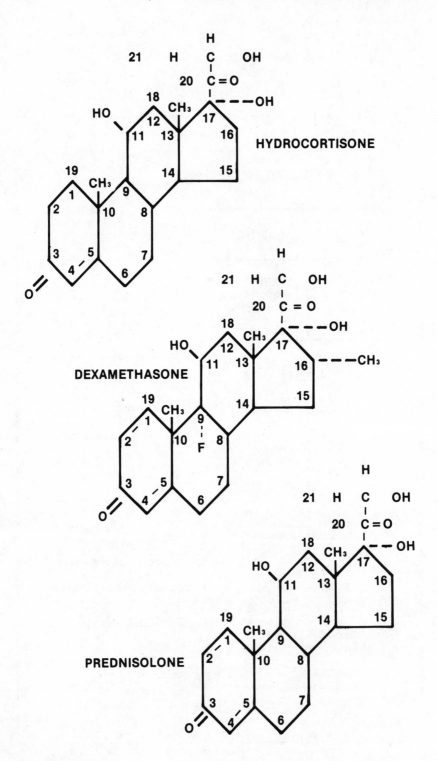

# Chemistry and Structure
## (Activity Relationships)

A. **BASIC COMPOUND IS HYDROCORTISONE** (*facing page*)

1. **Must have a functional oxygen group, OH, at carbon 11 to have anti-inflammatory and glucogenic ability**

2. **Must have a functional OH at carbon 21 and carbon 17 to be active** — this is called the alcohol form of the steroid.

3. **Prednisone is converted in the body to prednisolone** to be active.

4. **The basic active steroid** with OH groups at carbon 21 and carbon 17 is insoluble in water and forms a suspension in water. The alcohol form is soluble in 40 to 50% propylene glycol.

B. **CHEMICAL MODIFICATIONS AND ADDITIONS TO HYDROCORTISONE** — the resulting differences:

1. **Esterification at carbon 21 links an organic acid group through the OH at carbon 21.**

Examples:

ACETATE

$$21 \quad H \quad \overset{\displaystyle H}{\underset{\displaystyle |}{C}} - O - \overset{\displaystyle O}{\overset{\displaystyle \|}{C}} - \overset{\displaystyle H}{\underset{\displaystyle H}{CH}}$$

$$20 \quad C = O$$

PHOSPHATE

$$21 \quad H \quad \overset{\displaystyle |}{\underset{\displaystyle |}{C}} - O - \overset{\displaystyle \nearrow O}{\underset{\displaystyle \overset{\displaystyle O}{\underset{\displaystyle H}{|}}}{P}} - OH$$

$$20 \quad C = O$$

A) Addition of succinate or phosphate will make the steroid water-soluble.

B) Adding acetate, butylacetate, acetonide, methylacetate, or dipropionate causes the steroid to be more slowly absorbed from a tissue injection. Thus the steroid's duration of action is prolonged.

2. **The ester link must be hydrolyzed and carbon 21 returned to the OH form to be active.**

A) Phosphate and succinate esters are rapidly converted to the active form. Dexamethasone phosphate is converted to dexamethasone OH form, which gives peak levels in man in 10 minutes.

B) Conversion of other esters probably takes longer.

C) Conversion takes place intracellularly.

3. **Alterations on the steroid rings**
    A) Dehydrogenation (double bonding) between carbons 1 and 2 (designated delta-1)

    Example — dehydrogenation of carbons 1 and 2 of hydrocortisone results in prednisolone. Prednisolone is then delta-1 hydrocortisone.
    B) Adding fluorine
    C) Adding methyl group
    D) Adding OH group
    E) Addition of these groups to the rings results in:
    1) Increased anti-inflammatory potency
    2) Increased glucogenic potency
    3) Decreased mineralo activity

---

# Formulary
# (with Chemical Nomenclature)

**CORTISONE**
    Cortone®(Merck, Sharp & Dohme)

**HYDROCORTISONE**
    Cortef®(Upjohn)
    Hydrocortone®(Merck, Sharp & Dohme)

**PREDNISONE** (delta 1 — cortisone)
    Deltra®(Merck, Sharp & Dohme)
    Meticorten®(Schering)
    Paracort®(Parke-Davis)
    Zenadrid®(Diamond)

**PREDNISOLONE** (delta 1 — hydrocortisone)
    Delta Cortef®(Upjohn)
    Hydeltra®(Merck, Sharp & Dohme)
    Predsem®(Beecham)
    Meticortelone®(Schering)
    Paracortol®(Parke-Davis)
    Cortitab®(Burns - Biotec)

**PREDNISOLONE SODIUM SUCCINATE**
    Solu-Delta-Cortef®(Upjohn)

**PREDNISOLONE SODIUM PHOSPHATE**
    Cortisate-20®(Burns - Biotec)

**PREDINISOLONE TERTIARY — BUTYLACETATE**
    Hydeltrone - T.B.A.®(Merck, Sharp & Dohme)

**METHYL PREDNISOLONE** (6 methylprednisolone)
    Medrol®(Upjohn)

**METHYLPREDNISOLONE ACETATE**
    Depo Medrol®(Upjohn)

**DEXAMETHASONE** (9 alpha F,16 alpha $CH_3$-prednisolone)
Azium®(Schering)
Decadron®(Merck, Sharp & Dohme)
Voren®— Dexamethasone, 21 isonicotinate (Norden)

**PARAMETHOSONE**
Haldrone®(Lilly)

**FLUDROCORTISONE**
Alflorone®(Merck, Sharp & Dohme)
Florinef®(Squibb)
F Cortef®(Upjohn)

**FLUOROPREDNISOLONE** (9-F prednisolone acetate)
Predef - 2X®(Upjohn)

**BETAMETHASONE** (9 alpha F,16 beta $CH_3$-prednisolone)
Celestone®(Schering)
Betavet Soluspan® — a combination of betamethasone acetate and betame-thasone sodium phosphate (Schering)
Betasone® — a combination of betamethasone dipropionate and betame-thasone sodium phosphate (Schering)

**TRIAMCINOLONE** (9 alpha F,16 alpha OH-prednisolone)
Vetalog®(Squibb)
Aristicort®(Lederle)
Kenacort®(Squibb)

**FLUMETHASONE** (6 alpha F,9 alpha F,16 alpha $CH_3$-prednisolone)
Flucort®, Anaprime®(Diamond)
Methagon®(Lilly)

**FLUOCINOLONE ACETONIDE** (16 alpha,9 alpha Di-F,16 alpha OH, predniso-lone-16, 17 acetonide)
Synalar®(Diamond)

## Relative Potencies by Arbitrary Groups

|  | Generic Name | Gluco Anti-Inflammatory | Sodium Retention |
|---|---|---|---|
| Group I | Hydrocortisone | 1 | 1 |
| Group II | Prednisone Prednisolone | 5 | 0.8 |
| Group III | Dexamethasone Betamethasone Flumethasone Fluoroprednisolone | 25 - 50 (up to 100) | 0 |

Recommended doses and critical clinical evaluation of responses are the best guides.

# Metabolism

A. **ABSORPTION**

   1. **Readily absorbed from gastrointestinal tract** — peak blood levels are reached within two hours.

   2. **Readily absorbed from IM or SC injection** — peak blood levels are reached within one hour if OH form is used. Carbon 21 esters (acetate) are more slowly absorbed.

   3. **Intraarticular injections diffuse very slowly into circulation.** They may bring about significant blood levels.

   4. **Very slowly absorbed, if at all, after topical application to skin**

   5. **Intravenous injections give the shortest duration of action** — yield the highest blood levels.

B. **BIOTRANSFORMATION AND EXCRETION**

   1. **Steriods are biotransformed by the liver** — some conjugation occurs with glucuronic acid and sulfate.

   2. **Polar metabolites are excreted chiefly by the kidney.**

   3. **Some excretion in bile.**

   4. **Synthetic additions to hydrocortisone delay the biotransformation and excretion of the drug** — prolongs their action.

   5. **Urinary excretion of dexamethasone, after injection into the horse, has been studied.**
      A) 60% of the dose was excreted in first 30 to 40 hours as free dexamethasone and several nonconjugated polar metabolites.
      B) Greatest concentration in the urine occurred between 2½ and 5 hours after IM injection.
      C) Little unchanged dexamethasone was present in the urine after 20 to 30 hours.
      D) Dexamethasone and/or its metabolites were still being excreted in the urine four days after administration.
      E) Organic esters of dexamethasone are all excreted longer than is the phosphate form.

C. **HIGHLY PROTEIN-BOUND** (up to 90% in plasma)

D. **DURATION OF ACTION**

   1. **Intravenous injection used for shock**
      A) Prednisolone sodium succinate lasts 30 to 60 minutes.
      B) Dexamethasone phosphate lasts 2 to 3 hours.

   2. **Slowly absorbed when given IM** — durations of actions have been measured in weeks.

# Responses

## A. ENERGY METABOLISM

1. **Depletion of protein** from extrahepatic tissue cells due to decreased protein synthesis and increased breakdown.

2. **Increased hepatic glucose synthesis** — occurs from amino acids (gluconeogenesis).

3. **Increased breakdown of body fat.**

4. **This could result in:**
   A) Increased blood glucose for short time. Studies (horse) indicate long-term use does not increase blood glucose.
   B) Urea production is increased. Can become a kidney load.
   C) Animal is in negative nitrogen balance.
   D) Blood levels of fatty acids and glycerol are increased.
   E) In horses, prolonged therapy produced no change in serum proteins.

5. **Prolonged therapy (weeks) could lead to:**  **because of**
   A) Muscle wasting and weakness        ⎫  INHIBITED
   B) Delayed wound and fracture healing  ⎬  PROTEIN
   C) Osteoporosis                      ⎭  SYNTHESIS

## B. WATER AND ELECTROLYTE RESPONSES

1. **Increased retention of sodium** — also increased excretion of potassium by the kidneys.

2. **Increased retention of water**

3. **Increased volume of extracellular fluid plus edema**

4. **Increased mobilization of $Ca^{++}$** as a result of the steroid-induced breakdown in the protein matrix of bone, followed by increased renal excretion of the $Ca^{++}$.

5. **Decreased intestinal absorption of calcium**

6. **If these responses are prolonged** they could lead to:
   A) Alkalosis with increased excretion of $H^+$ in exchange for increased resorption of $Na^{++}$ in cells of the kidney tubules.
   B) Polyuria (increased urine flow) and polydipsia (increased water consumption)
      1) Proposed mechanisms
         a) Polydipsia
            (1) Increased sodium in plasma ———→ stimulates osmoreceptors in the hypothalamus.
            (2) Receptors sense hemoconcentration —→ stimulates thirst.
         b) Polyuria
            (1) Direct action of steroid on kidney tubule cells

        (2) Antagonism of antidiuretic hormone action in kidney

        (3) Water diuresis occurs because increased water intake results in increased water load in the plasma and the kidney excretes it.

    C) Decreased blood level of K

    D) Net loss of body calcium, the result of steroid-induced osteoporosis and decreased $Ca^{++}$ absorption, may lead to secondary hyperparathyroidism.

## C. ANTI-INFLAMMATORY EFFECT

1. Supresses tissue response to injury

2. Prevents, decreases or inhibits the acute, and often undesirable, reactions of tissue cells to insult
   A) Trauma and crush
   B) Toxins from bacteria, viruses, or fungi
   C) Toxins released as a result of the allergic reaction (histamine and others)
   D) Toxic substances released by cell destruction

3. Mechanisms and actions that affect the anti-inflammatory ability of steroids:
   A) Increase the stability of cell membranes and lysosomal membranes
      1) Decrease the release of inflammation - enhancing toxic products from injured cells and from lysosomes
      2) Decrease the cellular insult of toxins
   B) Enhance the integrity of capillary walls and decrease "capillary leakiness" and loss of fluids, electrolytes, and plasma proteins
   C) Inhibit the biosynthesis of prostaglandins by stabilizing cell membranes. Prevent the activation of lipases and phospholipases, thus preventing the supply of arachidonic acid that triggers the formation of prostaglandins. The release of prostaglandins is also inhibited. The untoward responses of prostaglandins, inflammation, pain and platelet aggregation are held in check.
   D) Production of prostaglandin by macrophages from inflammatory exudates is inhibited by dexamethasone. Response is dose-related. Relative potencies of prostaglandin inhibition are consistent with clinical anti-inflammatory ranking.

### E) Schematic of Anti-Inflammatory Action of Steroids

"This hormone appears not to extinguish the fire or to act like a carpenter to repair the damage of the fire. Instead, it appears to 'dampen the fire', or to provide, as it were, an asbestos suit behind which the patient, like some Biblical Shadrach, Meshach or Abednago, protects his tissues from the fire. If this protection is removed prematurely, before the fire has spent itself, the patient and his tissues will react again to the burning. But, if the protection is not discarded until the natural duration of the fire is over, the patient remains largely free of symptoms and apparently 'well'." (Hench, 1952)

## D. EFFECTS OF GLUCOCORTICOSTEROIDS ON THE BLOOD AND LYMPHATIC SYSTEM

1. **Decreased production of lymphocytes** — with involution of lymphoid tissue

2. **Reduced eosinophil count**

3. **Increased neutrophil count**

4. **Normal or increased white cell count**

5. **Decreased phagocytosis by neutrophils and reticuloendothelial cells**

6. **Increased RBC production is possible if production is already depressed**

7. **Long-term use and/or large doses may:**
   A) Produce an anemia
   B) Decrease hematocrit
   C) Decrease hemoglobin

E.  **IMMUNE RESPONSE TO CORTICOSTEROIDS**

1.  **Antibody production may be inhibited.** This response depends on species, antigen involved, steroid level, and steroid given.

2.  **A study has shown that canine distemper and hepatitis immunization are not adversely affected.**

3.  **Antigen-antibody reaction is not affected if antibodies are already present.**

F.  **INHIBIT VIRAL INTERFERON SYNTHESIS**

G.  **CARDIOVASCULAR RESPONSES IMPORTANT TO TREATING SHOCK**

1.  Corticosteroids cause:

    A) Increased strength of heart-muscle contraction
    B) Possibly increased blood pressure
    C) Maintenance of plasma volumes because:
       1) Capillary leakiness is decreased.
       2) Shift of fluids from extracellular space into intracellular spaces is prevented
    D) Increased perfusion, which opposes stasis
       1) Open capillary beds
       2) Open venules
       3) Prevent sludging
       4) Increase venous return
       5) Reduce peripheral resistance
    E) Increased cardiac output
    F) Increased urine output
    G) Protection of cells from insult and lysis which maintains the integrity of cell membranes.
    H) Maintenance of membrane transport mechanisms.
    I) Above responses require *massive* doses and are dependent upon fluid replacement.

H.  **CORTICOSTEROIDS EFFECT ON THE CENTRAL NERVOUS SYSTEM**

1.  **Enhanced excitability of neurons** — at the recommended dosages, the overall effect is CNS stimulation.

2.  **Lowered threshold for convulsions** — must use care

3.  **Production of a euphoria-like state** — a sense of well being and less response to pain

4.  **Reduction or prevention of cerebral edema**

## I. ENDOCRINE INTERACTIONS AFTER PROLONGED THERAPY

1. **There is decreased secretion of** ACTH — via the negative feedback control scheme. This results in atrophy of the portion of the adrenal cortex that biosynthesizes and releases hydrocortisone. After long-term therapy with a steroid, functional recovery of the pituitary-adrenal axis may take 2 to 9 months.

2. **Anti-insulin action** — leads to need for more insulin

3. **Tendency toward an androgenic (masculinizing) effect**

4. **May induce parturition** — in late stages of gestation in some species and with certain steroids.
   A) Cattle
      1) Inject in last 2 to 3 weeks of gestation
      2) Dexamethasone (20 mg) or flumethasone (10 mg)
      3) Induces parturition within 36 to 60 hours
      4) Live, healthy calves
      5) Increases incidence of retained placenta
      6) Animals should be carefully observed
   B) Sheep — inject ewe after 130th day of pregnancy to induce parturition. Retained placenta usually is not a problem.
   C) Mare
      1) 20 mg dexamethasone given IM to 5 pony mares during the last third of pregnancy did not induce parturition.
      2) Dexamethasone (10 to 80 mg/day from about 300 days of gestation) did not appear to cause parturition or alter duration of gestation.
      3) Dexamethasone, given in a dose of 100 mg daily from day 321 to day 324, induced premature parturition within $4 \pm 1.6$ days from the last injection. Foals from induced parturition were weaker at birth than control animals but improved after 7 to 10 days and then grew normally. Complications and dystocia have been encountered.
      4) In another study, dexamethasone in doses up to 80 mg/day was given during the second and third trimester of pregnancy. Doses were at levels usually used in clinical practice. They did not appear to alter the duration of gestation or to induce parturition in mares.

5. **Prolonged administration of large doses inhibits spermatogenesis and ovulation.**

6. **Hypothyroidism may be brought about.**

## J. EFFECTS OF CORTICOSTEROIDS ON EXOCRINE GLANDS

1. **Decreased milk production in cattle**

2. **Increased secretion of gastric juice, pepsin, and hydrochloride**

3. Possibly increased secretions by sweat glands, salivary glands, and sebaceous glands
4. Decreased formation of mucus in the gastrointestinal tract and respiratory tract

K. MAY IMPROVE PERFORMANCE OF MUSCLE WORK

# Adverse Reactions

A. SINGLE DOSE OR MULTIPLE DOSES OF STEROIDS —
cause no adverse side effects for 24 to 48 hours, even when given at very high levels.

B. SHUT-DOWN OF ADRENAL CORTEX BY NEGATIVE FEEDBACK
   1. Steroid let-down, negative feedback, and Addison's disease — caused by rather high levels of steroids given for a long period of time; *e.g.* a horse on the racetrack, or a dog on long-term therapy for arthritis or allergic dermatitis.
   2. One to two weeks at usual anti-inflammatory levels will not significantly suppress the pituitary adrenal axis — longer periods or larger doses for shorter periods, however, will cause suppression.
   3. Clinical signs
      A) Dullness
      B) Mental depression
      C) Easy fatigability
      D) Incoordination
      E) General unthriftiness and weight loss
   4. Results of the steroid-induced nonfunctional cortex
      A) Decreased serum sodium
      B) Increased serum potassium
      C) Muscle weakness
      D) Hypoglycemia
      E) Deterioration of muscle mass
      F) Osteoporosis
   5. An injection of dexamethasone in a pony — reduced plasma hydrocortisone from 8 $\mu$g/100 ml to 2 $\mu$g/100 ml in 24 hours.

C. IMPAIRED BODY-DEFENSE MECHANISMS
   1. Corticosteroids decrease emigration of leukocytes to infected sites — decrease phagocytosis.
   2. Corticosteroids decrease phagocytosis — by tissue macrophages and those of the reticuloendothelial system.
   3. Corticosteroids depress interferon production — reducing the first line of defense against concurrent viral disease.

4. Certain corticosteroids reduce the immune response to certain antigens (varies with animal species).

5. Corticosteroids may decrease connective-tissue ground substance — this is conducive to bacterial invasion.

D. **HAVE BEEN SHOWN TO REACTIVATE CERTAIN VIRUSES** (Herpes type)

1. **Horses**
   A) Horses that remained asymptomatic for a few months to a few years after the last recurrence of equine infectious anemia (EIA) gave a typical febrile response after treatment with dexamethasone.
   B) EIA virus was propagated.
   C) It was inferred that the febrile response was due to propagation of an immunological variant virus. This virus might have been produced as a result of decline in cell-mediated immunity.

2. **Cattle**
   A) Recurrent infection by *infectious bovine rhinotracheitis* (IBR) virus was induced in calves given dexamethasone (0.1 mg/kg IV, daily for 5 days) five months after the primary infection.
   B) IBR virus is reactivated in cattle by dexamethasone (20 mg/head/day IV for 6 days).

E. **DELAYED WOUND AND FRACTURE HEALING**

F. **BEHAVIORAL DISTURBANCES**

G. **LOOSE STOOLS**

H. **MAY PRECIPITATE BORDERLINE DIABETES MELLITUS**

I. **EYE** — Changes (glaucoma in man, cataracts in dogs) will occur if large doses are given or if the corticosteroid is given for a long period of time.

J. **CLEFT PALATE**

1. Administration of corticosteroids to human females in early pregnancy has been associated with cleft palates in the newborn.

2. A total cleft palate occurred in the foal of a purebred Arabian mare that was badly broken-winded. At various times during pregnancy, including the first few months, the mare was given corticosteroids *per orum* by the owners.

K. **CORTICOSTEROID-INDUCED ARTHROPATHY**

L. **CORTICOSTEROID-INDUCED LAMINITIS** — the incidence is

said to be greater with agents other than prednisolone.

M. **STEROIDS MAY CAUSE RECURRENCE OF BABESIASIS** — may be a problem in horses.

N. **INJECTION OF CORTICOSTEROID INTO TENDONS** — may reduce the tensil strength of the tendon, predisposing it to rupture.

# Rational Use of Corticosteroids

## Clinical Pharmacology of Corticosteroids

Considerable controversy seems to surround the clinical usefulness of this group of drugs. Some veterinarians swear by them, others swear at them, and still others seem confused and to wonder if there are any appropriate uses for steroids.

1. Drugs in this group have been inappropriately used in many situations.

2. The group has been unjustly condemned because of generalizations and/or inappropriate extrapolations from the literature.

3. Nothing is wrong with the corticosteroids; they are a valuable therapeutic tool.

In an effort to clarify this therapeutic dilemma, two areas for thought and study must be identified before these drugs are used. First is the careful study of the clinical pharmacology of these drugs. Second is the establishment of a proper therapeutic regimen.

To arrive at a proper approach to therapy, first one must understand the pathophysiology of the disease (in this case inflammation, shock, etc.). The specific objectives of therapy are then determined. The use of steroids for treating musculoskeletal inflammations or allergy requires a different regimen than is used for treating shock. A proper therapeutic regimen requires:

1. Choice of drug(s) based upon:
   A) Efficacy of the drug to meet the desired objectives
   B) Evaluation of possible adverse effects

2. Choice of dose, route of administration, frequency of administration, and duration of administration needed to achieve the objectives of treatment.

These decisions must be based on pharmacological research and clinical experience rather than hearsay or wishful thinking.

Most misuse of, and hence the negative feeling toward, the

steroids relates to errors in judgment regarding indications for use and treatment regimens.

1. Use only after a diagnosis has been reached.
2. Use to accomplish *specific objectives* of drug therapy.
3. Use appropriate *dose* and *frequency* and *duration* of treatment.
4. Corticosteroids are neither curative nor chemotherapeutic.
5. The dose needed to achieve a desired therapeutic effect must be determined by the art of medicine (trial and error) and must be constantly reevaluated.
6. Prolonged therapy — use the smallest dose possible to achieve the desired effect. Prolonged therapy increases the likelihood of adverse effects.
7. Intermittent therapy (alternate days, every third day) — has been effective for chronic treatment. There is less likelihood of pituitary inhibition and side effects.
8. Abrupt cessation of medication after prolonged administration of high doses is associated with a significant risk of adrenal insufficiency that could be life-threatening.
9. Large doses of steroids are definitely indicated for initial therapy in acute, debilitating, septicemic conditions, but they may be harmful later in the course of the disease. Antibiotics and sulfonamides depend heavily on the body defense mechanism to effect a cure of a bacterial disease; the steroids seriously inhibit the body's defense mechanism. Steroids probably should not be used more than 1 or 2 days in the presence of infectious disease.
10. In the presence of diagnosed or suspected bacterial disease, appropriate antibiotic therapy should accompany steroid therapy.
11. May mask the usual signs of disease.
12. Steroids are contraindicated in, or should be used with great care, in:
    A) Cushing's syndrome
    B) Diabetes mellitus
    C) Late stages of pregnancy — specific species and steroids involved have not been completely defined.
    D) Animals predisposed to epileptic-like seizures
13. Steroids with mineralo activity are contraindicated in:
    A) Congestive heart failure
    B) Renal insufficiency
14. Long-term therapy should include dietary additions of:
    A) High-quality protein

      B) A source of potassium
      C) Vitamin D and vitamin A supplements

# Drug Interactions

A. **MANY DRUGS CAN STIMULATE INCREASED ACTIVITY** of
the microsomal drug-metabolizing enzymes in the liver. This increased activity means that certain drugs will inactivate even
themselves at a faster rate, thus bringing about lowered blood
levels and shorter duration of action.

  1. **Drugs known to be potent stimulators of drug metabolism are**

| | |
|---|---|
| A) Phenobarbital | D) Insecticides |
| B) Pentobarbital | E) Phenylbutazone |
| C) Chlorinated hydrocarbon | F) Diphenylhydantoin |

  2. **If an animal has been pretreated with, or is currently receiving,
any of the above agents, the corticosteroids will be more rapidly
inactivated.**

  3. **Corticosteroids are capable of enzyme induction and therefore
enhance their own inactivation. They may also enhance the inactivation of other steroid hormones such as estrogens, androgens, progestins and anabolics; and even barbiturate
anesthetics.**

  4. **High levels of corticosteroids, administered acutely,** may compete for and overwhelm the drug-metabolizing enzyme
systems, thus inhibiting the inactivation of other steroids.

B. **THIAZIDES AND FUROSEMIDE** are additive with the corticosteroids in depleting potassium from the body.

C. **OPPOSE THE EFFECT OF INSULIN** — increased dosage of insulin is required by diabetic patients.

D. **USE WITH CARE** — in animals concurrently medicated with
drugs that may predispose an animal to seizures, such as:

  1. CNS stimulants

  2. **Local anesthetics, when large amounts may become systemic**

  3. **Phenothiazine-derivative tranquilizers**

  4. **Chloramphenicol, penicillin**

# Clinical Indications

A. **REPLACEMENT THERAPY**
   1. **Adrenal insufficiency** (Addison's disease)
   2. **After adrenalectomy**

B. **THERAPY FOR METABOLIC ABNORMALITIES** — Use for:
   1. **Functional hypoglycemia**
   2. **Bovine ketosis**
   3. **Canine eclampsia** (puerperal tetany)
   4. **vonGierke-like syndrome**

C. **THERAPY FOR NEOPLASTIC DISEASE**
   1. **Malignant lymphoma**
   2. **Mastocytoma**

D. **TISSUE INSULT** — from physical, chemical or biological agents
   1. **Anti-inflammatory and/or anti-immune responses**
      A) *Skin*
         1) Dermatitis related to parasitism infestation, contact with irritants, food or inhalant allergy, seborrhea, or infection
         2) Acral lick granuloma
         3) Otitis externa
         4) Acanthosis nigricans
      B) *Respiratory*
         1) Chronic obstructive pulmonary disease in horses
         2) Cough or dyspnea associated with laryngeal edema, neck injury, or chronic bronchitis
         3) Asthma
         4) Puppy strangles (lymphadenitis)
      C) *Cardiovascular*
         1) Treatment or prevention of shock associated with anesthesia, colic (in horse), hemorrhage, trauma, endotoxic shock, and acute pancreatitis. Believed to be most effective in endotoxin shock.
      D) *Gastrointestinal*
         1) Granulomatous colitis
         2) Eosinophilic gastroenteritis
         3) Restored integrity of mucosae
      E) *Musculoskeletal*
         1) Arthritis
         2) Bursitis
         3) Eosinophilic myositis
         4) Laminitis

       5) Lameness of various other types

       6) Treat either systemically or by intraarticular injection

F) *Renal* — glomerulonephritis (chronic)

G) *Eye* (except where associated with viral infection)

       1) Chemosis

       2) Pannus

       3) Uveitis

       4) Keratitis — except for ulceration of the central cornea

H) *Blood and blood-forming organs*

       1) Autoimmune hemolytic anemia

       2) Autoimmune thrombocytopenia

       3) Aplastic anemia

I) *Other*

       1) Acute septicemias, severely depressed animal

       2) Cerebral edema

       3) Coonhound paralysis syndrome

       4) Venom toxicoses

       5) Termination of pregnancy

       6) Suppression of excessive formation of granulation tissue

CHAPTER

# 5

# Gonadotropins and Gonadal Hormones

## Basic Principles

A. FEEDBACK CONTROL MECHANISM
1. The hypothalamus, the pituitary gland and the gonads all contribute to an interrelationship — can either stimulate or inhibit gonadal activity.
2. Gonadal activity and release of steroid hormone influence other tissues in the body.
3. Feedback may be either positive or negative.
4. The environment, the central nervous system, the endocrine system and reproductive organs interrelate via a neuro-endocrine communication system that functions to make reproduction as efficient as possible.
5. Successful therapy of reproductive disorders depends upon the identification of alterations in this scheme and the judicious use of all forms of therapy directed toward restoring the proper functional balance to the scheme.
6. These are discretely controlled schemes in which:
   A) Environmental factors are important
   B) The CNS should not be unduly influenced by undesirable stresses.
   C) The chemical messengers (hormones) are active and effective after small *physiological* amounts are given; *i.e.*, nanograms ($10^{-9}$ grams) per ml of plasma are the usual.
7. Massive doses are counterproductive in treatment of disorders of reproduction. Exceedingly high doses may defeat the pur-

pose of the therapy.

8. **Pharmacological responses** — many of the hormones to be discussed act upon tissues other than the reproductive organs, inciting physiological responses that may make larger doses necessary. The use of diethylstilbestrol to induce abortion in feedlot heifers is an example.

## Schematic of Gonadal Hormones
## (FEMALE)

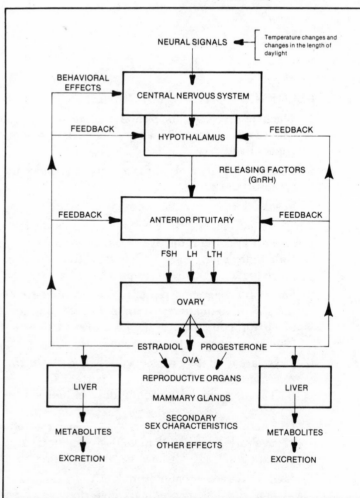

## Schematic of Gonadal Hormones
## (MALE)

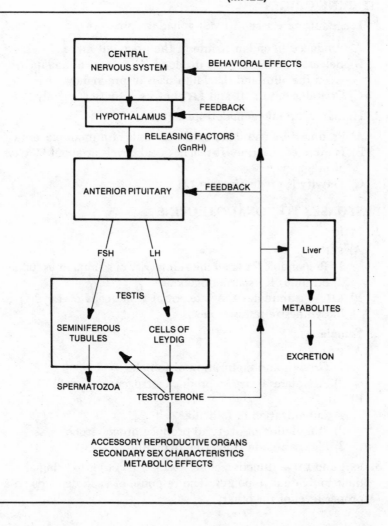

# Gonadotropins

A. **PITUITARY ORIGIN**

1. **Prepared from the pituitary glands of slaughtered animals**
2. **Some preparations are "purified" — they are either FSH or LH.**
3. **Some preparations are extracts — *i.e.*, mixtures of FSH and LH.**
4. **Species variations — relative concentrations of FSH and LH in the anterior pituitary vary with the animal used as the source.**

   A) *Horse and ox* — relatively high amounts of LSH and less LH
   B) *Sheep* — relatively high amounts of LH

B. **UTERINE ORIGIN**

1. **Pregnant mare serum (PMS) gonadotropin**

   A) Produced in endometrium of the pregnant mare
   B) Released and circulates in blood. It is most abundant between the 40th and the 140th days of pregnancy.
   C) Contains both FSH and LH, but its activity is mainly FSH

2. **Human chorionic gonadotropins (HCG)**

   A) Produced by chorionic epithelial cells of human placenta
   B) Is excreted in urine. It reaches peak levels at about 50 days of pregnancy.
   C) Activity is predominately LH

C. **RESPONSES TO GONADOTROPINS**

1. **Male**
   A) FSH
      1) Responsible for anatomical integrity of seminiferous tubules
      2) Stimulus for spermatogenesis
   B) LH — stimulates the interstitial cells (cells of Leydig) to biosynthesize testosterone

2. **Female**
   A) FSH
      1) Growth and maturation of follicles
      2) Stimulates ovary to produce estrogen (estradiol)
   B) LH
      1) Luteinization of follicular cells
      2) Stimulation of ovary to produce progesterone
      3) Plays a role in triggering ovulation

3. **FSH and LH** — function closely with each other to bring about their individual responses. The response of each depends on a proper level of the other.

D. **METABOLISM**
  1. **Parenteral use only** — IV, IM, and SC forms are available.
  2. **Biotransformed by liver**
  3. **Rapid disappearance from blood**
     A) FSH and LH have shortest durations.
     B) Chorionic gonadotropin endures a little longer.
     C) PMS has the longest duration of activity.

E. **FORMULARY**
  1. **Pituitary Gonadotropins**
     A) F.S.H.-P® (Burns-Biotec)
     B) P.L.H.® (Burns-Biotec)
     C) Vetrophin® (ovine origin) (CEVA)
     D) Gonadovet® (equine origin) (Jen-Sal)
     E) A.P. Godin-5® (Haver-Lockhart)
  2. **Non-Pituitary Gonadotropins**
     A) Chorionic gonadotropin (Med-Tech)
     B) Follutein® (chorionic) (Squibb)
     C) Gonamone® (chorionic) (Fort Dodge)
     D) Gonadin® (PMS)
     E) Chortropin® (chorionic)

# Principles of Gonadal Hormones

A. **CHEMISTRY**
  1. Most are steroids, with some exceptions; *e.g. diethylstilbestrol.*
  2. Each group has a characteristic molecule — provides an inherent structure-activity relationship.
  3. These molecules can be manipulated to retain, emphasize or even eliminate certain responses.

B. **METABOLISM**
  1. **Absorption**
     A) Oral
        1) Subject to degradation in the gastrointestinal tract
        2) Via portal circulation. Subjected to hepatic biotransformation which is very important with natural steroids.
        3) Absorption is slower than with parenteral administration.
     B) Parenteral
        1) Intravenous is fast and subject to fewer variables, but is of short duration.
        2) Absorption from intramuscular sites can be delayed by al-

tering the vehicle and molecular makeup of the drug with esters and repositol forms and oil.

C. **BIOTRANSFORMATION AND EXCRETION**

 1. **Natural steroids are biotransformed quickly** — by the hepatic microsomal systems. Progesterone has a T½ of less than 10 minutes.

 2. **Steroids with molecular alterations** — are more slowly biotransformed and excreted, have longer durations of action.

 3. **Nonsteroid compounds** — are biotransformed and excreted at about the same rate as other synthetic steroids.

 4. **Steroids are excreted as metabolites** — excreted principally in the urine.

 5. **Biotransformation may be stimulated** by enzyme inducers such as phenobarbital and phenylbutazone.

 6. **Biotransformation may be inhibited** by several means; *e.g.* by high levels of estrogen.

# Estrogens

A. **NATURAL SOURCES**

 1. **Plants** — many clovers have high estrogen content.

 2. **Mammalian tissues** — ovary, testicle, adrenal cortex, placenta, urine, and blood contain estrogen.

B. **COMMERCIAL PREPARATIONS**

 1. **Synthetic** — diethylstilbestrol (DES) and synthetic steroids.

 2. **Natural** — gathered and purified from tissues. Conjugated estrogens come from:
    A) Stallion urine
    B) Human pregnancy urine
    C) Equine pregnancy urine

C. **RESPONSES**

 1. **Needed for maturation, growth and development of reproductive organs** — also secondary sex characteristics of females

 2. **Required for development and growth of ductile components of the mammary gland**

 3. **Stimulate normal physiological processes of the tubular reproductive tract (proliferative)**
    A) Growth of the uterine muscle

B) Development of the endometrial lining of the uterus

C) Increase the vascularity of the uterus

4. **Induce behavioral estrus (heat)** — by acting on the CNS.

5. **Induce edema in folds of the mucosa at the junction of the oviduct and uterus** — zygotes, if present, may be locked in the oviduct, where they may degenerate. This is the basis for use of estrogens in mismating in bitches.

6. **Dilate the cervix**

7. **Metabolic**
   A) Enhance water retention
   B) Increase the blood level of calcium, phosphates, sodium and nitrogen
   C) Favor protein build-up, but not as potent as the androgens
   D) Alter the fatty components of the blood; decrease cholesterol
   E) Increase fat deposition

8. **Play role in the normal health and function of the skin**

9. **Uterus shows increased motility and is more sensitive to oxytocin**

10. **Render the uterus less susceptible to infection**

11. **May inhibit some activities of the liver** — decrease the microsomal-enzyme activity of the endoplasmic reticulum

12. **Cause anterior pituitary inhibition** — via a negative feedback mechanism; high levels of estrogen inhibit the release of FSH and LH.

## D. FORMULARY

1. **Estrogens (therapy)**
   A) Diethylstilbestrol
   B) Repositol™ diethylstilbestrol (Pitman-Moore)
   C) Dinol® (dienestrol)
   D) Dinogen® (dienestrol)
   E) Estradiol
   F) Conjugated estrogens
   G) Estriol
   H) Estrone
   I) Theelin® (Parke-Davis)
   J) Estinyl® (ethinyl estradiol) (Schering)
   K) Estradiol cyclopentylpropionate
   L) Estrovarin®

2. **Estrogens** (feed additive and implants)
   A) Esmopal® (estradiol past implant)................Poultry
   B) Synovex-S® (progesterone & estradiol
      implant) (Diamond)...........................Steers
   C) Synovex-H® (testosterone and estradiol
      implant) (Diamond)..........................Heifers

# Progestins

A. **NATURAL SOURCES** — from mammalian tissue; *i.e.* ovary, testicle, adrenal cortex, placenta, and blood.

B. **COMMERCIAL PREPARATIONS** — mostly synthetic

C. **RESPONSES**
   1. **Uterine changes** — secretory in nature
      A) Myometrium hypertrophies
      B) Secretions increase in the endometrial glands, vagina and cervix
      C) Motility of uterine muscle reduced
   2. **Play a role in maintenance of pregnancy or pseudopregnancy**
   3. **Play a role in ovulation** — may trigger ovulation if other hormone levels are normal
   4. **Metabolic**
      A) Increase urinary excretion of nitrogen
      B) Increase sodium retention
   5. **Development of secretory system in mammary gland**
   6. **Inhibit smooth muscle of the uterus** — render the uterus *less* sensitive to oxytocin
   7. **Uterus becomes more susceptible to infection**
   8. **Anterior pituitary inhibition** — occurs via negative feedback.

D. **FORMULARY**
   1. **Progestins** (therapy)
      A) Progesterone
      B) Repositol™ (progesterone — Pitman-Moore)
      C) Repogest® (repository progesterone — Burns-Biotec)

2. **Progestins** (heat synchronization)
   A) Repromix® (medroxyprogesterone acetate). Feed additive for cattle and sheep. (No longer available)
   B) Syncro-Mate® (flurogestone) — pessaries for sheep
3. **Progestins** (growth promotion): melengestrol acetate (MGA) — suppresses heat and improves the rate of gain in heifers.
4. **Progestin** (control of estrus): megestrol acetate (Ovaban® — Schering)
   A) Control or postpone estrus
   B) Alleviate false pregnancy
      1) For oral use in dogs only
      2) Toxicity
         a) When given for long periods, cystic endometrial hyperplasia was observed.
         b) When given during the last half of pregnancy, litter size and viability of the pups was reduced.
         c) In clinical studies pyometra was reported in 0.6% of the cases.
      3) Mechanism of action is by negative feedback on the anterior pituitary.
      4) Contraindications:
         a) Must not be used in dogs if there is evidence of disease of the uterus or any reproductive organ.
         b) Should be not used in dogs before or during the first estrous cycle.
         c) Should not be used in pregnant dogs.
         d) Should not be used in dogs with mammary tumors.
      5) Transient side effects that are occasionally seen
         a) Mammary enlargement    d) Increased appetite
         b) Lactation                      e) Change in temperament
         c) Listlessness

# Androgens

A. **NATURAL SOURCES**
   1. **Testicle**    2. **Ovary**    3. **Adrenal cortex**

B. **COMMERCIAL PREPARATIONS** — mostly synthetic

C. **RESPONSES**
   1. **Maturation, growth, and development of reproductive organs and secondary sex characteristics of the male**
   2. **Increase libido or sex drive**

3. **Metabolic**
   A) Increase protein anabolism
   B) Decrease urinary excretion of nitrogen
   C) Increase retention of potassium and phosphorus
   D) Favor the formation of dense bone tissue
4. **Stimulate erythropoeisis**
5. **Maintain the secretory responses of accessory sex organs** — provide the fluid component of semen
6. **Inhibit anterior pituitary** — via negative feedback

D. **PROTEIN ANABOLIC STEROIDS** — androgens in which the molecule has been changed to:
   1. **Diminish or remove the masculinizing effects and effects upon the reproductive organs**
   2. **Enhance the protein anabolic effect**
   3. **Increase size of muscle fibers** (not the numbers)

E. **FORMULARY**
   1. **Androgens**
      A) Testosterone, aqueous and in oil
      B) Repositol™ testosterone (Pitman-Moore)
      C) Methyl testosterone
      D) Testosterone propionate
      E) Testosterone cyclopentylpropionate
   2. **Anabolic steroids**
      A) Probolic® (methandriol dipropionate — Hickam)
      B) Winstrol-V® (stanozolol — Winthrop)
      C) Norethandrolone
      D) Ralgro® (zeranol — IMC). Not related chemically to the androgen implants.
      E) Equipoise® (boldenone undecylenate — Squibb)
   3. **Androgen** — for control of estrus
      A) Cheque® (mibolerone — Upjohn). For oral administration to dogs
         1) Chemistry — closely related chemically to testosterone
         2) Mechanism of action
            a) Inhibits the anterior pituitary via negative feedback
            b) Follicles develop to a certain point, then no further.
            c) There is no rapid increase in estradiol levels; hence there is no LH surge from the anterior pituitary.
            d) Without the LH surge, there is no ovulation or development of corpora lutea.
            e) The result is suppression of the estrous cycle.

    3) Metabolism
      a) Well absorbed from the intestine
      b) Rapidly biotransformed (more than ten metabolites)
    4) Toxicity
      a) Safe; no adverse effects have been reported.
      b) 10,000 times the recommended dose caused:
        (1) No toxic effects in clinical tests
        (2) Thickening of myometrium and endometrium
        (3) Inhibition of spermatogenesis
      c) Side effects observed:
        (1) Clitoral enlargement in 20%
        (2) Vaginal discharge in 1%
        (3) Riding behavior in 1.6%
      d) When mibolerone was given to pregnant bitches, gestation and parturition were normal, but female pups were masculinized.
      e) Should not be given to any animal with a history of liver or kidney disease.

# Prostaglandins

A. **INTRODUCTION**
    1. **They are a group of compounds synthesized in the body from arachidonic acid.**
    2. **They have been arranged into four major series according to chemical make up: A, B, E, or F.** There may be different prostaglandins within a series.
    3. **Many different physiological and pharmacological actions reportedly affect the following systems:**
      A) Central nervous system    D) Gastrointestinal
      B) Cardiovascular system     E) Respiratory
      C) Urinary system         F) Reproductive
    4. **Certain prostaglandins** are involved in the inflammatory reaction and allied adverse reactions of the body to injury.

B. **BIOLOGICAL ACTIVITY ASSOCIATED WITH REPRODUCTION**
    1. **E and F series**
      A) Involved as a messenger and/or a stimulator of parturition
      B) May induce abortion or parturition
    2. **$F_2$ alpha** — stimulates luteolysis

C. **F$_2$ ALPHA PROSTAGLANDINS APPROVED FOR HORSES**

1. **Dinoprost tromethamine** — prostaglandin F$_2$ alpha (Prostin F2 Alpha® — Upjohn)

2. **Prostalene** — analogue of F$_2$ alpha (Synchrocept® — Diamond)

3. **Actions**
   A) The fully formed corpus luteum regresses.
   B) Progesterone levels fall immediately after luteolysis.
   C) Anterior pituitary increases FSH and begins follicular development in the ovaries.
   D) Normal estrus and ovulation ensue, usually within 4 to 6 days.

4. **Toxicity**
   A) Safe, causing no organ pathology

5. **Side effects** — reported with Prostin F2 Alpha®
   A) *Sweating* — starts within 15 minutes after administration and lasts about 90 minutes.
   B) *Body temperature drops* to 97.5 F. Begins one-half hour after administration and lasts up to five hours.
   C) *Occasional and transient signs* — may last 1 to 1½ hours.
      1) Mild colicky symptoms and diarrhea
      2) Impaired motor coordination

6. **Precautions**
   A) Do not administer to pregnant mares; may induce abortion or parturition.
   B) Do not administer intravenously.
   C) Do not use concurrently with nonsteroidal anti-inflammatory drugs.
   D) Use with caution in mares with acute or subacute diseases of the vascular, gastrointestinal, respiratory or reproductive systems.

7. **Precautions in man**
   A) Avoid direct contact between solution and skin.
   B) Should not be handled by:
      1) Pregnant women
      2) Asthmatics or persons with respiratory problems

D. **PROSTAGLANDIN F$_2$ ALPHA (Lutalyse® —Upjohn)**

1. **Approved for synchronization of heat** in cattle.

2. **Mechanism of action is via luteolysis.** For this reason, the timing of treatment in relation to the cow's estrual cycle is extremely important. Cows must be cycling.

3. **Treatment neither increases nor decreases fertility.**

# Gonadorelin (Cystorelin® —Ceva)

A. **APPROVED FOR TREATMENT OF CYSTIC OVARIES IN DAIRY CATTLE**

   1. **Chemistry** — gonadorelin diacetate tetrahydrate, a synthetic ester of a polypeptide (10 amino acids).

   2. **Gonadorelin**
      A) Gonadotropin-releasing hormone (GnRH)
      B) The hypothalamic-releasing factor that stimulates the anterior pituitary to release FSH and LH

   3. **Action**
      A) Increases release of FSH **and** LH from the anterior pituitary.
      B) In cows aids in correcting improper cycling resulting from ovarian follicular cysts (retained follicles).
      C) Stimulates the follicular cells to change to luteal cells; forms a corpus luteum.
      D) Corpus luteum regresses normally; the cow begins a new, normal, cycle.

   4. **Toxicity**
      A) No adverse effects reported
      B) Nonantigenic

# Therapeutic Principles
# (Gonadotropins and Gonadal Hormones)

A. **PROPER BLOOD LEVEL IS IMPORTANT**

   1. **Replacement therapy** — use low physiological levels.

   2. **Pharmacological responses** — use larger doses.

   3. **Common tendency is to overdose.**

B. **INDICATIONS**

   1. **For improved weight gain and feed efficiency in feedlot cattle and lambs**
      A) Alone: melengestrol acetate (MGA)
      B) Combinations: progesterone and estradiol
      C) Implants: pellets or paste
      D) In feed

   2. **For synchronization of heat periods in breeding animals to achieve closely spaced breeding, hence uniform times of parturition.** Use a progestin.
      A) Administer agent in feed or as vaginal insert.

    B) Estrual cycling is halted because of pituitary inhibition.
    C) Simultaneously remove source of agent from all animals.
    D) In a few days (less than 7) cycling will begin again.
    E) Breed animals at next heat.
    F) Best suited to artificial insemination programs.

3. **To induce abortion in feedlot heifers:**
    A) Use an estrogen such as estradiol (ECP® — Upjohn).
    B) Animals should not be more than six months pregnant.
    C) Animals should be closely watched.

4. **To induce temporary periods of anestrus mostly in racing, show, or performance animals:**
    A) Synthetic progestins are used.
    B) Fertility is not affected.

5. **To treat certain endocrine imbalances and upsets that impair the reproductive performance of males and females.**
    Examples:
    A) Cystic ovaries     D) Silent heat
    B) Nymphomania     E) To increase sex drive
    C) Late ovulators

6. **To prevent pregnancy in mismated bitches:**
    A) Use an estrogen.
    B) Treat within 2 days of mating and continue for 6 to 7 days.

7. **Exerts antineoplastic effect on certain tumors** — primarily tumors in the prostate and mammary glands.

8. **Estrogen** — used in certain skin conditions, such as dermatitis of spayed bitches.

9. **Estrogen** — used in urinary incontinence in spayed bitches.

10. **Estrogen** — used to aid in the removal of retained placentas.

11. **Used as an oral contraceptive in human medicine**
    A) These are combinations of an estrogen and a progestin.
    B) Ovulation is prevented.
    C) Anterior pituitary inhibition occurs.
    D) They may be given simultaneously or sequentially.

12. **To control or postpone estrus** — in dogs:
    Ovaban® (Schering) or Cheque® (Upjohn).


C. **THERAPY PROBLEMS** (possible causes of failures)
    1. **Improper timing** — should relate to natural cyclic nature of endocrine control of reproduction and environmental influences whenever possible. Drug response should be correlated with the body response.

2. **Antagonistic influences** — may be an important factor in the less-than-acceptable response(s) to gonadal hormone therapy.
   A) Concurrent disease
   B) Hypothyroidism
   C) Poor nutritional status
   D) Emotional disturbances (fear, fright, apprehension, etc.)
   E) Antihormones. With continued use of gonadotropins (proteins) the recipient's body produces antihormones capable of neutralizing the gonadotropin (endogenous also).
   F) Some drugs inhibit secretion of gonadotropin and ovulation — hypothalamic inhibition. These drugs are:
      1) Pentobarbital          4) Atropine
      2) Chlorpromazine      5) Alpha blockers
      3) Morphine

3. **Improper dosage** — for replacement therapy physiological levels are needed versus pharmacological levels, which are sometimes used for a specific organ response.

## D. PRECAUTIONS AND POSSIBLE TOXIC MANIFESTATIONS

1. **High doses and chronic administration of gonadal hormones** — may cause chemical castration in which the negative feedback leads to gonadal atrophy and cessation of function.

2. **Overdosage of estrogens may produce aplastic anemia** — a single dose of 5 mg of ECP® (Upjohn) has produced anemia.

3. **Excessive doses of PMS or FSH-P ®** (Burns-Biotec) — will bring about hyper-ovarian activity and possibly follicular cysts.

4. **Chronic progesterone or progestin administration** — maintains the uterus in a secretory state. This may cause cystic hyperplasia of the endometrium. Progestins also favor closure of the cervix, hence poor drainage of the uterine glandular secretions. This condition favors development of chronic endometritis and pyometra.

5. **High plasma levels of estrogen** — have inhibitory influence on the hepatic excretory processes.

6. **High chronic doses of methyltestosterone** — may produce cholestatic hepatitis with jaundice (demonstrated in man).

CHAPTER

# 6

# Muscle Relaxants

## General Principles

A. **THREE GENERAL DRUG GROUPINGS CAPABLE OF RELAXING MUSCLES:**

1. **Central nervous system depressants** — depress the motor output from the cerebral cortex and spinal cord, thereby reducing the tone of skeletal muscle.

   A) *General anesthetics* — include ether, barbiturates.

   B) *Narcotics* and *hypnotics* — include morphine (Demerol — Winthrop), xylazine (Rompun® — Haver Lockhart), M-99.

   C) Degree of affect varies among different compounds, depending upon their actions on the motor area of the cortex and spinal cord.

   D) Production of extensive muscle relaxation with this group also causes depression of the respiratory and vasomotor centers because extensive relaxation requires deep surgical anesthesia.

2. **Local anesthetics**

   A) Injected around the motor nerve(s) supplying the muscles

   B) Injected directly into the muscle

3. **Muscle relaxants** — there are two groups according to their site of action:

   A) Act at *myoneural junction*
      1) Curare
      2) Succinylcholine chloride — Sucostrin® (Squibb); Anectine® (Burroughs-Wellcome).

   B) *Central acting* — spinal cord
      1) Mephenesin
      2) Glyceryl guaiacolate or guaifenesin; Gecolate® —Summit Hill; Glycodex—Burns-Biotec)
      3) Chlorphenesin carbamate — Maolate® (Upjohn)
      4) Methocarbamol — Robaxin-V® (A. H. Robins)

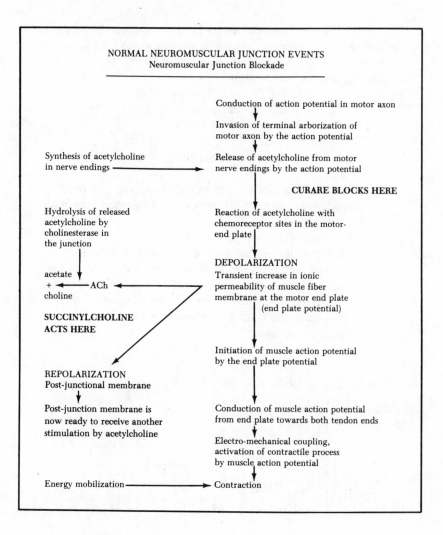

NORMAL NEUROMUSCULAR JUNCTION EVENTS
Neuromuscular Junction Blockade

Conduction of action potential in motor axon

Invasion of terminal arborization of
motor axon by the action potential

Synthesis of acetylcholine
in nerve endings

Release of acetylcholine from motor
nerve endings by the action potential

**CURARE BLOCKS HERE**

Hydrolysis of released
acetylcholine by
cholinesterase in
the junction

Reaction of acetylcholine with
chemoreceptor sites in the motor-
end plate

acetate
+ ◄——ACh
choline

DEPOLARIZATION
Transient increase in ionic
permeability of muscle fiber
membrane at the motor end plate
(end plate potential)

**SUCCINYLCHOLINE
ACTS HERE**

Initiation of muscle action potential
by the end plate potential

REPOLARIZATION
Post-junctional membrane

Post-junction membrane is
now ready to receive another
stimulation by acetylcholine

Conduction of muscle action potential
from end plate towards both tendon ends

Electro-mechanical coupling,
activation of contractile process
by muscle action potential

Energy mobilization ——————► Contraction

# Myoneural Junction Blocking Agents

A.  **CURARE GROUP.** Curare is also known as South American arrowhead poison. It has many active principles. d-Tubocurarine is the active principle used medically.

1.  **Chemistry**
    A) Fairly large molecule
    B) Two quaternary ammonium structures separated by a distance of 14 angstroms
    C) Stable in solution

2. **Paralysis of skeletal muscle occurs from nondepolarization**
   A) Mechanism: Receptor blockade or competitive antagonism prevents acetylcholine from meshing with receptors and initiating muscle contraction.
   B) Muscles are affected in the following order:
      1) Short muscles of toes, ears, and eyes
      2) Muscles of the head and neck
      3) Muscles of the limbs
      4) Respiratory muscles: first the thoracic muscles and then the diaphram
   C) To reverse or antagonize the curare paralysis use neostigmine, physostigmine, or edrophonium chloride (Tensilon® — Roche).
      1) Mechanism of reversal or antagonism is:
         a) Direct excitatory action upon the skeletal muscle
         b) An indirect increase in the concentration of acetylcholine by an anticholinesterase action. The increase in acetylcholine may override the curare blockade.
         c) Antagonization of the respiratory-muscle paralysis caused by curare

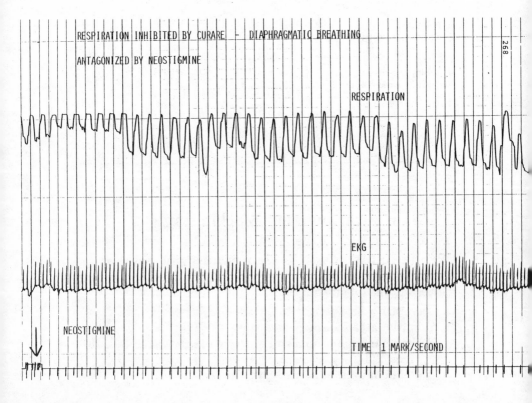

RESPIRATION INHIBITED BY CURARE — DIAPHRAGMATIC BREATHING
ANTAGONIZED BY NEOSTIGMINE

RESPIRATION

EKG

NEOSTIGMINE

TIME 1 MARK/SECOND

3. **Central nervous system**
   A) No narcosis, no analgesia occurs
   B) Does not enter brain to any great extent

4. **Cardiovascular**
   A) Tendency to cause hypotension resulting from vasodilation, which is due to:
      1) Blockade of autonomic ganglia. This causes reduced vasomotor tone and a lesser stimulus for vasoconstriction.
      2) Histamine release. This in turn causes vasodilation.

5. **Respiration** — Tendency toward respiratory paralysis via inhibition of the muscles of respiration. May cause death.

6. **Not effective orally** — poorly absorbed from the GI tract

7. **Fate**
   A) Biotransformed by liver
   B) Metabolites eliminated via the bile and kidney

8. **Does not cross placental membranes to any significant degree.**

B. **GALLAMINE TRIETHIODIDE** (flaxedil triethiodide)

1. **Nondepolarizer, curare-like action** — competitive antagonist to acetylcholine

2. **Less potent than d-tubocurarine;** 7 mg gallamine is equivalant to 1 mg d-tubocurarine.

3. **Vagal block** — tendency to tachycardia

4. **No histamine release in dog**

5. **Tendency to hypotension in cat**

6. **Excreted unchanged by kidney**

C. **SUCCINYLCHOLINE CHLORIDE** — Sucostrin® (Squibb), Anectine® (Burroughs Wellcome), Quelicin® (Abbott)

1. **Chemistry**
   A) Diacetylcholine is a condensation of two molecules of acetylcholine.
   B) Solutions are not stable. They should be kept in a refrigerator and their expiration dates observed.

2. **Skeletal muscle response** — initial twitch and muscle tremors occur, followed by paralysis.
   A) Mechanism
      1) Postjunctional membrane (receptors) are depolarized. This produces the muscle tremors.
      2) Succinylcholine remains on receptors and does not allow repolarization to occur.
      3) The end plate is refractory.

       4) There is no end plate potential.

       5) There is no initiation of muscle action potential.

       6) Paralysis is then produced.

  B) Order of muscles affected depends on dosage.

       1) Limbs are affected first.

       2) Respiratory muscles are affected last.

  C) Fast onset of action — 20 to 60 seconds after IV injection.

  D) Fate

       1) Biotransformed rapidly by hydrolysis via a nonspecific cholinesterase

       2) Mostly in plasma

  E) Duration of action

       1) Varies with species and breed according to levels of plasma cholinesterase

       2) Horse has high levels of cholinesterase, thus duration is short; *i.e.* 3 to 10 minutes.

       3) Ruminants have low levels of cholinesterase, thus duration is long. Very dangerous in ruminants.

       4) Duration in dogs, cats and swine is intermediate.

  F) No known pharmacological antagonist. Action will be potentiated by cholinesterase inhibitors such as organophosphate insecticides.

3. **Central nervous system** — enters the brain poorly, therefore causing little effect.

  A) No narcosis or analgesia

  B) Patient remains conscious

4. **Cardiovascular responses**

  A) Blood pressure may increase drastically.

  B) Heart rate increases.

  C) Mechanisms for cardiovascular response:

       1) Release of epinephrine caused by fright of restraint

       2) Compensatory to hypoxia and hypercapnia

       3) Ganglionic stimulation occurs with a sympathetic output of epinephrine and norepinephrine.

  D) May induce arrythmias, which can be prevented by administration of atropine.

5. **Respiratory response** — hypoventilation or apnea

6. **Muscarinic stimulation as follows:**

  A) Intestinal hypermotility

  B) Micturition

  C) Salivation

  D) May be blocked by atropine

# Muscle Relaxants
# Acting Centrally

A. **SPINAL CORD**

1. **Chemistry**
   A) All are chemically related interneuron-blocking drugs.
   B) Mephenesin could be termed the parent drug.
   C) Benzene ring group-O-glycerol derivatives

2. **Mephenesin** (Tolserol® —Squibb)
   A) Not used extensively in veterinary medicine
   B) Has been used with pentobarbital as a fixed drug combination (Somnevet®; Myotal®; Myothesia®— Beecham)
   C) Irritating to tissues
   D) Large doses given IV may produce hemolysis.

3. **Glyceryl guaiacolate or guaifensin** (Gecolate® —Summit Hill; Glycodex® —Burns-Biotec)
   A) Acts at interneurons of brain stem and spinal cord
   B) Some hypnosis and analgesia occur due to action upon the brain stem.
   C) Biotransformed in the liver. The glucuronide metabolite is then excreted by the kidneys.
   D) Relatively short duration of action when given IV
      1) Intravenous — 10 to 30 minutes
      2) Longer duration in stallions.
   E) Little respiratory depression
   F) Capable of producing hemolysis
      1) The addition of 5% dextrose apparently reduces this action. The action appears not to depend on total dose but on the concentration of the injected solution.
      2) Use of a solution greater than 5 or 6% is not recommended.
   G) Precautions
      1) Avoid perivascular leakage which may cause an irritating response.
      2) Use with care in anemic or hypovolemic animals.
   H) The use of physostigmine or neostigmine with guaifenesin is contraindicated.

4. **Chlorphenesin carbamate** (Maolate®— Upjohn)
   A) Acts at interneurons of the spinal cord
   B) Oral use only
   C) Dog only
   D) Has some ability to depress the CNS — sedative or tranquilizing action.
   E) Not a true analgetic

    F) Readily absorbed; peak blood levels are reached within 2 to 3 hours.

    G) Biotransformed by liver to glucuronide and sulfate which are excreted in the urine.

  5. **Methocarbamol** (Robaxin-V® — A. H. Robins)

    A) Acts at interneurons of the spinal cord — interrupts abnormal impulses.

    B) Intravenous — administer slowly (2 ml/min).

    C) Dog and cat — intravenous or oral use.

    D) Large doses are hynotic.

    E) Relatively nontoxic

  6. **Meprobamate** (Equanil® — Wyeth; Miltown® — Wallace)

    A) Minor tranquilizer

    B) Acts at interneurons of the spinal cord

    C) Not used extensively in veterinary medicine

B. **TRANQUILIZERS AND NARCOTIC GROUP** — used for muscle relaxation

  1. **Valium®** (Roche) — a minor tranquilizer that acts at presynaptic sites. It enhances or prolongs the action of the inhibitory transmitter (GABA). Motor output is therefore depressed.

  2. **M-99** (Etorphine)

    A) A controlled drug (Schedule II), it is available for use by veterinarians in zoo or exotic animal practice.

    B) Related chemically and pharmacologically to morphine. It is a derivative of the opium alkaloid, thebaine.

    C) More potent than morphine
      1) For restraint — 850 times more potent than morphine
      2) For analgesia — 1000 times more potent than morphine

    D) Wider margin of safety than morphine: therapeutic index is 9,000 times that of morphine.

    E) May produce dependence

    F) After IM injection, the onset of action is 3 to 4 minutes. The sequence of action is:
      1) Salivation        3) Ataxia
      2) Stiff gait, arched back  4) Recumbent for 7 to 8 minutes

    G) Duration of recumbency is dose-dependent. Dose may be repeated.

    H) Nalorphine (Nalline® — Merck, Sharp & Dohme), naloxone, and other morphine antagonists will also antagonize M-99. This allows rapid reversal of the effects.

    I) M 50-50 is a specific antagonist — a controlled drug with same restrictions as for M-99.

# Clinical Uses
# for Muscle Relaxants

A. **INDICATED FOR MUSCLE RELAXATION DURING SURGERY WITH A GENERAL ANESTHETIC**

1. **Tubocurarine chloride** — as single injection or drip
2. **Glyceryl guaiacolate** — as single injection
3. **Succinylcholine chloride** — as a drip

B. **CHEMICAL RESTRAINT**

1. **Succinylcholine chloride**
   A) Capture of animals      B) Minor surgery in horses
2. **M-99 (Etorphine)**
   A) Potent and relatively safe for capture of free-roaming animals
   B) Can be used with phenothiazine-derivative tranquilizers
   C) Has been used on many species, both wild and domestic
   D) Availability is limited
3. **Nicotine sulfate**
   A) Muscle paralysis      B) Toxic and dangerous

C. **ALLEVIATION OF MUSCLE-ORIENTED DISORDERS** such as myositis, muscle sprains, traumatic injuries, and intervertebral disc syndrome.

   1. **Maolate®** (Upjohn)    2. **Robaxin-V®** (A. H. Robins)

D. **THERAPY OF STRYCHNINE POISONING**

1. **Robaxin-V®** (A. H. Robins)

   A) Apparently less chance for toxicity as compared to repeated administration of barbiturates
   B) No respiratory depression
   C) Is additive with barbiturates in regard to CNS depression
   D) Not as quick or reliable as pentobarbital
   E) Useful as a follow-up therapy after light pentobarbital anesthesia

E. **MAKE ABDOMINAL PALPATION EASIER** — relax abdominal muscles with Valium® (Roche) given IV.

F. **MAY BE INDICATED IN THERAPY OF TETANUS** for the control of muscle spasms: Robaxin-V® (A. H. Robins), guaifenesin

G. **GLYCERYL GUAIACOLATE** — used for surgical anesthesia in the horse.

1. Produces "general anesthesia" of sorts when used alone.

2. **Usually given with other agents**
   A) Before administering glyceryl guaiacolate give: phenothiazine-derivative tranquilizers and/or narcotics such as Demerol® (Winthrop) or Rompun® (Haver-Lockhart).
   B) Can be used simultaneously with Surital® (Parke-Davis) or Dipentol® (Diamond) mixed in the solution

H. **DRUG INTERACTIONS OF MUSCLE RELAXANTS**
   1. **Group acting on the central nervous system** — all are additive with CNS depressants.
   2. **Antibiotics that can block the myoneural junction and therefore are additive:**

   | | |
   |---|---|
   | A) Neomycin | D) Polymixin |
   | B) Streptomycin | E) Viomycin |
   | C) Kanamycin | |

I. **CURARE AND SUCCINYLCHOLINE** — should never be given without availability of means for administering oxygen.

# Suggestions for the Use of Succinylcholine Chloride

### from the
### American Association of Equine Practitioners

A. **COMPLICATIONS MAY ARISE** — even under the best circumstances. Discretion should be used in selecting this method of restraint. Provision should be made to handle whatever emergencies arise. The suggestions below may be helpful.

   1. **Vials of succinylcholine chloride should be refrigerated.**
   2. **It is prudent to inform the owner or agent that succinylcholine chloride is to be used as a restraining agent, not as an anesthetic** — some risk to life is always involved with any type of restraint, either physical or chemical.
   3. **Before using the drug** — a thorough history of previous sickness or drug administration should be obtained. Use of the drug is contraindicated if any of the following have been given or applied within 30 days.
      A) Any organophosphate anthelmintic
      B) Any antibiotic with a generic name ending in "mycin" (*i.e.* the aminoglycosides)
      C) Any organophosphate insecticide

D) Any other cholinesterase inhibitor

E) Procaine

4. **The drug should not be given to debilitated horses.**

5. **The drug should not be given to excited or exhausted horses.**

6. **When possible, food should be withheld for 4 to 6 hours before the drug is administered.**

7. **Dosage**
   A) A normal, healthy horse can be restrained with 0.04 mg succinylcholine chloride per pound of body weight, given IV. The objective should be to paralyze skeletal muscles without depressing respiration. Overdosing, leading to paralysis of thoracic musculature, is certain to cause apnea and possibly death.
   B) The dosage can usually be reduced if the drug is used in conjunction with a preanesthetic agent such as a tranquilizer. Such combinations are especially useful in horses that tend to be unruly or excitable.

8. **Some precautions to observe after the administration of succinylcholine chloride:**
   A) Have the horse held by someone familiar with reactions to the drug so that the horse does not fall forward on its nose sustaining damage to its mouth and causing hyperflexion of the occipitoatlantal articulation. The latter trauma may cause rupture of the intervertebral artery, with death ensuing rapidly. The horse should also be prevented from falling in any other way that might result in injury. Turning the horse slowly as it collapses should be conducive to a safe fall.
   B) Be prepared with oxygen and the expertise to give artificial respiration if apnea occurs.

9. **In case of death after the administration of succinylcholine chloride** — a necropsy should be performed. Death could be unrelated to the drug. Any form of restraint, chemical or physical, can lead indirectly to death from some physical problem such as a chronic diaphragmatic defect or a verminous aneurysm.

**NOTE:** These suggestions were prepared by the Research Subcommittee of the Professional Liability Insurance Committee, American Association of Equine Practitioners, September 1970. They are recommended by the AAEP and the AVMA Liability Insurance Trust.

CHAPTER

# 7

# Urinary System

## General Principles

The kidney plays an important homeostatic role in maintaining the volume and composition of the body fluids.

A. **FUNCTIONS CAN BE SUMMARIZED:**
   1. **Elimination of nitrogenous wastes**
   2. **Elimination of excess inorganic salts**
   3. **Elimination of excess water**
   4. **Elimination of nonvolatile, soluble foreign substances**
   5. **Aids in the regulation of acid-base balance**
   6. **Conservation of water, electrolytes and base when necesary**

B. **A DYNAMIC AND DISCRETELY CONTROLLED ORGAN SYSTEM** — especially sensitive to:
   1. **Alterations in plasma composition**
   2. **Cardiovascular changes:** In proportion to their weight, the kidneys receive the greatest blood flow of any organ in the body. When the animal is at rest, renal blood for amounts to 20 to 25% of cardiac output; renal weight is only 0.4% of body weight. High blood flow is obviously related to the function of regulation of body-fluid composition.
   3. **Certain drugs**

C. **GENERAL CONCEPTS OF URINE FORMATION**
   1. **Glomerulus filtration**
      A) Removal of water and dissolved substances from the plasma by mechanical filtration
      B) The effective filtration pressure (EFP) is the controlling factor in the formation of the filtrate. EFP = blood pressure minus (plasma osmotic pressure + capsule pressure).

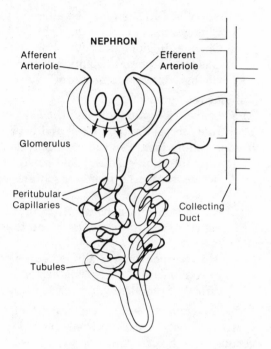

**NEPHRON**

Afferent Arteriole

Efferent Arteriole

Glomerulus

Peritubular Capillaries

Collecting Duct

Tubules

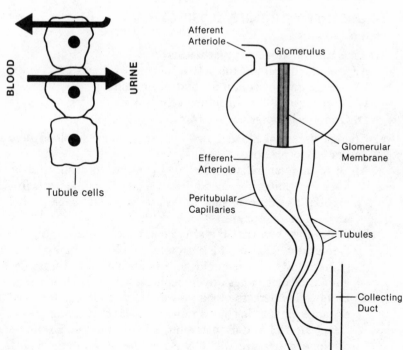

BLOOD

URINE

Tubule cells

Afferent Arteriole

Glomerulus

Efferent Arteriole

Glomerular Membrane

Peritubular Capillaries

Tubules

Collecting Duct

C) Glomerular filtration may be altered by:
   1) Changes in blood flow through the glomerulus
   2) Changes in glomerular blood pressure
   3) Changes in plasma osmotic pressure
   4) Changes in capsule pressure

2. **Tubular resorption**
   A) Selective resorption of the needed substances from the filtrate, across the tubule cell and back into plasma
   B) Controlling factors in tubular resorption are:
      1) Concentration gradients and passive transport
      2) Active transport systems for sodium, chloride, and bicarbonate
      3) Antidiuretic hormone (ADH) from the posterior pituitary enhances resorption of water and thus reduces urine formation.
      4) Aldosterone from the adrenal cortex enhances resorption of sodium, thus decreasing excretion of sodium and indirectly (osmotically) decreasing urine formation.

3. **Tubular secretion** — active transport of certain endogenous substances, potassium, hydrogen, and uric acid, and many exogenous substances

D. **DRUGS INFLUENCE RENAL FUNCTION** — by altering control factors.

1. **Alter tubular transport mechanisms**
   A) Specifically inhibit the active transport systems
   B) Interfere with sodium for hydrogen exchange
   C) Alter permeability of tubule cells to ions
   D) Osmotically alter passive transport of water

2. **Change the renal blood flow** — alter glomerular blood flow and/or blood pressure
   A) Drugs may cause systemic blood pressure to drop, thereby lowering glomerular blood pressure and reducing urine formation. Examples of such drugs are vasodilators, carbachol and organophosphates.
   B) Drugs may constrict the afferent arterioles that supply the glomerulus. The result is a drop in the blood pressure in the glomerulus and a reduction in the formation of urine. Examples of such drugs are epinephrine and norepinephrine.
   C) Drugs may increase blood pressure and cardiac output and enhance glomerular blood flow without constricting the afferent arterioles, thus increasing urine formation. Examples of these drugs are digitalis glycosides, isoproterenol and dopamine.

3. Change osmotic pressure of plasma
4. Influence levels of antidiuretic hormone
5. Alter the load of water and/or sodium in plasma to be filtered

# Diuretic Drugs

**Diuresis** — the action produced by a diuretic agent that increases the flow of urine.

**Saluresis** — the action produced by a saluretic agent that increases the excretion of salts; *i.e.* sodium.

**Diuretic drugs** — usually increase both urine flow and sodium excretion to remove excess extracellular fluid (edema).

A. CLASSIFICATION OF DIURETIC DRUGS

   1. **Drugs that act upon the cardiovascular system:**

      A) Digitalis and xanthine derivatives — improve strength of heart
      B) Colloidal plasma expanders
         1) Better blood flow
         2) Increase plasma osmotic pressure
      C) Glucocorticosteroids

   2. Osmotic drugs:

      A) Large osmotically active molecules
      B) Low kidney-threshold salts

   3. **Inhibitors of sodium resorption:**

      A) Organic mercurials
      B) Carbonic anhydrase inhibitors
      C) Benzothiadiazides (thiazides)
      D) Anthranilic acid derivatives
      E) Aldosterone antagonists
      F) Acidifying agents

   4. **Inhibitors of ADH release:**

      A) Decrease ADH ➡ decreased resorption of water in tubules ➡ increased excretion of water.
      B) Examples: water and ethyl alcohol

# Mercurial Diuretics

**Organic mercurials** — mercury bonded to an organic group

> **Mersalyl**
> **Mercaptomerin** — Thiomerin® (Wyeth)
> **Chlormerodrin** — Neohydrin® (Lakeside)
> **Meralluride** — Mercuhydrin® (Lakeside)

Both inorganic and organic mercury can produce diuresis. Historically, calomel (mercurous chloride) was first to be used. Because it caused too much tubular damage, it is no longer used. The organic mercurials used today cause much less tubular damage.

A. **MECHANISM OF ACTION**

1. **Reduce tubular reabsorption of sodium** — increase sodium in the filtrate and osmotically decreases resorption of water

2. **Minute quantities of mercuric ions are released intracellularly** — an increase in cellular acidity enhances this release, whereas alkalosis inhibits it.

3. **Thought to act in tubule cells by tying up sulfhydryl groups of enzymes** — these enzymes are vital to the furnishing of energy for the active transport of sodium.

4. **Results in increased excretion of water, sodium and chloride.**

B. **MAY EXHIBIT SYNERGISM** — with ammonium chloride and theophylline. May be antagonized by alkalinizing salts or systemic alkalosis.

C. **MERCURIALS** — tend to cause metabolic alkalosis after extended use because less bicarbonate is lost and its accumulates. This renders use of mecurials somewhat self-limiting.

D. **METABOLISM**

1. **Slow and irregular absorbtion follows oral administration.**

2. **Well absorbed after parenteral administration**

3. **Excreted predominately in urine**

E. **ONSET OF ACTION** — within 10 to 20 minutes after IM injection.

1. **Duration of action is up to six hours**

F. **TOXIC MANIFESTATIONS**

1. **Excessive use may lead to electrolyte imabalances.**

2. **High levels are toxic to kidneys, causing tubular necrosis.**

3. High levels can induce cardiac arrhythmias and, ultimately, ventricular fibrillation.

4. Hypersensitivity in man has been reported.

G. **CONTRAINDICATED** — in renal insufficiency and acute nephritis.

1. Decreased excretion causes an accumulation of toxic amounts of mercury.

2. May aggravate an existing renal lesion by causing further tubular necrosis.

# Methyl Xanthines

A. **CHEMISTRY**
1. **Caffeine sodium benzoate** — 1, 3, 7, trimethyl xanthine, sodium benzoate salt
**Theophylline** — 1, 3 dimethyl xanthine
**Aerolate®** (**Fleming**) — sustained-release capsule of theophylline
**Theobromine** — 3, 7 dimethyl xanthine

2. **Alkaloids have poor solublility in water** — they form water-soluble sodium salts; *i.e.:*
A) Caffeine sodium benzoate
B) Theophylline with ethylene diamine (aminophylline)

B. **SUMMARY OF THEIR ACTIONS**
1. **Cerebral stimulation** — caffeine is the most potent.

2. **Diuresis** — theophylline is the most potent diuretic, followed by theobromine and then caffeine.

3. **Smooth-muscle relaxation** — vasodilator and bronchodilator action; theophylline and aminophylline are used.

C. **MECHANISM OF ACTION** — mechanism for diuretic activity is not well understood.

1. **Inhibit tubular resorption of sodium**

2. **Increase renal blood flow and increase glomerular filtration because of slight stimulatory effect upon the heart**

D. **WELL ABSORBED ORALLY AND PARENTERALLY**

# Carbonic Anhydrase Inhibitors

**Acetazolamide — Vetamox®**

A. **CHEMICALLY RELATED TO SULFONAMIDES**
1. **Well absorbed by oral route**
2. **Used parenterally, intramuscularly, or intraperitoneally**

B. **MECHANISM OF ACTION**
1. **Inhibition** (noncompetitive) of the tubule-cell carbonic anhydrase (CA) enzyme. Also inhibits carbonic anhydrase of the eye.
2. **Inhibition of carbonic anhydrase** — reduces the supply of cellular hydrogen available to exchange for the sodium in the sodium resorption scheme. (*See* below.)
3. **Result is less sodium resorbed.**
4. **Intracellular potassium may substitute to some extent for the**

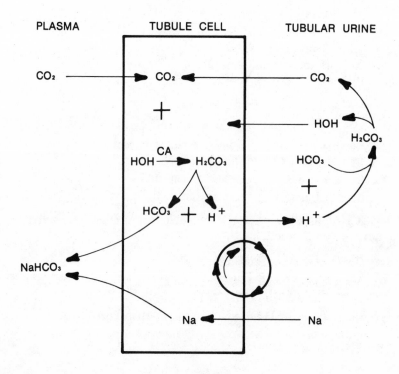

hydrogen — exchanges for sodium, thus enhancing excretion of potassium.

5. Bicabonate is trapped in the urine and less is returned to the plasma.

C.  NET RESULTS OF KIDNEY ACTION

1.  Saluresis and diuresis

2.  Increased loss of potassium

3.  Increased loss of bicarbonate in urine

4.  Increased urine pH

5.  **Less bicarbonate resorbed into the plasma.** A tendency toward acidosis occurs because buffering ability is lost.

D.  **RENAL ACIDOSIS INHIBITS ACTION** — supplies free hydrogen to exchange for the sodium. Since acetazolamide produces a systemic acidosis, its action is self-limiting for continual use.

E.  ELIMINATED UNCHANGED IN URINE

F.  **A UNIQUE ABILITY TO REDUCE INTRAOCULAR PRESSURE** — inhibits the rate at which aqueous humor is formed. Used in treatment of glaucoma.

# Benzothiadiazides and Thiazides

Chlorothiazide — Diuril® (Merck)
**Hydrochlorothiazide** — Hydrozide® (Merck), Esidrix® (Ciba)
**Cyclothiazide** — Renazide® (Lilly)
**Trichlormethiazide** — Naqua® (Schering)

A.  **GROUP CAME ABOUT AS A RESULT OF RESEARCH IN 1957** — used newly synthesized carbonic anhydrase inhibitors.

B.  MECHANISM OF ACTION

1.  **Inhibit the tubular resorption of sodium, chloride (in nearly equimolar amounts) and water.**

2.  **Significantly increase the excretion of potassium in amounts sufficient to produce hypokalemia.**

3.  **Specific cellular mechanism is not well understood** — it may include an inhibition of the transport system as well as a slight inhibition of carbonic anhydrase.

C. **ACTION** is independent of alterations in the acid-base balance.

D. **MAJOR DIFFERENCES** among members of the group is in potency, which is accounted for by dosage; *e.g.* hydrochlorothiazide is 5 to 20 times more potent than chlorothiazide.

E. **METABOLISM**

   1. **Well absorbed from oral or parental routes** — onset of action is within one hour after administration *per orum*.

   2. **Uniform distribution** — concentrated in the kidney

   3. **Cross the placental barrier**

   4. **Excretion from the kidneys is by tubular secretion**

   5. **Duration of action is 12 to 24 hours**

F. **TOXIC MANIFESTATIONS**

   1. **Relatively nontoxic at therapeutic levels**

   2. **May produce a trend toward electrolyte imbalance** — primarily *hypokalemia*. Patient should be carefully observed and monitored if therapy is prolonged.

   3. **Borderline renal and hepatic insufficiencies may be aggravated by thiazides** — mechanism not known.

   4. **May produce a trend toward hyperglycemia and aggravate diabetes mellitus**

# Derivatives of Anthranilic Acid

**Furosemide** — Lasix® (American Hoechst)
**Ethacrynic acid** — Edecrin® (Merck, Sharp and Dohme)

A. **RESEMBLE THE SULFONAMIDES CHEMICALLY**

B. **MECHANISM OF ACTION**

   1. **Inhibit tubular resorption of sodium**

   2. **Resorption of sodium is inhibited throughout the nephron** — in the proximal and distal tubules as well as in the ascending limb of the loop of Henle. This may account for a high degree of efficacy and the rapid onset of actions.

   3. **Increase the excretion of sodium, chloride, potassium, and water** — excretion of bicarbonate is not altered.

   4. **Carbonic anhydrase activity is not affected.**

C. **ACTION** — independent of alterations in the acid-base balance.

D. **WELL ABSORBED** — from oral or parenteral routes.

E. **RAPID ONSET OF ACTION** — is 10 to 20 minutes after IV or IM injection and within one hour after oral administration.

F. **RAPID RENAL EXCRETION (UNCHANGED)** — poor lipid solubility and no cumulative effect.

G. **SHORT DURATION OF ACTION** — 5 to 6 hours by oral route; 3 to 4 hours by intravenous route.

H. **A RELIABLE DOSE-RESPONSE RELATIONSHIP** over a wide range of dosages — large doses cause excretion of more water and sodium than can be attained with other veterinary diuretics.

I. **RELATIVELY NONTOXIC** — can excrete tremendous amounts of potassium. When dogs on a normal, balanced diet and eating well were given furosemide orally for extended periods, no clinical signs of hypokalemia were evident.

J. **LASIX®** (American Hoechst) — used to prevent epistaxis in race horses. The mechanism for this action is not well understood.

# Aldosterone Antagonists

A. **SPIRONOLACTONE** (Aldactone® - Searle)
   1. **Chemically** — steroids, analogues of aldosterone
   2. **Mechanism of Action**
      A) Competitive antagonism of aldosterone
      B) No action in an adrenalectomized animal
      C) Increased excretion of sodium and water
      D) Reduced excretion of potassium.
   3. **Therapy should be limited to refractory cases and cases in which aldosterone output is increased.**
   4. **Action may be synergistic with other diuretics.**

# Osmotic Diuretics

A. **MANNITOL, SORBITOL, DEXTROSE**
   1. **Osmotically active molecules**
   2. **Mechanism of action**
      A) Pass through the glomerular membrane and exert high osmotic pressure in the tubule. Tubular resorption is limited.

B) Draw water into the filtrate, thus diminishing the resorption and increasing the excretion of water.

C) May cause a similar force and response between extra-cellular fluid of tissues and plasma. This is the basis for use of these agents in edema (specifically cerebral edema).

D) Pharmacologically inert except for the osmotic actions cited in B and C

3. The same attributes that account for the limited tubular resorption are responsible for poor absorption from the gastro-intestinal tract.

4. Must be given parenterally — usually IV.

B. **LOW KIDNEY-THRESHOLD SALTS**

1. **Potassium nitrate, sodium sulfate, and urea**

2. **Not widely used therapeutically**

# Acidifying Agents

A. **AMMONIUM CHLORIDE, SODIUM ACID PHOSPHATE**

1. **Mechanism of action**

A) Ammonium chloride is absorbed from the GI tract and is converted by the liver to urea and hydrochloric acid.

B) Hydrochloric acid ionizes to hydrogen and chloride.

C) Hydrogen combines with bicarbonate buffer to form car-bonic acid which converts to carbon dioxide and water or is excreted, giving an acid urine.

D) Carbon dioxide is expired and chloride is left in extracellular fluid.

2. **Increased chloride load to the tubules and appreciable amounts of chloride escape resorption.** An equivalent amount of cation (initially sodium) and an isosmotic quantity of water also escape.

3. **Action is of short duration (1 or 2 days)** — the tubule cells respond to acidosis by forming ammonia to react with hydrogen to yield ammonium. The ammonium then replaces sodium as the equivalent cation for excretion of chloride. Loss = intake and no diuretic action.

4. **Used to intensify mercurial diuretics**

5. **Used to acidify the urine**

# Antidiuretics

A. **REDUCE URINE OUTPUT** — vasopressin or antidiuretic hormone (ADH) (Pitressin® — Parke-Davis)

B. **RELEASE OF ADH IS STIMULATED BY CERTAIN DRUGS:**

1. Nicotine    2. Morphine    3. Acetylcholine

C. **REDUCE RENAL BLOOD FLOW**

1. **Lowers systemic arterial pressure** — due to release of cholinergics or histamine.

2. **Constricts renal afferent vessels** — due to release of epinephrine and norepinephrine.

D. **DELAY ABSORPTION OF WATER FROM THE GUT** (ether)

E. **REDUCE THIRST AND WATER INTAKE** (amphetamine)

# Clinical Applications of Diuretics

A. **DIURETIC DRUGS** are used to remove excess extracellular fluid (edema).

B. **CHOICE OF AND PROPER ADMINISTRATION OF DIURETIC DRUGS** depend on a thorough understanding of the cause of the edema.

C. **ACCUMULATION OF EXCESS FLUID AND/OR SODIUM IN THE TISSUES** may be brought about by a local or systemic mechanism or a combination of many mechanisms. The following are examples of conditions that may lead to edema:

1. **Increased capillary blood pressure, hypertension**

2. **Decreased plasma osmotic pressure**

3. **Increased tissue-fluid content of protein,** leading to increased osmotic pressure of interstitial fluid, as occurs with inflammation and traumatic swelling.

4. **Increased plasma levels of aldosterone**

5. **Renal insufficiency** (chronic)

6. **Liver disease** (chronic)

7. **Congestive heart failure**

8. **Endocrine disorders**

9. **Impaired lymph flow**

10  Nutritional deficiencies, especially protein deficiencies

D.  OBJECTIVES OF DIURETIC THERAPY

 1.  Mobilization of surpluses of salt and water from the interstitial fluid compartment

 2.  Restoration of a balance between the daily intake and excretion of electrolytes and water

E.  CLINICAL INDICATIONS FOR DIURETICS

 1.  Relief of edema and/or ascites associated with:
   A) Prepartum and postpartum mammary edema in cows and mares
   B) Congestive heart failure
   C) Cirrhosis
   D) Tissue insult from trauma of crush, fractures, or surgical manipulation
   E) Cerebral edema (osmotic diuretics)
   F) Stocking-up in lower limbs of horses
   G) Allergic reactions
   H) Enterotoxemia (gut edema) of swine

 2.  Adjunctive therapy in laminitis (founder) of horses

 3.  Adjunctive therapy in myositis or myopathy (tying up) in horses

 4.  Adjunctive therapy in azoturia (Monday-morning disease) in horses

 5.  Reduction of intraocular pressure
   A) For therapy of glaucoma and to reduce danger of prolapse of the vitreous humor after lens or cataract surgery.
   B) Carbonic anhydrase inhibitors or osmotic diuretics should be used.

 6.  Postoperative renal failure
   A) Use an osmotic diuretic such as mannitol. In dogs: 0.25 to 0.5 g 20% mannitol/kg body weight in lactated Ringer's solution (10 to 15 ml/kg) by slow IV injection.

 7.  Uremia — use osmotic diuretics such as dextrose. Rehydrate the animal with lactated Ringer's solution. Give 10% glucose IV at a rate of 2 to 10 ml/min for 10 to 15 min.

 8.  Reduction of generalized inflammation — a combination of a diuretic and a corticosteroid may be used (trichlormethiazide plus dexamethasone [Naquasone® — Schering]).

F.  ELECTROLYTE AND ACID-BASE DISTURBANCES RESULTING FROM DIURETIC THERAPY — requires chronic administration.

1. **Depletion of extracellular fluid** results from excessively rapid, heavy diuresis. May induce orthostatic hypotension or shock.

2. **Sodium depletion (hyponatremia)** in absence of edema it results from excessive continuous administration of a diuretic, inducing true depletion of body stores of sodium.

3. **Hypokalemia** results from accelerated distal exchange of sodium for potassium. It is increased by the greater delivery of sodium to exchange sites and by an elevated level of circulating aldosterone.

4. **Hyperkalemia** may occur when aldosterone antagonists are administered with potassium supplements or to patients with renal disease.

5. **Metabolic acidosis** may result from reduced exchange of sodium for hydrogen brought on by aldosterone antagonists or by urinary losses of bicarbonate after administration of carbonic anhydrase inhibitors.

6. **Hypochloremia** may result from disproportionate urinary losses of chloride caused by administration of mercurials, thiazides, ethacrynic acid, furosemide. In salt-restricted patients, hypochloremia may induce inappropriate urinary losses of hydrogen and perpetuate a diuretic-induced metabolic alkalosis.

CHAPTER

# 8

# Gastrointestinal System

## General Principles

A. **CONTROL SYSTEMS OF GASTROINTESTINAL MOTILITY**

1. **Nervous System**

    A) Extrinsic — includes ANS and nonadrenergic inhibitor fibers.

    B) Intrinsic — includes myenteric and submucosal plexuses.

2. **Gastrointestinal hormones**

3. **Substances liberated from specialized cells of the gut:**

    A) Histamine                    B) Serotonin

4. **Hormones or humoral substances other than those from the gut**

B. **SUMMARY OF DRUGS THAT AFFECT GASTROINTESTINAL MOTILITY**

1. **Drugs affecting neurotransmission, in the ANS, to the smooth muscles of the gastrointestinal tract**

    A) Stimulate the GI tract:

        1) Direct cholinergics — carbachol

        2) Cholinesterase inhibitors — neostigmine

        3) Increases the synthesis of acetylcholine — dexpanthenol

    B) Inhibit the GI tract:

        1) Cholinergic blocker — atropine

        2) Direct adrenergic — epinephrine

        3) Prevent release of acetylcholine — neomycin, streptomycin, kanamycin, ether, halothane, digitalis, barbiturates

2. **Direct action on smooth muscle** (not via ANS receptors)
   A) Stimulate the GI tract:
      1) Histamine
      2) Coherin
      3) Angiotensin
      4) Coecolysin®
      5) Vasopressin
      6) Prostaglandins
   B) Inhibit the GI tract:
      1) Opiates — morphine, paregoric
      2) Antispasmodics — Oct-Vet® (Summit Hill), Jenotone® (Jen-Sal), Neopavrin® (Savage), Novin® (Haver-Lockhart)
      3) Glucagon
3. **Reflex action via intrinsic nervous mechanisms**
   A) Increase stretch
      1) Hydrophilic colloids
      2) Hypertonic salts
      3) Lubricants
      4) Softening and wetting agents
   B) Irritate
      1) Emodin group
      2) Phenolphthalein
      3) Castor oil
      4) Resinous compounds

C. **TREATMENT PRINCIPLES**
   1. **Treatment is directed at the relief of symptoms and restoration of optimal physiological function.**
   2. **Drugs useful in treating disorders of the GI tract do not effect many cures.**
   3. **The underlying cause(s) of the disorder must first be recognized and properly alleviated.**
   4. **Use of the potent drugs may eliminate a specific complaint — may mask a sign needed for an accurate diagnosis and, in turn, proper regimen of therapy.**
   5. **Most of the drugs to be discussed also have actions on organ systems other than the GI tract.**

# Stimulants of Gastrointestinal Tract

A. **CHOLINERGICS** (muscarinic)

   1. **Acetylcholine is the prototype but it is not used clinically.**
   2. **Carbachol (Lentin®)**
   3. **Indirect cholinergics**
      A) Neostigmine
      B) Physostigmine

4. **Alkaloids**
   A) Pilocarpine        B) Arecoline (Nemural® — Winthrop)
   C) Muscarine
5. **Summary of action**
   A) Increase motility
   B) Increase salivation, which may be profuse and watery
   C) Slightly increase bile flow (questionable)
   D) Increase flow of pancreatic juice
   E) Increase secretion of intestinal mucus

B. **LAXATIVES** — other terms: cathartic, purge or purgative
   1. **Irritant laxatives**
      A) Increase motility by irritating the gut wall, resulting in increased stimulation of smooth-muscle wall.
      B) Emodin (botanical origin)
         1) Contains an inert glycoside which decomposes gradually in the intestine to form the active substance, *emodin.*
         2) Substances in which emodin is the active agent:
            a) Aloe, senna — oral
            b) Cascara sagrada — oral and injectable
               (1) Excreted in urine, turning the urine to a yellowish to brown color.
               (2) Excreted in milk, may discolor the milk.
      C) Castor oil
         1) Castor oil itself does not irritate the GI tract.
         2) Contains an unsaturated triglyceride of ricinoleic acid which, when exposed to the alkaline medium of the intestine, is saponified to the irritating sodium ricinoleate.
         3) Can be extremely harsh
      D) Resinous irritants
         1) Gamboge        3) Podophyllum
         2) Jolap          4) Colocynth
      E) Phenolphthalein
         1) Is irritating to intestine when given orally
         2) Is absorbed and reenters the gut via enterohepatic circulation through the bile, prolonging its action.
         3) Turns red in alkaline urine
   2. **Bulk-producing laxatives**
      A) Their general mechanism of action is to increase bulk in the lumen of the intestine by:
         1) Holding and preventing the absorption of imbibed water and pulling body water into the gut lumen from the surrounding tissues

2) Increasing the fluidity of feces
3) Increasing the bulk of the intestinal contents which causes distention of the gut wall. This increases stimuli for greater propulsive motility.

B) Hydrophilic colloids and undigestible fiber laxatives

1) Psyllium — Metamucil® (Searle)
2) Plantago — Siblin® (Parke-Davis)
3) Agar
4) Bran
5) Methylcellulose

C) Saline laxative

1) Hypertonic salt solutions are poorly absorbed; hence they remain in the intestine where they are osmotically active and draw water into the lumen from surrounding tissues.
2) They will dehydrate the animal.
3) Their action and the severity of the dehydration they cause depends on dosage.
4) Some saline laxatives:
    a) Magnesium sulfate (Epsom salts)
    b) Sodium sulfate (Glauber's salts)
    c) Sodium phosphate
    d) Magnesium hydroxide (milk of magnesia)
    e) Magnesium oxide
    f) Sodium and potassium tartrate (Rochelle salt)
    g) Sodium biphosphate and sodium phosphate (Fleet® Enema — Pitman-Moore)
    h) Cosert®, a suppository form of laxative containing potassium bitartrate, sodium bicarbonate and polyethylene glycols.

D) Lubricants

1) Increase bulk in the intestine
2) Lubricate and soften fecal mass so that it moves more easily through the tract
3) Mineral oil (liquid petrolatum) — several grades and sources available. Chronic use may interfere with the absorption of lipids and the fat-soluble vitamins (A, D, E, & K), thus leading to nutritional dificiencies.
4) Raw linseed oil
    a) Lubricates in addition to its irritating action
    b) Only the raw form (not boiled or treated) should be used.

E) Softening agents
   1) Surface-active emulsifying and wetting agents
   2) Mix with feces — increase water retention, soften, lubricate, and add bulk
   3) Dioctyl sodium sulfosuccinate (Colace® — Mead Johnson; Doxinate® — American Hoechst)
   4) Dioctyl calcium sulfosuccinate (Surfak® — American Hoechst)
   5) Slow onset of 1 to 3 days

## C. CHOLERETICS

1. **Stimulate the flow of bile**
2. **Bile salts** — given orally
   A) Act via enterohepatic circulation. When bile salts are absorbed and go to the liver via the portal blood, they stimulate liver cells to secrete more bile.

## D. MISCELLANEOUS

1. **Histamine**
   A) Stimulates motility
   B) A potent stimulator of the flow of gastric juices, particularly hydrochloric acid
   C) Stimulates the flow of pancreatic juice
   D) These actions cannot be blocked by either atropine or antihistamines.
2. **Caffeine** — stimulates the flow of gastric juices and increases the acidity of the stomach.
3. **Ethyl alcohol** — also stimulates the flow of gastric juices.
4. **Meperidine** (Demerol® — Winthrop). Given IV has been shown to stimulate the flow of pancreatic juice in dogs.
5. **Vasopressin** — Pitressin® (Parke-Davis)
   A) Has been shown in man to be of benefit in treating intestinal distention caused by gas
   B) Suggested to be beneficial in correcting ileus in dogs
6. **Dexpanthenol** — Ilopan® (Warren-Teed)
   A) An alcoholic analogue of the vitamin, pantothenic acid
   B) A coenzyme precursor claimed to enhance the formation of extra acetylcholine
   C) The extra acetylcholine increases intestinal motility.
7. **Coherin**
   A) Postulated release from the posterior pituitary
   B) Inhibits the GI tract for a few minutes, then stimulates it

8. **Prostaglandins**
    A) Released from the intestinal wall
    B) Clinical use is questionable
9. **Coecolysin**
    A) Claimed to stimulate secretions and peristalsis and to relieve existing spasms. Efficacy is questionable. Its action may be attributable to histamine in the preparation.
    B) Not approved in the United States

E. **EMETICS** (*See* facing page.)

1. **An emetic is a drug capable of inducing vomiting.**

2. **Vomiting is a complex reflex act under the control of an emetic center** — center located in the medulla of the brain.

3. **Adjacent to the emetic center is an area of nervous tissue. It contains receptors sensitive to many chemicals that reach this area via the bloodstream** — this highly specialized area is called the *chemoreceptor trigger zone* (CRTZ).

4. **Stimulation of the CRTZ stimulates the emetic center.**

5. **Impulses reach the emetic center from four main sources:**
   A) From *higher centers* of the brain. Stimuli that are applicable here are pain, fear, taste, and intracranial disease.
   B) Disturbances of motion and equilibrium may be channeled through the *cerebellum* into the emetic center, but more probably from the *cerebellum* to the CRTZ and then to the emetic center in dogs and cats.
   C) From *afferent sympathetic* and *parasympathetic nerves* from the *viscera*. These nerves receive their stimuli from inflammation and disease of visceral organs and from local irritation of the mucosa of the pharynx and GI tract.
   D) From *drugs* or *toxins* that stimulate the CRTZ

6. **Centrally-acting or direct-acting emetics** — drugs that act via the CRTZ. This may be their therapeutic purpose; *e.g.* apomorphine given IV or SC. Emetic action might be a side effect of a drug used for another purpose, such as digitalis.

7. **Local-acting or indirect emetics** — drugs that act by irritating the mucosa of the gastrointestinal tract
   A) Irritant emetics are given orally, preferably by a stomach tube.
   B) Irritant emetics found to be effective include:
      1) Copper sulfate, 1%
      2) Sodium chloride in warm water
      3) Ipecac

## Schematic Representation of Emesis

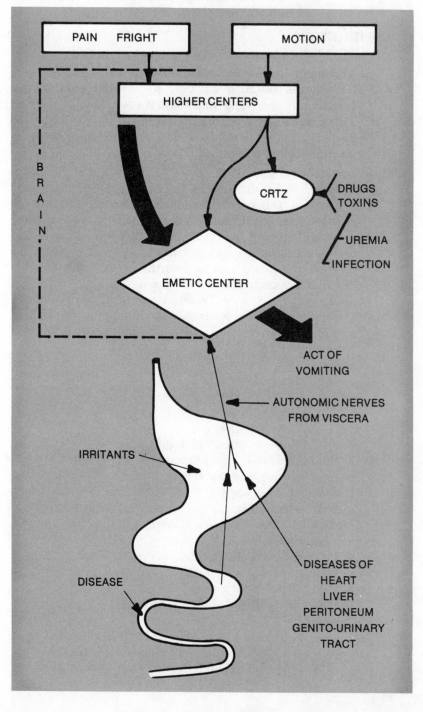

# Inhibitors of the
# Gastrointestinal Tract

A. **ANTIEMETICS**

  1. **General principles**
     A) Antiemetics are used to control nausea and vomiting.
     B) Nausea and vomiting are only signs and should not be treated until the underlying cause is determined.
     C) Antiemetic therapy is usually empirical.
     D) The drugs recommended for antiemetic therapy belong to several different groups.

  2. **Antiemetic drug groups**
     A) Sedatives and hypnotics
        1) Drugs in this group exert their antiemetic action by a sedative action upon the higher centers of the brain and by inhibition of the emetic center in the medulla.
        2) The barbiturates (phenobarbital, pentobarbital, and secobarbital) are most noteworthy in this group.
        3) Chloral hydrate may also be used.
        4) Morphine is unique. When given SC, it first initiates vomiting (in about 5 minutes) by stimulating the CRTZ. It then prevents vomiting by inhibiting the CRTZ and the emetic center.
        5) Meperidine (Demerol® — Winthrop) inhibits vomiting but does not stimulate it.
        6) Recognized side effects include:
           a) Respiratory depression
           b) Excessive sedation
           c) Tendency to reduce blood pressure
     B) Antihistamines — The mechanisms by which the antihistaminic drugs exert antiemetic action are not completely understood. They apparently do not block the CRTZ. A suggested mechanism an ability of these drugs to depress certain areas of the higher centers. Examples of effective drugs in this group are:
        1) Promethazine — Phenergan® (Wyeth)
        2) Diphenhydramine — Benadryl® (Parke-Davis)
        3) Dramamine® (Searle)
        4) Bonamine® (Pfizer), Bonine® (Roerig)
     C) Tranquilizers
        1) The phenothiazine-derivative tranquilizers are the most effective antiemetics in small animal medicine.
           a) They can inhibit both the CRTZ and the emetic center in dogs. Chlorpromazine prevents vomiting in a dog

when five times the effective dose of apomorphine is given IV.

b) These tranquilizers are effective in preventing car sickness in dogs and cats.

c) They are not especially effective against irritant emetics.

d) A noted side effect is their ability as adrenergic blockers to cause a tendency toward hypotension.

2) Another tranquilizer with considerable antiemetic ability is trimethobenzamide (Tigan® — Beecham).

a) It is not a phenothiazine derivative.

b) It blocks the CRTZ and is effective in preventing apomorphine-induced vomiting. It does not protect against local irritant emetics.

c) Compared to the phenothiazine-derivative drugs, trimethobenzamide causes less CNS depression and less tendency toward hypotension.

D) Local-acting antiemetics

1) This group of drugs has limited therapeutic value.

2) They diminish the irritant stimuli that may begin in the stomach by:

a) Anesthetizing the gastric mucosa (*e.g.* butacaine and benzocaine)

b) Soothing and protecting the gastric mucosa (*e.g.* kaolin, pectin, bismuth)

## B. CHOLINERGIC (MUSCARINIC) BLOCKERS

1. **Classic cholinergic blockers**

   A) Belladonna alkaloids      D) Methscopolamine

   B) Atropine                  E) Robinul-V®

   C) Scopolamine               F) Centrine®

2. **Mechanism of action: competitive antagonism of acetylcholine at parasympathetic (motor) nerve endings to the GI system.**

3. **Normal stimulatory impulses are removed, reducing activity.**

4. **Inhibition is more pronounced in the presence of hypermotility or increased secretions, as in diarrhea.**

5. **Pharmacodynamic responses of the GI system to the atropine group:**

   A) Decreased intestinal motility and tone

   B) Decreased gastric secretions

   C) Little or no decrease in flow of pancreatic juice and intestinal juice

   D) Marked decrease in salivary secretions

   6.  Side effects of this group:
       A) Dryness of mouth
       B) Tendency toward increased heart rate (tachycardia)
       C) Dilated pupils
   7.  Fixed drug combinations containing members of this group are commonly used.
       A) One such compound (Darbazine® — Norden) combines isopropamide (a synthetic cholinergic blocker) with prochlorperazine (a phenothiazine-derivative tranquilizer).
       B) Methscopolamine combined with neomycin is available as Biosol-M® (Upjohn).

C.  OPIUM DERIVATIVES AND SYNTHETICS
   1.  **Opium** — a time-honored remedy for treating diarrhea.
   2.  **Morphine** — an opium derivative. Initially it stimulates, later inhibits, propulsive movements of the intestine.
   3.  **Defecation after injection of morphine is common.** This is followed by increased tone of the smooth muscle, a state of *spastic paralysis* with no propulsive movements in the tract, and contracted sphincter.
   4.  **Paregoric** (camphorated tincture of opium) contains the alkaloids, morphine and codeine, together with certain alkaloids (papaverine) that inhibit the smooth muscle of the hypermotile intestine. This group of drugs is efficient in relieving pain of visceral origin.
   5.  **Morphine is contraindicated in liver and pancreatic inflammatory disease because it raises the pressures in biliary and pancreatic duct systems.**
   6.  **Diphenoxalate (Lomotil® — Searle)** — a synthetic narcotic that slows intestinal motility.

D.  SMOOTH-MUSCLE RELAXANTS
   1.  **A miscellaneous group of drugs** — all relax the smooth muscle of the intestine.
   2.  **Mechanism of action** — they are believed to inhibit cellular function directly rather than via ANS receptors.
   3.  **These drugs are sometimes called antispasmodics** — an often confusing term.
   4.  **Examples of this group:**
       A) Isometheptene — Oct-Vet® (Summit Hill)
       B) Dipyrone — Novin® (Haver-Lockhart)
       C) Aminopropazine — Jenotone® (Jen-Sal)

D) Ethaverine — Neopavrin® (Savage) or Myoquin-65V® (Hickam)

5. Care must be observed when hypotensive patients are treated with smooth-muscle relaxants.

# Drugs that Modify Contents of the Intestinal Tract

A. INHIBITORS OF MICROORGANISMS IN THE TRACT
  1. Frequently the need arises to employ the chemotherapy of pathogenic enteric microorganisms.
  2. Antibiotics and sulfonamides are frequently chosen, not just for their efficacy in inhibiting bacterial organisms, but because they are not absorbed from the intestine.
  3. This allows greater concentrations of the drug to remain in the tract for longer periods of time.
  4. Antibiotics that are poorly absorbed when given orally are streptomycin, neomycin, and bacitracin.
  5. Enteric sulfonamides include sulfaguanidine, phthalylsulfathiazole, and sulfaquinoxaline.

B. CHANGE IN THE FLORA
  1. Cultures of *Lactobacillus* — may be used to treat refractory enteritis and colitis. *Lactobacillus* should be given orally.
  2. Mechanism of action — *Lactobacillus* changes the pH of the tract media to one unfavorable to the offending organisms and/or in competition with the offending organisms for nutrient factors needed for growth and multiplication, thus inhibiting the offenders.

C. ADSORBENTS AND PROTECTANTS
  1. This is a group of inert, insoluble compounds of varying chemical make-up.
  2. They are used to protect against the mucosal irritation and/or adsorption of various toxic compounds that arise from disease processes in the intestine (enteritis) or from ingested matter (garbage toxemia).
  3. They are common ingredients in antidiarrheal preparations.
  4. Mechanism of action:
     A) Coat the mucosa of the tract
     B) Adsorb or bind to the noxious agents; *e.g.* 1 g of activated

charcoal can remove 100 mg of strychnine from 50 ml of an aqueous solution.

5. Examples
   A) Kaolin (aluminum silicate)
   B) Pectin (a carbohydrate from fruit rinds)
   C) Activated charcoal
   D) Insoluble bismuth salts

D. Antacids
   1. There is little clinical evidence that they are useful in small animal medicine.
   2. Their duration of action is short.
   3. Hourly dosing may be necessary.
   4. Antiacids may be valuable supportive treatment of pancreatitis in small animals and digestive upsets in ruminants.
   5. Antacids will neutralize the pH of stomach contents, reducing the amount of free acid that is emptied into the duodenum.
   6. The acidity of ingesta in the duodenum causes the release of secretin. This stimulates increased secretion of pancreatic juice. The reduction of free acid by an antacid would then indirectly reduce the flow of pancreatic juice.
   7. Common antacids
      A) Calcium carbonate     C) Magnesium hydroxide
      B) Magnesium oxide       D) Various aluminum salts

# Replacement Compounds

The role of many of the drugs of this group has been questioned.

A. DIGESTANTS
   1. Dilute HCl (10%) — may aid digestion and may aid in the absorption of iron.
   2. Enzymes — will generally aid in digestion.
      A) Pepsin
      B) Rennin
      C) Pancreatin — amylase, lipase, and trypsin.
      D) Whole pancreas — Viokase-V® (A. H. Robins)
      E) Diastase — Taka® (Parke-Davis)

B. CARMINATIVES
   1. Aids in expelling gas from stomach — action is questionable
   2. Capsicum, ginger and oil of turpentine

C. **BITTERS**
   1. **Reputed to aid in stimulating digestion and motility.**
      A) Nux vomica (strychnine)   C) Quassia
      B) Gentian root              D) Absinth

# Drugs that Act on the Rumen

A. **RUMINATORICS**
   1. **Of questionable value in increasing rumen motility**
   2. **Reputed to stimulate an atonic rumen; this action has not been shown experimentally.**
      A) Tartar emetic   C) Barium chloride
      B) Nux vomica      D) Ammonium carbonate

B. **ANTIFERMENTIVES**
   1. **Used to control bloat caused by free gas**
      A) Salicylic acid       D) Soluble pine oil
      B) Oil of turpentine    E) Ethyl alcohol
      C) Creolin              F) Formaldehyde

C. **ANTI-FROTHING AGENTS**
   1. **Used to control frothy (legume) bloat**
      A) Oil of turpentine
      B) Polymerized silicones
      C) Detergents
      D) Emulsified oils; an example is Turcapsol™ (Pitman-Moore) containing salicylic acid, methyl salicylate, camphor, and oil of turpentine.
   2. **Poloxalene**
      A) *For prevention:* daily while animals are on legume pasture, administer Bloat Guard® (SmithKline); very effective.
      B) *For treatment:* Therabloat® (Norden) may be effective if bloat is not too far advanced.

D. **CHOLINERGICS**
   1. **Stimulation — slight to none**
   2. **Neostigmine or carbachol is used**

# Drug Interactions and
# Gastrointestinal Function

A. **MOST OBSERVATIONS ARE FROM HUMAN MEDICINE** —
but they may also apply to veterinary medicine.

B. **INTERFERENCE** — certain drugs interfere with the absorption,
efficacy and/or safety of certain other drugs. The following table
outlines the specific effects of a few of these drugs that might be
applicable to veterinary medicine.

| THERAPEUTIC AGENT | RESPONSES | MECHANISMS |
|---|---|---|
| Antacids | Lower the rate of absorption of acidic drugs such as phenylbutazone, nitrofurantoin, pentobarbital, and some sulfonamides | Change pH of contents and thus change drug to a less absorbable form |
| Cathartics | Reduce amount of slowly and erratically absorbed drugs such as digitoxin and tetracyclines | Speed the passage through the intestine |
| Milk products; oral compounds containing calcium, aluminum or magnesium | Erratic and incomplete absorption of tetracyclines | Tetracyclines chelate metals and form insoluble complexes |
| Antihistamines | Enhance effect of cholinergic blockers | Antihistamines have anticholinergic activity |
| Antihistamines | Enhance effect of sedatives | Antihistamines may be CNS depressants |
| Lomotil® (Searle) | Enhance effect of sedatives | Lomotil® is a CNS depressant |
| Dioctyl sodium sulfosuccinate | May increase the absorption of mineral oil | Surface-active agent allows greater ease of absorption |

C. **INTERFERENCE WITH ABSORPTION** — certain drugs interfere with the absorption of some nutrients from the digestive tract. The following are examples that might be applicable to veterinary medicine.

| THERAPEUTIC AGENT | RESPONSES | MECHANISMS |
|---|---|---|
| Chronic administration of antibiotics or sulfas | Blood coagulation problems | Sterilize the gut; Inhibit vitamin K synthesis by intestinal bacteria |
| Diphenylhydantoin (Dilantin® — Parke-Davis) | Anemia | Decrease absorption of folic acid and/or vitamin $B_{12}$ |
| Neomycin | Steatorrhea, electrolyte loss, free fatty-acid loss | Mucosal injury and binding of bile salt |
| Carbonates, long term | Anemia | Decrease absorption of iron |
| Mineral oil | Deficiencies of: lipid nutrients vitamins A,D,E,K | Decrease absorption |

CHAPTER

# 9

# Blood
# and
# Blood-Forming System

## Agents that Affect
## Coagulation of Blood

### A. SUMMARY OF BLOOD-CLOTTING MECHANISM

TISSUE TRAUMA $\longrightarrow$ THROMBOPLASTIN

PLATELET DISINTEGRATION $\longrightarrow$ THROMBOPLASTIN
AHF  rapid disintegration (lipid)

THROMBOPLASTIN + PROTHROMBIN + SPECIFIC FACTORS  + $CA^{++}$ $\longrightarrow$ THROMBIN
               formed in liver       catalysts                 (A protein)
               vitamin K necessary   formed in liver

THROMBIN + FIBRINOGEN $\longrightarrow$ FIBRIN (clot formed by
           (plasma protein)                      fibrin threads)

### B. HEMOSTATIC — enhance blood clotting

1. **Local application**
   A) Acts by constricting or closing vessels
      1) Mechanical pressure and cold applications
      2) A vasoconstrictor such as epinephrine may be used
   B) Aids in providing a network favorable to clotting
      1) Cotton and gauze
      2) Absorbable materials form a network and then are absorbed
         a) Gelfoam® (Upjohn)
         b) Solusponge®
         c) Surgicell® (Johnson & Johnson)

    C) Fibrin foam

    D) Thrombin, thromboplastin of mammalian origin

    E) Astringents such as styptics and hemostatic powders and solutions coagulate protein in the blood and begin the formation of a clot.

        a) Monsel® (Wade) solution (ferric subsulfate)

        b) Iron subsulfate, ferrous sulfate

        c) Silver nitrate

        d) Alum

2. **Systemic hemostatics** — efficacy has been questioned and is not considered reliable.

    A) Vitamin K — enhances the formation of prothrombin

    B) Conjugated estrogens — increase factor V and prothrombin

    C) Klot® — n-butyl alcohol in saline (not available)

    D) Koagamin® — oxalic and malonic acid (not available)

    E) Hemostop® — adrenochrome (not available)

    F) Gelatin solutions (Intragel® )

    G) Brain-tissue extracts — containing impure cephalins and kephalins; *e.g.*, caprine-origin rabies vaccine

    H) Formalin — IV, oral or intramammary

C. **ANTICOAGULANTS** — sometimes needed:

    A) To maintain donated blood for transfusion

    B) To treat and prevent thrombophlebitis and embolism

    C) For experimental techniques, blood sampling, etc.

1. **Heparin**

    A) Naturally occurring from mast cells of the liver and the lung

    B) Chemically, a polysaccharide esterified with sulfuric acid; use sodium salt.

    C) Standardized — 1 mg = 100 USP units.

    D) Mechanism of action

        1) Prevents conversion of prothrombin to thrombin

        2) Inactivates thrombin

        3) Prevents disintegration of platelets

        4) Anti-thromboplastin effect

    E) Active *in vivo* and *in vitro* on enzyme systems

        1) Not active orally

        2) Rapidly leaves the blood stream

            a) From blood to tissue

            b) Renal excretion

            c) Tissue destruction by heparinase

    F) May be antagonized by protamine sulfate and toluidine blue

2. **Dicumarol** (dicoumarin) — warfarin

    A) The offending agent in sweet-clover poisoning in cattle.

Moldy sweet-clover hay contains dicumarol, which causes internal hemorrhage leading to death.
B) Mechanism of action
   1) Prevents formation of prothrombin
   2) Prevents formation of factor VII (and other factors) in the liver
   3) Antimetabolite of vitamin K (indirect anticoagulants). This is a form of biological antagonism.
C) Metabolism
   1) Active orally
   2) Degraded to inactive compounds by the liver
D) Slow onset of action. It is an indirect action. Requires 24 hours for inhibition of coagulation. Prothrombin is already formed.
E) Action continues after therapy is discontinued. Time is required for biosynthesis of prothrombin to reach an effective level.
F) Not active in shed blood; *in vivo* use only.
G) Vitamin K is the antidote for dicumarol poisoning.
   1) Reversal occurs in 30-60 minutes.
   2) Administer IV
      a) For dogs: 5 mg/kg
      b) For cattle: 2 g; for calves: 50 to 100 mg
      c) For horses: 250 to 500 mg

3. **Chemicals that tie-up calcium**
   A) Sodium citrate binds calcium in a *complex*, leaving no free ionic calcium to act in the coagulation scheme. For *in vitro* use only. A combination of citric acid, citrate and dextrose (ACD solution — Squibb) is used for blood storage.
   B) Ethylene diamine tetra acetic acid (EDTA)
      1) EDTA (uncombined) — a chelating agent that chelates calcium. For *In vitro* use only.
      2) Combined with calcium it is used as a detoxifying agent; *e.g.* lead poisoning can be treated.
         a) EDTA exchanges its calcium for lead and forms a stable, non-ionic, water-soluble complex that can be excreted, thus eliminating the lead from the blood.
         b) An example is Havidote® (Haver-Lockhart) containing calcium disodium ethylene diamine tetra-acetate, 6.6%.

# Blood Substitutes

## Plasma Expanders

A. **THEORETICAL REQUIREMENTS OF AN IDEAL PLASMA SUBSTITUTE**

1. **Does not pass readily into the tissue fluids or is not rapidly excreted by the kidney** — should have a molecular weight of at least 70,000 (the same as serum albumin). Should not be rapidly biotransformed or removed by the tissues but eventually be excreted or biotransformed.

2. **Exert an osmotic pressure and have viscosity similar to that of plasma**

3. **Stable composition** — easily sterilized

4. **Nontoxic** — does not induce fever (nonpyrogenic).

5. **Nonantigenic** — causes no hypersensitivity reactions

6. **Not stored in tissues for long periods**

7. **Does not act as a diuretic**

8. **Pharmacodynamically inert** — does not adversely affect any visceral function

B. **FUNCTION OF MACROMOLECULAR COLLOID**

1. **Maintains volume** — also maintains blood pressure

2. **Maintains osmotic blood pressure** — important for proper balance of fluid between blood and tissues

C. **PLASMA EXPANDERS OR BLOOD SUBSTITUTES**

1. **Gelatin** (Intragel® ) from pigskin; contains 8 g gelatin per 100 ml.

2. **Dextrans** — many different varieties
   A) Polysaccharide — long-chain polymer of glucose
   B) Naturally formed from bacteria
   C) Molecular weight is over 75,000
   D) Fate
      1) Eliminated as dextran in urine
      2) Catabolized to glucose, to carbon dioxide, and energy
      3) Leaves blood stream in about 12 hours
   E) Damage to the liver and kidneys of dogs has been reported.

3. **Polyvinylpyrrolidone** (PVP)
   A) High molecular-weight polymer
   B) Nontoxic. In man it remains in body tissue for extended periods of time.
   C) Histamine release in dogs

D) Gives plasma-expanding action that persists 12 hours
E) Is excreted via the kidneys (75%), bile and feces
F) Binds other drugs (detoxification), causing slow release

4. **Plasmanate®** (Cutter)
   A) Contains plasma protein fraction from human sources
   B) Selected plasma proteins plus sodium chloride and sodium acetate
   C) Plasma protein percent:
      1) Albumin - 88%
      2) Alpha globulin - 7%
      3) Beta globulin - 5%

5. **Electrolyte solutions** — Ringer's solution, lactated Ringer's solution, and balanced electrolyte solutions.

# Hematinics

They enhance erythropoeisis. Their efficacy is usually assessed in terms of their ability to increase the PCV and hemoglobin value. They are used to treat anemia. Many preparations, composed of many combinations, are used. The major compounds are listed below.

A. **IRON**
   1. **Oral** — ferrous sulfate, ferric pyrophosphate
   2. **Injectable** — iron complexed with an organic molecule such as dextran
   3. **Sorbitol reportedly increases the oral absorption of iron**

B. **COPPER AND COBALT** (oral)

C. **VITAMINS**
   1. $B_{12}$              3. **Folic acid**
   2. **Pyridoxine**        4. **Riboflavin**
                               A) Oral
                               B) Injectable

D. **LIVER EXTRACT** (oral and injectable)

CHAPTER
# 10
# Cardiovascular System

## Cardiotonic Glycosides

Digitalis group
  Digoxin — Lanoxin® (Wellcome/Jen-Sal), Cardoxin® (Evsco),
    Digitone® (Med-Tech)
  Digitoxin

A. **HISTORY**
  1. **Squill** — Ebers Papyrus, — 1500 BC
  2. **Purple foxglove** — William Withering in 1785 described its medical use and response in the human heart.

B. **PHARMACOGNOSY** — plants containing cardiotonic glycosides:
  1. **Digitalis**
  2. **Strophanthus**
  3. **Squill**
  4. **Apocynum**
    A) *Digitalis pupurea* (purple foxglove) glycosides contain:
      1) Digitoxin    2) Gitoxin    3) Gitalin
    B) *Digitalis lanata* glycosides contain:
      1) Digoxin    2) Digitoxin    3) Gitoxin
    C) *Strophanthus* glycosides contain:
      1) Ouabain    2) Strophanthin

C. **CHEMISTRY**
  1. **Steroid nucleus** — has the activity and causes the efficacy
  2. **Lactone ring** — determines the affinity
  3. **Sugar group** — increase solubility, potency, and duration of action

D. **ACTIONS ON THE HEART**
1. **Summary of responses**
   A) Force of contraction — greater
   B) Rate — reduced
   C) Excitability — greater
   D) Automaticity — greater
2. **Increase the force of myocardial contractions** (positive inotropic effect) in a failing heart. Increase the efficiency of utilization of ATP, causing a greater force but the same utilization of oxygen. Mechanisms proposed:
   A) Direct facilitating action upon contractile protein
   B) Increased efficiency of the excitation-contraction coupling mechanism. Free calcium establishes a link between excitation and contraction. Digitalis increases free calcium in heart cells and interferes with normal exchange of sodium and potassium. Potassium is prevented from entering the cell to exchange with sodium.

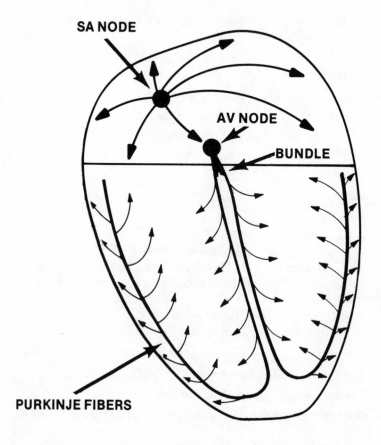

3. **Heart rate is slowed** (negative chronotropic effect). This is especially true when the rate is very rapid, as in congestive heart failure.
   A) Decreased rate of discharge from the sino-atrial (SA) node due to:
      1) Stimulation of vagus, centrally
      2) Direct depression of the SA node
   B) Refractory period of the atrio-ventricular (AV) node is prolonged.
   C) AV conduction is slowed.

4. **Excitability of the myocardium is increased** — the ability to respond to an electrical stimuli is enhanced.

5. **Automaticity of all areas of the heart muscle is increased** — is especially marked in the ventricles. Formation of ectopic impulse is increased. Pacemaker activity can be initiated in Purkinje fibers of the ventricles instead of being paced via the SA and AV nodal areas.

6. **Degree of excitability and automaticity is related to dosage** — an increase in plasma levels of digitalis will increase both.

7. **Toxicity** — the progressive sequence of events is an important factor in toxicity. (*See* physiograph on next page.)
   A) Ventricular ectopic beats (arrhythmia due to increased automaticity).
   B) Incomplete AV block (arrhythmia due to slowed AV conduction).
   C) Extrasystoles (arrhythmia due to increased automaticity).
   D) Ventricular tachycardia (arrhythmia due to increased automaticity and excitability).
   E) Ventricular fibrillation (arrhythmia due to increased automaticity).

8. **Progressive changes in ECG that reflect the toxic alterations in heart function:**
   A) Increased P-R interval
   B) Inverted T waves
   C) Biphasic and inverted monophasic QRS intervals
   D) AV block
   E) Bizarre, barely identifiable waves
   F) Fibrillation

E. **ACTIONS ON OTHER ORGANS**
   1. **Constriction of arterioles** — this direct action results in a slight and transient rise in blood pressure.
   2. **Stimulation emesis** — by a central action on the CRTZ.

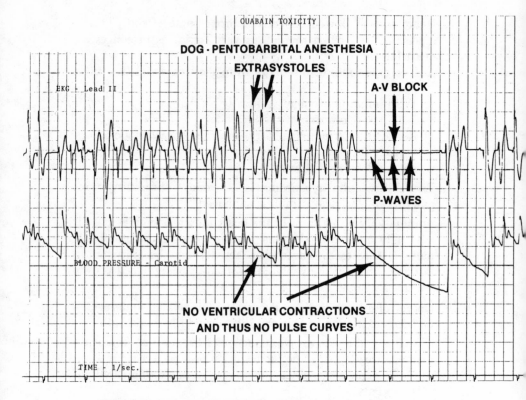

## F. DIGITALIS AND CATIONS

1. **Inhibit the active transport of sodium out of cells and reduce the entry of potassium into the cell** — *pump*-interference results in a net *loss* of intracellular potassium. This mechanism may be involved in toxicity.

2. **Calcium and digitalis may be synergistic.**

## G. METABOLISM

1. **Absorption** — varies among glycosides when given orally. The nonpolar compounds are more readily absorbed.
    A) Digitoxin — in the dog, tincture of digitoxin is well and completely (95%-100%) absorbed.
    B) Digoxin in the dog is well absorbed (65%-75%).
    C) Ouabain — is poorly absorbed.
    D) In ruminants, bacterial degradation causes variable absorption.

2. **Biotransformed in liver** — eliminated by urinary excretion and/or biliary excretion. Digoxin is eliminated primarily by urinary excretion. Digitoxin is excreted primarily by biliary excretion, some unchanged and as metabolites.

3. **Onset of action** — ouabain is most rapid, followed by digoxin, then digitoxin.

4. **Duration of action** — ouabain is shortest, then digoxin. Digitoxin is longest.

5. **Plasma t$_{1/2}$**
   A) *Digoxin* — 39 hours in dogs
   B) *Digitoxin* — 49 hours
   C) Horse — Digoxin t$_{1/2}$ is 17 hours.
   D) Cat — Digoxin t$_{1/2}$ is 21 to 25 hours.

H. **CLINICAL MANIFESTATIONS OF TOXICITY**

1. **Gastrointestinal tract** — off feed, diarrhea, emesis (good clinical guide to early toxicity in a patient)

2. **Muscular weakness** — may be due to loss of potassium; patient is lethargic and weak.

3. **Central nervous system** — disorientation, confusion, depression, and visual disturbances

4. **Cardiac**
   A) Dropped beats caused by partial or complete AV block
   B) Ventricular arrhythmias including fibrillation
   C) Myocardial necrosis — may be related to loss of intracellular potassium

5. **Drug interactions related to toxicity:**
   A) Estrogens protect against digitalis toxicity.
   B) Tylosin may increase the toxicity of cardiac glycosides. The cause is postulated to be the increased loss of potassium from the cell.
   C) Diuretics that deplete body potassium increase the toxicity of digitalis.

6. **Treatment of digitalis toxicity** (*temporarily withdraw the drug*)
   A) Cage rest and administration of CNS depressants such as pentobarbital, Dilantin® (Parke-Davis), phenobarbital
   B) Potassium salts; bananas, unsalted nuts or raisins
   C) EDTA to decrease available free calcium; extreme care must be exercised.
   D) Anti-arrhythmia drugs — quinidine, lidocaine, propanolol, phenytoin

I. **DRUGS THAT INCREASE THE EFFECTS OF THE DIGITALIS GROUP**

   1. Calcium salts     3. Isoproterenol     5. Thyroid preparations
   2. Diuretics         4. Resperpine        6. Chloramphenicol

J. DRUGS THAT DECREASE THE EFFECTS
   OF THE DIGITALIS GROUP
   1. Sodium EDTA       3. Primidone
   2. Phenobarbital     4. Spironolactone


# Glucagon

A. PHYSIOLOGY
   1. Produced in the pancreas
   2. Increases blood sugar by increasing glycogenolysis; epineph-
      rine-like mechanism.

B. PHARMACOLOGICAL RESPONSE — requires larger doses
   1. Gluconeogenesis
   2. Stimulates release of free fatty acid from adipose tissue
   3. Increases secretion of insulin
   4. Cardiac responses — has been used to treat shock in man.
      A) Increased heart rate because of a direct effect on SA node
      B) Increased contractile force (positive inotrope)
      C) Increased myocardial consumption of oxygen
      D) Increased rate of AV conduction
      E) Little or no effect on automaticity
      F) Decreased peripheral resistance
      G) Increased cardiac output (65% in dogs)
      H) Little change in blood pressure
      I) Increased coronary blood flow


# Therapy of Congestive Heart Failure

A. DIGITALIS
   1. Slow or rapid digitalization
   2. Oral
      A) Digoxin and tincture of digitoxin (Yes)
      B) Digitoxin (Questionable)
      C) Ouabain (No)
   3. Parenteral (intravenous)
      A) Digoxin
      B) Digitoxin
      C) Ouabain

# CONGESTIVE HEART FAILURE

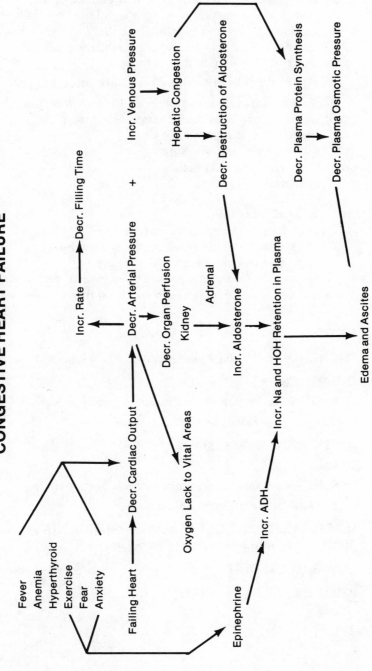

4. **Onset of action**

　A) Occurs in 1.5 to 2 hours after oral administration. Time of onset is about the same for digoxin and tincture of digitoxin.

　B) Intravenous: very rapid for ouabain, usually in 15 to 30 minutes. With digoxin and digitoxin, the maximum action occurs within 60 minutes.

5. **Actions of digitalis in a failing heart** (*See* preceding page.)

　A) Slower heart rate causes increased filling time (diastole)

　B) Increases efficiency and strength of contractions

　C) Increases cardiac output

　　1) Reduces venous pressure

　　2) Increases arterial pressure

　　3) Increases organ perfusion

　　4) Increases oxygen to tissues

　　5) Removes edema

　　　a) Proper tissue hemodynamics

　　　b) Eliminates improper retention of sodium

　　　c) Restores plasma oncotic pressure

　　6) Diuresis (indirect) is caused by increased cardiac output. This results in increased renal blood flow and glomerular fillration rate.

B. **OXYGEN**

C. **BRONCHODILATORS** — aminophylline (also is a light diuretic).

D. **DIURETICS**

　1. **Thiazides or furosemide are most commonly used.**

　2. **They may increase loss of potassium.**

E. **RESTRICTED EXERCISE**

　1. **Cage rest**

　2. **Sedatives are indicated (pentobarbital, phenobarbital).**

　3. **Tranquilizers are contraindicated.**

F. **MORPHINE, DEMEROL®** (Winthrop), **NUMORPHAN®** (Endo)— to control dyspnea and to sedate.

G. **LOW-SODIUM DIET**

H. **PARACENTESIS** — with care

# Anti-Arrhythmic Drugs, Cardiac Depressants

Quinidine
Procainamide (Pronestyl® — Squibb)
Lidocaine (Xylocaine® — Astra)
Propanolol (Inderal® — Ayerst)
Meperidine (Demerol® — Winthrop)
Antihistamines
Phenytoin (Dilantin® — Parke-Davis)

A. **GENERAL PRINCIPLES**
   1. The ability to generate impulses (automaticity) is a basic property of cardiac muscle.
   2. A pacemaker depolarizes more rapidly than other myocardial areas.
   3. Depolarization of pacemaker initiates an impulse.
   4. The usual pacemaker is the SA node.
   5. If other conductive tissue depolarizes more rapidly, an abnormal focus generates the impulse, possibly causing *arrhythmia*.
   6. Drugs favoring rapid depolarization:
      A) Digitalis  B) Catecholamines  C) Diuretics (hypokalemia)
   7. Drugs favoring slow depolarization:
      A) Lidocaine          C) Quinidine
      B) Propanolol         D) Procainamide

B. **CARDIAC ACTIONS OF THE ANTI-ARRYTHMIA DRUGS**
   1. Depress excitability of heart muscle — increases the threshold to stimuli.
   2. Refractory period of the myocardium is increased.
   3. Depress contractility of the myocardium (negative inotrope).
   4. AV conduction is slowed — similar to digitalis.
   5. Depress spontaneous discharge of pacemaker tissue, making ectopic beats less likely.
   6. Depress frequency of spontaneous discharge of the SA node.
   7. Cause vagal blockade.
   8. Large doses lower blood pressure via vasodilation.

C. **THERAPEUTIC APPLICATIONS**
   1. To treat digitalis toxicity.

2. **To treat cardiac arrhythmias** — lidocaine is the most useful of the group because it decreases automaticity (reverse arrhythmias) with less suppression of contractility.

## Summary of ECG Changes

|  | Digitalis | Anti-Arrhythmic Drugs |
|---|---|---|
| P-R interval | Increased | Increased |
| QRS time | Decreased | Increased |
| Q-T interval | Decreased | Increased |
| T wave | Flattened or inverted | Flattened or inverted |

# Vasodilators

A. **SMOOTH—MUSCLE RELAXANTS**
   1. **General body responses:**
      A) Vasodilation
      B) Bronchodilation
      C) Suppression of spasms of:
         1) GI tract          3) Urinary tract
         2) Biliary tract     4) Uterus
   2. **Two mechanisms for the smooth-muscle relaxing action:**
      A) Direct action on smooth-muscle cells
      B) Action meshing with ANS receptors

B. **DIRECT-ACTING VASODILATORS** — act on cells of the smooth muscles
   1. **Nitrites and nitrates**
      A) Smooth-muscle relaxant to the vessel wall
         1) Other sites:
            a) Biliary tract
            b) Ureter
            c) Bronchial smooth muscle
      B) Sodium nitrite; amyl nitrite; octyl nitrite; glyceryl trinitrate; mannitol hexanitrate; erythrityl tetranitrate (Cardilate® —Burroughs Wellcome)
   2. **Aminophylline** (theophylline plus ethylene diamine) is a more

potent bronchodilator; is also a mild diuretic.

3. **Papaverine** — isoquinoline group of opium alkaloids

4. **Ethyl alcohol**

5. **Histamine**

C. **ANS VASODILATORS**

1. **Act via an action on the ANS receptors**
   A) Cholinergics — Lentin®
   B) Beta adrenergics
      1) Isoproterenol — Isuprel® (Winthrop)
      2) Nylidrin — Arlidin® (USV Pharmaceuticals)
   C) Dopamine, low doses

CHAPTER

# 11

# Anthelmintics

## Internal Parasiticides

The term *anthelmintic* means *against worms*. The control of internal parasites in food animal medicine, equine medicine, small animal medicine and laboratory and zoo animal medicine is *extremely* important both economically and medically.

A. PROPERTIES OF AN IDEAL ANTHELMINTIC
   1. **Reaches the proper site in the GI tract** — enables the drug to contact the specific worm
   2. **Effective in removing the worm** — preferably by killing it
   3. **Minimal absorption and wide safety margin**
      A) Highly toxic to parasite, but nontoxic to host
      B) Does not adversely affect mucosae of GI tract
   4. **Easy to administer** — especially by clients
      A) The drinking water or in feed are easy means of administration by clients.
      B) One-dose treatment is preferable if it is active.
   5. **Causes minimal upset in animal's routine**
      A) No starving or fasting
      B) No removal of water
   6. **Causes minimal upset or set-back** (loss of appetite, diarrhea)

B. GENERAL MECHANISMS OF ACTION
   1. **Kills the parasite** *(vermicide)* — interferes with enzyme systems of the parasite.
   2. **Paralysis or relaxation of parasite** *(vermifuge)* — causes the parasite to be expelled, sometimes alive.

3. Increases the motility of intestines via a harsh laxative action — expels the worms. This means is not widely used today.

C. **ALL ARE POTENTIALLY TOXIC.**

D. **READ PACKAGE LITERATURE CAREFULLY** — follow directions and observe precautions.

# Antinematodal Drugs

A . PHENOTHIAZINE

1. **Chemistry**

   A) Two phenyl rings joined by an amine group and sulfur
   B) Almost insoluble in water
   C) Stable in dry form but deteriorates in water

2. **Administration** (orally)

   A) Drench — suspension in water, or oblet or tablet form
   B) Low-level administration in feed or salt blocks
      1) Palatability has been a problem.
      2) Reportedly interrupts life cycle of flies in manure from treated animals.

3. **Metabolism**

   A) Small amounts are absorbed into blood.
   B) It is biotransformed by the liver.
   C) Metabolites are excreted primarily in the urine — some metabolites are *red* and will discolor the urine and milk.

4. **Kills the adult parasites**

   A) Interferes with parasite anaerobic energy schemes
   B) Relatively ineffective against immature worms that are in the migrating or somatic form
   C) Activity is inversely proportional to particle size

5. **Relatively nontoxic in some species** — but very toxic to others.

   A) Order of increasing susceptibility to toxic effect:

   |            |           |
   |------------|-----------|
   | 1) Sheep   | 4) Cattle |
   | 2) Birds   | 5) Swine  |
   | 3) Goats   | 6) Horses |

   B) Toxic to dogs
   C) May produce photosensitization
   D) May produce RBC hemolysis in horses and cases of anemia

B. **PIPERAZINE**

1. **Chemistry**
   A) Freely soluble in water
   B) Is a strong base which forms such salts as hydrochloride, citrate, and tartrate
   C) The strength of piperazine compounds should be judged on the basis of milligrams of free base and not weight of total salt. Molecular weights of salt forms vary.

2. **Administration** (oral)
   A) Drench       C) In the drinking water
   B) Solution     D) In feed

3. **Paralyzes worms** — does not kill them.
   A) Worms are expelled alive.
   B) Some immature worms are expelled if they are present in the digestive tract.

4. **Relatively nontoxic**
   A) Probably less chance of toxicity as compared to phenothiazine
   B) Occasional vomiting and diarrhea

C. **THIABENDAZOLE** (Thiabenzole®, Equizole®, TBZ6®, Omnizole® — Merck)

1. **Chemistry**
   A) Insoluble in water
   B) A benzimidazole compound

2. **Administration** (oral)
   A) Drench — suspension in water or as oblets or boluses
   B) In feed — as wormer pellets
   C) Pig-wormer paste; paste form for horses

3. **Kills the parasites**

4. **Good margin of safety** — has been used successfully in pregnant animals

5. **Has been recommended as treatment for migrating larvae in horses** (verminous aneurism) — give at ten times the usual dose with proper antibiotic and corticosteroid therapy.

6. **30-day withdrawal period for animals to be slaughtered**

7. **Equizole B®** (Merck) — thiabendazole with trichlorfon (See D, 3.)

8. **Equizole-A®** (Merck) — thiabendazole with piperazine

9. **Thiabendazole is reported to have antifungal properties** — specifically against *Microsporum canis*. It is one of the ingredients in Tresaderm® (Merck), which contains thiabendazole, dexamethasone, and neomycin.

D. ORGANOPHOSPHATES

1. Good margin of safety when used properly
   A) Have been used in pregnant animals
   B) Use with *extreme care or not at all with any other organo-phosphates, cholinesterase inhibitors, succinylcholine, or phenothiazine-derivative tranquilizers.*

2. Dichlorvos (DDVP) — (Atgard V®, Equigard®, Task®, Equigel® — Squibb)
   A) Chemistry
      1) Organophosphate-impregnated resin pellets or paste (Equigel® — Squibb)
      2) Organophosphate concentration and special vehicle vary with each preparation
      3) Formulated for the gastrointestinal tract of each species
   B) Administration (oral)
      1) Rice-shaped resin pellets are mixed with feed or are put in gelatin capsules for administration to individual animals.
      2) Paste is placed in the mouth a with special syringe.
   C) Metabolism
      1) Drug is absorbed.
      2) Resin pellet or vehicle releases drug at a rate low enough that the drug absorbed into the blood does not exceed the animal biotransformation capacity.
   D) Kills the parasites
   E) Will kill adult heartworms

3. Trichlorphon — Dyrex® (Ft. Dodge), Combot® (Haver-Lockhart), Equi-Verm®
   A) For horses
   B) Granules, bolus, or stomach tube
   C) Dyrex® Tube Formula contains trichlorphon, piperazine, and phenothiazine.

4. Coumaphos — Baymix® (Haver-Lockhart)
   A) Lactating dairy cows can be dewormed and their milk sold. No withdrawal period.
   B) Treat once daily for six days as a top dressing on feed.

5. Butonate (T-113® — Vet-Kem), a tube formulation for horses

6. Haloxon (Halox® — Wellcome/Jen-Sal), for oral administration to cattle

E. LEVAMISOLE (Ripercol® — American Cyanamid; Levasole™ — Pitman-Moore)

1. Chemistry — imidazothiazoles
   A) HCl salt is highly water-soluble.

　　　B) Phosphate salt is used parenterally.

　2. **Available for oral and parenteral use**

　3. **Approved for use in cattle, sheep, swine, poultry. For horses, a product is available containing Ripercol L® and piperazine.**

　4. **Metabolism**
　　　A) Tissue residues are insignificant.
　　　B) Excretion is both urinary and fecal.

　5. **Action**
　　　A) Paralytic action on nematode; worm is expelled alive.
　　　B) Drug interferes with energy metabolism of worm.

　6. **Adverse reaction**
　　　A) Transient froth and foam at mouth
　　　B) Administer accurately. Do not overdose.

　7. **Has been used in dogs as a microfilaricidal agent** — three weeks after thiacetarsamide therapy for canine dirofilariasis. (Not approved by FDA.)
　　　A) Dosage is 10 mg/kg orally, in gelatin capsules.
　　　B) Clears microfilariae from circulation in 7 to 11 days.
　　　C) Causes transient vomiting, diarrhea, and inappetance.
　　　D) May be used concurrently with diethylcarbamazine citrate.

　8. **Other pharmacodynamic actions**
　　　A) Antiviral activity
　　　B) Anti-inflammatory activity
　　　C) Stimulatory effect on the immune system

F.　**MEBENDAZOLE** (Telmin™; Telmintic™ — Pitman-Moore)
　　**FENBENDAZOLE** (Panacur® — American Hoechst)
　　**CAMBENDAZOLE** (Camvet® — Merck)
　　**OXFENDAZOLE** (Benzelmin® — Diamond)

　1. **Chemistry**
　　　A) All are relatives of thiabendazole and are benzimidazoles.
　　　B) All are slightly soluble in water.

　2. **Metabolism**
　　　A) Only small amounts are absorbed, but residues have been found in liver up to two weeks after administration.
　　　B) Mebendazole is excreted unchanged in the feces.
　　　C) Cambendazole is rapidly metabolized to degradation products and is excreted in feces.

　3. **Mode of action** (vermicidal)
　　　A) Inhibits glucose uptake of nematodes, resulting in slow expulsion of worms.
　　　B) Effective against mature, and some immature, worms. Ovicidal to many nematodes.

4. **Adverse reactions**
   A) Free from side effects
   B) Can be given to sick and debilitated animals
   C) Contraindicated in early gestation of sheep; *i.e.*, before 4 weeks. It has been shown to be teratogenic.

G. **PYRANTEL**
   **Pyrantel tartrate** (Banmith® —Pfizer) for swine
       Strongid-T® (Pfizer) and Imathal® (Beecham) for horses
       Nemex® (Pfizer) for dogs
   **Pyrantel tartrate**

1. **Chemistry and metabolism**
   A) Chemistry related to that of levamisole
   B) Tartrate salt
      1) Fairly water-soluble
      2) Well absorbed from the gut of the pig and dog
   C) Pamoate salt
      1) Less soluble in water
      2) Absorption from the gut is greatly reduced; thus more drug stays in the intestinal tract to give anthelmintic action further down the tract.
   D) If pyrantel becomes systemic, it is quickly biotransformed for both urinary and fecal excretion.

2. **Action**
   A) Removes adult worms from the tract by producing a tetanic type of paralysis. Worms are then expelled.
   B) Kills larvae as they are hatched from eggs in the intestinal tract. The larvae do not enter the animal's body; thus the liver and lungs are not damaged by migrating larvae.

3. **Adverse reactions**
   A) Safe when used as directed
   B) Safe for use in horses of any age; can be used in pregnant mares.
   C) Toxic signs (if any)
      1) Increased respiratory rate
      2) Profuse sweating
      3) Incoordination

H. **THENIUM CLOSYLATE:** Canopar® (Wellcome/Jen-Sal) — for dogs only

1. **Chemistry**
   A) Insoluble in water
   B) Extremely bitter taste

2. **Not absorbed when given orally** — fat in the diet will,

however, facilitate absorption.

3. **Mode of action:** effective against adult and immature worms in the gut.

4. **Adverse reactions** — vomiting occurs occasionally. If vomiting is delayed two hours, the efficacy of the drug is not impaired.

5. **Should not be given to suckling puppies or recently weaned puppies weighing less than 5 lb** — fat in the milk will facilitate absorption.

I.   **DISOPHENOL** (DNP® — American Cyanamid) is available in 0.9% and 4.5% concentrations.

1. **Modes of action**
   A) Unknown. Parasite is affected only after it has consumed drug-laden blood. Systemic effects.
   B) No effect on histotropic larval stages. Effective primarily against adults.

2. **Adverse reactions**
   A) Signs
      1) Increased heart rate
      2) Increased respiratory rate
      3) Increased metabolic rate
      4) Increased body temperature
      5) Vomiting
      6) Early rigor mortis
      7) Transient lens capacity — changes occur in young dogs under 4 months of age.
   B) Possible mechanisms
      1) Uncoupling reaction of oxidative phosphorylation
      2) Poor biotransformation, plus sequestering or possible enterohepatic circulation, leading to accumulation of high levels of disophenol in the body.

3. **Precautions**
   A) Use with care in very young animals.
   B) Use with care in animals with liver or kidney damage or dysfunction.
   C) Use with care in high ambient temperatures.
   D) Do not heavily exercise treated animals.
   E) Weigh and dose animals accurately, especially small animals. Toxicity is dose-dependent. **Do not overdose!**
   F) Use extreme care in repeating doses. DNP® accumulates in the body. Do not repeat the full dose within 21 days.
   G) Intramuscular injection is painful.
   H) This product will stain permanently.

4. **Proposed treatment of toxicity**
   A) Lower the body temperature (by cooling; not with antipyretics).
   B) Correct dehydration and metabolic acidosis.
   C) Provide supplemental oxygen.

J. **PHTHALOFYNE** (formerly available for use in dogs)
   1. **Intravenous and oral administration**
   2. **Intravenous solution**
      A) Not for routine use. It should be used only when oral treatment is not feasible.
      B) More toxic than oral route. There is no specific antidote.
         1) Anaphylactic-like reactions have been seen.
         2) Severe depression, vomiting, respiratory distress, coma, and shock have occurred.
      C) Dog should be observed for several hours after treatment.
   3. **Oral** (tablets)
      A) Is absorbed, reaches significant blood levels
      B) Fewer adverse effects than when given IV
      C) Drowsiness, ataxia, vomiting
   4. **Care should be taken** — especially when older animals, debilitated animals and animals with mixed parasitic infections are treated.
   5. **Contraindicated** — in animals with chronic nephritis, hepatitis or cardiac insufficiency.

K. **GLYCOBIARSOL** (Milibis® — Winthrop)
   1. **Chemistry** — an odorless and tasteless powder that is slightly soluble in water. Easily mixed with feed.
   2. **Less than 2% absorbed**
   3. **Adverse reactions** — occasional vomiting, especially in dogs less than 1 year old
   4. **In man** — widely used to treat amebiasis and trichomoniasis

L. **TETRACHLOROETHYLENE**
   1. **Adverse reactions**
      A) A fat diet increases the absorption of drug and frequency of toxic reactions.
      B) It causes dizziness, incoordination, liver damage and death.
   2. **Contraindicated** — in tapeworm-infected dogs, in febrile or debilitated patients.

M. **TOLUENE** — methyl benzene (Methacide® — Beecham); many manufacturers
1. **Only slightly absorbed**
2. **Mild laxative action**
3. **Adverse reactions**
   A) Older dogs and puppies are most susceptible to toxic dosages
   B) Irritates the digestive mucosa
   C) Muscle tremors, unsteady gait, and vomiting

N. **N-BUTYL CHLORIDE**
1. **A rather ineffective over-the-counter medication**
2. **Adverse reactions**
   A) Vomiting      B) Diarrhea

O. **CARBON DISULFIDE**
1. **Indicated for treatment of bot infestation in horses**
2. **Irritating** — use care in administration.

P. **CYANACETHHYDRAZINE**
1. **For treatment of lungworm infection in cattle, sheep, goats, swine**
2. **Used subcutaneously**

Q. **PARVEX®** (Upjohn) — a suspension containing piperazine plus carbon disulfide.

R. **PARVEX® PLUS** (Upjohn) — a suspension containing piperazine, carbon disulfide, and phenothiazine

S. **VERMIPLEX™** (Pitman-Moore), **PARACIDE®** (Norden) — dichlorophene with methylbenzene (toluene reagent)

T. **THENATOL®** (Wellcome/Jen-Sal) — piperazine with thenium closylate

U. **BUTAMISOLE** — Styquin® (American Cyanamid)
1. **Chemistry**
   A) A benzimidazole compound with an added isobutylamido group
   B) In solution in 70% propylene glycol
2. **Administered subcutaneously** — IM injection causes pain
3. **Low therapeutic ratio**
4. **Primarily effective against adult hookworms** — minimal effect on larvae. Also effective against whipworms.

5. **Toxicity**
   A) Concurrent use of Styquin® and Scolaban® (Wellcome/Jen-Sal) is contraindicated. Toxicity from simultaneous use has been reported.
      1) Muscle weakness
      2) Paresis
      3) Ataxia
      4) Muscle tremors
      5) Respiratory difficulty and cyanosis
      6) High mortality
   B) Toxic manifestations, similar to those above have been reported after administration of six times the recommended dose of Styquin® given alone.

U. **FEBANTEL** — Rintal® (Haver-Lockhart) for horses
   1. **Chemistry**
      A) A phenylquanidine
      B) Not an organophosphate
      C) Not a benzimidazole
   2. **Is in paste form and very palatable**
      A) Can be placed in mouth on back of tongue or can be incorporated in the grain ration
      B) Approved for use in horses
   3. **Very safe**
      A) Has been given to horses and to nursing foals less than 1 month old in doses 40 times the clinical dose without causing adverse signs or effects clinically or in the laboratory.
      B) In a multiple-dose trial it was given daily at 4 times and 8 times the clinical dose for 10 days with the following results:
         1) Diarrhea after four days at 8 times the clinical dose
         2) No other adverse signs, clinical pathology changes or gross or tissue pathology
   4. **Can be given to breeding mares and stallions and to pregnant mares.**

V. **HISTORIC IMPORTANCE** — drugs used in the past include:
   1. **Oil of chenopodium**　　4. **Copper sulfate**
   2. **Sodium fluoride**　　　 5. **Santonin**
   3. **Cadmium salts**　　　　 6. **Carbon tetrachloride**

# Anticestodal Drugs

A. **DROCARBIL** (Nemural® —Winthrop) for dogs and cats

   1. **Chemistry**
      A) Combination of arecoline and acetarsol
         1) *Arecoline* — an alkaloid, direct-acting cholinergic.
         2) *Acetarsol* — an organic arsenical compound.
      B) Freely soluble in water

   2. **Actions**
      A) Vermifuge     B) Purgative

   3. **Some absorption occurs**

   4. **Adverse effects**
      A) Occasional vomiting
      B) Overdosage leads to
         1) Salivation    3) Ataxia
         2) Restlessness   4) Labored breathing
      C) Antidote is atropine

   5. **Administer without prior fasting**

B. **BUNAMIDINE** (Scolaban® — Wellcome/Jen-Sal) — for cats and dogs

   1. **Action**
      A) A *complete* taeniacide
      B) The whole tapeworm is killed and disintegrates, usually before leaving the intestine.
      C) The tapeworm may not be seen in the feces.

   2. **Some absorption occurs, which can result in toxicity.**

   3. **Adverse effects**
      A) Slight, transient changes in the ECG have been noted after administration of three times the normal dose.
      B) Reduced spermatogenesis in male dogs has been reported.
      C) Sudden-death syndrome is an idiosyncratic reaction. It may be related to dosage.

   4. **Give on an empty stomach** — fast for 3 to 4 hours.

   5. **Administer with care to animals with heart conditions.**

   6. **Do not give concurrently with Styquin® — (American Cyanamid)**

C. **NICLOSAMIDE** (Yomesan® — Haver-Lockhart) — for cats and dogs

   1. **Action**
      A) A true taeniacide    C) Scolex and neck disintegrate
      B) Removes entire worm   D) May not be seen in feces

2. Little absorption

3. Few adverse effects reported

4. Overnight fast is recommended

5. Not reported to be as effective against *Dipylidium caninum* as is bunamidine

D. **DICHLOROPHENE** (Di-phenthane-70)

1. Insoluble in water

2. Aids in the removal of tapeworms

3. Other actions
   A) Fungicidal     B) Antimicrobial     C) Coccidiostatic

E. **OTHER AGENTS**

1. **Quinacrine** (atabrine)

2. **Nicotine sulfate**

3. **Lead arsenate**

4. **Kamala**

5. **Di-n-butyl tin dilaurate** (Butynorate®)

6. **Oleoresin of aspidium**

# Anti-Fluke Drugs

A. **HEXACHLOROETHANE** (taken off the market; declared carcinogenic; illegal to use or ship)

B. **CARBON TETRACHLORIDE** (too toxic for clinical use; not approved)

C. **RAFOXANIDE** (experimental) kills immature and adult flukes

D. **DIAMFENATHIDE** (experimental) kills immature and adult flukes

E. **ALBENDAZOLE**

1. The only legally available drug for the treatment of liver flukes

2. May be used under strict conditions as an emergency investigational drug.

3. The following states have been granted permission to use albendazole: Arkansas, California, Florida, Hawaii, Idaho, Louisiana, Montana, Oregon, Texas, Utah, Washington, New Mexico, Nevada, and Mississippi.

# Coccidiostats

A. **AMPROLIUM** — Amprol® and Corid® (Merck) for cattle. Available as 9.6% solution, 1.25% crumbles, 20% soluble powder
1. **Chemistry** — a structural analogue of vitamin B₁ or thiamine (antifolate)
2. **Anticoccidial, coccidiostat mechanism**
   A) Starves coccidia to death by biological antagonism with vitamin B₁ or thiamine
   B) Retards development of first-generation schizonts in the cells of the intestinal wall
3. **Safe when used as directed**
   A) Interferes with absorption and may interfere with activation of thiamine in mammals
   B) Excessive dosages for extended periods have produced thiamine deficiency in sheep and puppies.
   C) Do not use more than 12 days in puppies.

B. **SULFONAMIDES** (kill mature coccidia)

C. **TETRACYCLINE ANTIBIOTICS** (kill mature coccidia)

D. **NICARBOZIN**

E. **NITROPHENIDE**

F. **ARSANALATES**

G. **NITROFURANS**

H. **DECOQUINATE** (Deccox®) for cattle
1. **Feed for 28 days**
2. **Kills parasites in the early stages (first six days)**
3. **Will not kill mature coccidia**

I. **MONENSIN SODIUM**
1. **Coban® (Elanco) for poultry**
2. **Rumensin® (Elanco) for cattle**
   A) Labelled for use as a feed additive
   B) Will increase weight gains but permitted dosage is too low to be effective as a coccidiostat.

# Antifilarial Agents
## Canine

Canine heartworm treatment

A. **GENERAL CONSIDERATIONS**

1. Treatment of dogs harboring adult heartworms or microfilariae can involve considerable risk. The treatment may be worse than the disease.

2. When adult heartworms are killed, pulmonary thromboemboli, with life-threatening sequelae, may result within 5 to 30 days.
   A) May occur after treatment with caparsolate
   B) May occur after administration of diethylcarbamazine citrate to an animal thought to be free of adult heartworms
   C) May occur when an animal not known to have adult heartworms is given dosage of an agent for treating intestinal parasites that produces systemic blood levels sufficient to kill adult heartworms, (*e.g.* Task® — Squibb).

3. **Drugs for treatment and control**
   A) Lethal to adult heartworms
      1) Thiacetarsamide
      2) Diethylcarbamazine citrate (slight)
      3) Levamisole
   B) Lethal to microfilariae
      1) Dithiazanine iodide
      2) Diethylcarbamazine citrate
      3) Levamisole
      4) Fenthion
   C) Lethal to migrating larvae (none available)
   D) Prevention
      1) Diethylcarbamazine citrate
      2) Styrylpyridinium chloride with diethylcarbamazine base
      3) Thiacetarsamide

B. **THIACETARSAMIDE SODIUM** (Caparsolate® — Diamond, CEVA)

1. **Chemistry** — an organic arsenical compound
2. **Mode of action** — vermicidal to adult heartworms
3. **Adverse reactions**
   A) Hepatotoxic and nephrotoxic
   B) Signs of arsenic toxicity
      1) Persistent vomiting    2) Icterus    3) Orange urine

C) Embolic shower of dead worms released into lungs may produce cardiovascular collapse.

C. **DITHIAZANINE IODIDE** (Dizan™ — Pitman-Moore)

1. **Chemistry**
   A) A cyanine dye
   B) Intense-blue powder

2. **Metabolism** — absorption from the intestinal tract is minimal, but may cause bluish discoloration of tissues.

3. **Mode of action**
   A) Assumed to inhibit uptake of glucose by microfilariae
   B) Microfilariae lose their motility, become trapped, and are phagocytized by the tissues.

4. **Adverse reactions**
   A) Vomiting and diarrhea are common
   B) May cause anorexia and asthenia
   C) Feces and vomitus turn blue-to-purple

D. **DIETHYLCARBAMAZINE CITRATE** (Dirocide® — Squibb; Caricide® — American Cyanamid; Filaribits® — Norden; D.E.C.® — BioCeutic; Decacide® —Professional Vet Labs; Diro-Form® — Vet-A-Mix)

1. **Chemistry**
   A) A colorless, odorless crystal
   B) Highly soluble in water

2. **Mode of action**: vermicidal to infective larvae and microfilariae

3. **Metabolism**
   A) Rapidly absorbed from GI tract and distributed to all tissues except fat
   B) Excreted by degraded products in the urine

4. **Adverse reactions**
   A) Irritates gastric mucosa at high levels
   B) Possibly fatal anaphylactic-type reaction may occur in microfilariae-positive dogs

E. **STYRYLPYRIDINIUM PLUS DIETHYLCARBAMAZINE BASE** (Styrid® -Caricide® — American Cyanamid)

1. **Liquid for administration** *per orum*

2. **For prevention of heartworms**

3. **For control of hookworms and roundworms**

4. **Nontoxic**

5. **Not to be given to dogs with established heartworm infection**

## PROCEDURES FOR THE TREATMENT AND PREVENTION OF CANINE HEARTWORM DISEASE

(Report prepared on behalf of the Council on Veterinary Service by R.F. Jackson, DVM, St. Augustine, FL, with the cooperation and assistance of Jack D. Noyes, DVM, Barrington, IL; J.W. Henderson, DVM, Port Arthur, TX; Dallen H. Jones, Roseburg, OR; and members of the AVMA Council on Veterinary Service.) *JAVMA 162*(8): 660; 1973.


Because canine heartworm disease has become widespread among dogs in the United States in recent years, and because its control involves administration of a variety of drugs and treatment regimens, the Council on Veterinary Service assumed the responsibility for providing guidelines for treatment and prevention that veterinarians could refer to with confidence. These guidelines are based on observations of clinicians who have successfully employed the methods described here, and on authenticated reports published in scientific journals.

### Diagnosis

Diagnosis of heartworm disease is made on the basis of finding microfilariae of the parasite in the peripheral blood. A concentration technique, such as the modified Knott's method, is recommended to avoid the possibility of missing a lightly infected dog. Since *Dipetalonema reconditum* is also widespread in the United States, it is necessary to differentiate between the microfilariae of this parasite and those of *Dirofilaria immitis*. Microfilariae of *D. immitis* undulate in one place in a fresh smear; those of *D. reconditum* have progressive movement. *Dirofilaria immitis* microfilariae are larger than those of *D. reconditum* and have a tapered head and straight tail; those of *D. reconditum* have a blunt head and button-hooked tail. Of infected dogs, 5 to 10% do not have any microfilariae, and in these dogs diagnosis must be made on the basis of history of exposure to infected mosquitoes, signs of coughing and tiring after exercise, and the typical radiographic signs of enlarged pulmonary conus, enlarged right ventricles, and dense and tortuous branches of the pulmonary artery.

### Pretreatment Examination

A complete physical examination and laboratory screening tests, such as complete blood count, urinalysis, and blood urea nitrogen and liver function determinations (SGPT and BSP tests), are recommended prior to initiating treatment. Any reversible condition not due to heartworm disease should be corrected before therapy is attempted. Chronic liver or kidney disease may preclude treatment. Radiography is most helpful in assessing pulmonary and cardiac changes due to heartworm disease.

### Elimination of Adult Worms

Thiacetarsamide is the only drug which consistently kills adult heartworms. The recommended dosage schedule is 0.1 ml/lb. (0.45 kg.) body weight intravenously (IV) twice daily for 2 days.

Vomiting occasionally follows administration of thiacetarsamide. If no other signs are present and if the dog's appetite remains good, treatment may be continued. Persistent vomiting, anorexia, or icterus following injections of thiacetarsamide are reason to suspend therapy. Thromboemboli from dead worms may create inflammatory reactions in the lungs from 5 to 30 days following thiacetarsamide therapy. Such reactions with signs of elevated temperature and cough may be kept to a minimum by enforced rest and by careful observation of the dog following chemotherapy. Rectal temperatures should be taken daily for 1 week, and if an elevation above 102F (38.9C) is observed, an injection of prednisone or similar steroid should be given.

### Elimination of Microfilariae

Four drugs have been used as microfilaricides: dithiazinine iodide, fenthion, diethylcarbamazine, and levamisole. None are without potential hazards.

**Dithiazinine iodide** is the only product presently available that is approved by the U.S. Food and Drug Administration (FDA) for use as a microfilaricide. It has been used in doses of 2 to 10 mg./lb. (0.45 kg.) per day orally. Vomiting and diarrhea often accompany the use of this drug and it is potentially nephrotoxic. To minimize these effects, the lower dose (2 mg./lb. (0.45 kg.)) is recommended.

To eliminate microfilariae give dithiazinine iodide, 2 mg./lb. (0.45 kg.) daily for 7 days.

Examine the blood for microfilariae on the 8th day. If microfilariae are still present, and if there has been little or no reaction to the drug, the dose may be increased to 5 mg./lb. (0.45 kg). This dose is given daily until the blood is free from microfilariae, but no longer than 10 days.

**Fenthion** was an effective microfilaricidal agent but it is no longer available commercially under this label.

**Diethylcarbamazine** given to dogs with microfilariae may cause severe reactions, some of which may be fatal. For this reason, it should not be used as a microfilaricide.

**Levamisole** recently has been successfully used as a microfilaricide. This preparation is sold commercially for use in cattle, sheep, and hogs, but has not been approved by FDA for use in dogs; therefore, it must be considered as an experimental drug.

Give 5 mg./lb. (0.45 kg.) of active ingredient of the levamisole preparation orally daily until the blood is free from microfilariae but give no more than 15 doses. In most dogs microfilariae will not be found after 6 to 10 doses; it is therefore advisable to make periodic examinations of the blood after the 6th day of therapy. Stop therapy as soon as the blood is free from microfilariae. The vomiting which frequently accompanies the use of this drug may be controlled by the administration of an anticholinergic agent such as atropine sulfate shortly before the levamisole is given. Occasionally signs of restlessness or nervousness develop following a dose of levamisole. When this occurs, treatment should be discontinued.

Fewer undesirable reactions will occur in connection with the use of any microfilaricidal agent if at least 6 weeks have elapsed since thiacetarsamide was given to kill adult worms.

Occasionally it is impossible to free a dog from microfilariae due to the fact that drug reactions may be severe enough to suspend treatment or to the fact that a particular dog may be refractory to treatment. When this occurs, the blood should be examined 1 year later. If microfilariae are still present, re-examine in another 3 months. If microfilariae are still present and more than 18 months have passed since thiacetarsamide therapy, reinfection may be assumed.

**Preventive Treatment**

Two methods of prevention have been shown to be effective.

1) Diethylcarbamazine citrate given at the rate of 2.5 mg./lb. (0.45 kg.) body weight (or diethylcarbamazine base given at the rate of 1.25 mg./lb. (0.45 kg.) body weight) daily, starting at the time a dog will be exposed to mosquitoes and continuing throughout the period of exposure (mosquito season) and for 2 months afterwards, will prevent heartworm disease. In places where mosquitoes may be active all year, medication must be given every day of the year. Dogs subjected to this routine must be microfilariae-free before it is initiated.

An infected dog must first be treated with thiacetarsamide to eliminate adult worms, and 6 weeks later treated with a microfilaricide. After that the dog can be started on prophylactic treatment with diethylcarbamazine. An adult dog with an unknown history of exposure and which is microfilariae-free may be started on a preventive regimen with diethylcarbamazine immediately. Its blood should be examined 3 months later and every 6 months thereafter. A dog on a preventive routine with diethylcarbamazine should be examined for presence of microfilariae every 6 months.

Occasionally in an enzootic area one may encounter some difficulty in keeping a dog free from heartworms after one treatment with thiacetarsamide and a microfilaricide, even though the dog is subjected to a preventive routine with diethylcarbamazine following therapy. Continuous exposure may create a condition wherein all stages of the parasite are present in the dog at the time of treatment. The thiacetarsamide kills the adult worms present, the microfilaricide eliminates the microfilarial stage. The diethylcarbamazine prevents development of larvae only after administration of the drug has started. Nothing yet known will kill the larvae already migrating through the tissues, and some of these larvae may go on to mature. Consequently, in such a circumstance, a second treatment with thiacetarsamide may be required some months after the first.

2) Thiacetarsamide, 0.1 mg./lb. (0.45 kg.), given IV twice daily for 2 days at 6-month intervals is an effective preventive method. Given with this frequency the drug eliminates the worms before a sufficient number have developed to cause clinical disorders.

Many dogs in urban areas have little exposure to mosquitoes and, therefore, need not be subjected to a preventive program. Such dogs should be examined for the presence of microfilariae when 1 year old and every 6 months thereafter. A concentration method (e.g., the modified Knott's technique) of microfilariae detection should always be used.

# Management of
# Canine Heartworm Disease

Adapted from "Recommended Procedures for the Management of Canine Heartworm Disease". In *Proceedings of Heartworm Symposium '77*. Veterinary Medicine Publishing Co., Bonner Springs, Kansas, 1978; and *JAVMA 173*(10), 1978.

A.  **CONTROLLING HEARTWORM** — The Council on Veterinary Service of the American Veterinary Medical Association (JAVMA 162[8]:660; 1973) and the Executive Committee of the American Heartworm Society (Proceedings of Heartworm Symposium '74:126-127, 1975) endorsed similar recommendations for controlling canine heartworm disease. In 1977 the American Heartworm Society reaffirmed these recommendations and reviewed and commented on recent developments. Four aspects were given special attention:

1. **The value of pretreatment with a microfilaricide** — it has been repeatedly suggested that pretreatment with a microfilaricide would reduce the risk of toxic reaction to the adulticide, thiacetarsamide. No one, not even the primary proponent of this procedure, has provided any evidence to justify this recommenda-

tion. It is based on the theoretic concept that the pathophysiologic responses induced by the microfilariae predisposes to a lower tolerance to the adulticide, thiacetarsamide.

On the contrary, controlled studies stimulated by the American Heartworm Society, have shown that the same pathophysiologic responses from thiacetarsamide occur regardless of presence or absence of a microfilaremia, regardless of the level of microfilaremia, and regardless of whether or not a microfilaricide was administered as a pretreatment. In an earlier study, it was demonstrated that it is difficult to eliminate microfilariae, and microfilaremia levels promptly increase when the microfilaricide precedes the adulticide. Hence, the pretreatment with a microfilaricide followed by the adulticide requires a repeated microfilaricide treatment before preventive medication with diethylcarbamazine (DEC) can be initiated. This complicates and adds cost to the treatment of heartworm infection, without any discernible value.

2. **Current status of thiacetarsamide** — the reduced potency and reduced therapeutic efficacy associated with thiacetarsamide in 1976 has been traced to one lot of one brand. This lot was withdrawn from the market, the formulation error was corrected, an improved assay method was developed, and the therapeutic potency of thiacetarsamide was verified in controlled studies, including necropsy in the determination of the effectiveness. There is some indication that the therapeutic efficiency is more consistent if the formerly recommended regimen of 0.1 mg/lb BID/2 days is extended to 3 days.

3. **The relation of DEC and/or styrylpiridinium-diethylcarbamazine to sterility in males** — so far, no one has succeeded in producing this phenomenon experimentally. Nevertheless, it is reliably reported in the routine use for prevention of heartworm infection. It appears to be rare, which suggests an individual idiosyncrasy rather than a common side reaction. At any event, full potency is restored after the daily medication is terminated; DEC remains as the best preventive medication.

4. **Role of levamisole in the management of heartworm disease** — this drug has not been approved by FDA for use against any stage of the heartworm in dogs. Any use must be technically treated as experimental and the practitioner using it or dispensing it for use will be well advised to require written approval from his client.

Nevertheless, levamisole has been widely and effectively used as a microfilaricide. It has one limitation in common with all other microfilaricides. There is no dose or regimen that will consistently and dependably eliminate the microfilariae, it must be given to effect and is not always effective. Both the daily dose and the duration of treatment should be restricted due to the toxicity of levamisole. A daily dose of 5 mg/lb has been widely used. Some experienced practitioners limit the number of daily doses to 15.

Levamisole also will kill some adult worms. Unfortunately at any and every dose and dosage schedule so far evaluated in controlled studies, including posttreatment necropsy, there have been very wide variations in the percentage of worms killed. The range is commonly from 0% to 100%. Since varying percentages of dogs have a persistent microfilaremia after the normal death of the adults, elimination of microfilaremia can provide a spurious indication of adulticidal action. Immediate but temporary apparent improvement in health due to extra care and rest during treatment can be equally misleading. It appears to be a basic error to use a potentially toxic drug without unequivocal evidence of activity.

Although there are 2 reports of activity against the developing stages, consideration of the toxicity precludes the continuous use for many months which would be required for effective preventive medication.

The American Heartworm Society in 1977 recommended that these medical management procedures be employed to assure the best possible control of canine heartworm disease:

A) **Diagnosis** — diagnosis is usually made by finding the microfilariae in the circulating blood. To reduce the chance of missing the microfilariae, it is desirable to use a concentration technique such as the Knott's method with 1.0 ml of blood and 10.0 ml of 2% formalin, or one of the filter techniques. Nevertheless, microfilariae may not be detected in 5% to 20% of infected dogs. Diagnosis must then be made on history, including exposure to mosquitoes in an enzootic area, clinical signs such as coughing and tiring on exercise plus radiographic signs such as enlarged pulmonary conus, enlarged right ventricle, and "pruning" of pulmonary branches.

It is necessary to differentiate between microfilariae of the heartworm (*Dirofilaria immitis*) and *Dipetalonema reconditum*. In the fresh blood smear, diluted with saline solution, those of the heartworm undulate in one place and never migrate, whereas those of *D reconditum* have intervals of progressive movement. In the modified Knott's method, those of *D immitis* are straight with a straight tail and tapered head while those of *D reconditum* are curved with a button-hooked tail and blunt head.

B) **Pretreatment Examination** — a complete physical examination and laboratory tests are recommended prior to treatment. The latter should include complete blood counts, urinalysis, blood urea nitrogen, and liver function tests. Since the adulticide, thiacetarsamide, is an arsenical and thus a potential nephrotoxin and hepatotoxin, kidney or liver disease may preclude treatment. Radiography is helpful in assessing pulmonary and cardiac changes and the resulting prognosis.

C) **Elimination of Adult Worms** — thiacetarsamide is the only available drug that consistently kills adult heartworms. The recommended dosage schedule is 0.1 ml/lb (0.45 kg) of body weight intravenously twice daily for 2 days and, on the basis of recent information, there appears to be some possible advantage in extending the schedule to 3 days.

Vomiting occasionally follows administration of thiacetarsamide. If no other signs are present and if the dog's appetite remains good, treatment may be continued. Persistent vomiting, anorexia, or icterus following injections of thiacetarsamide are reason to suspend therapy.

The dead worms as emboli may induce extensive inflammatory reaction in the lungs from 5 to 30 days after thiacetarsamide therapy. The clinical signs of elevated temperature and cough may be kept at a minimum by enforced rest. Rectal temperatures should be taken daily for 1 week after treatment. If there is a temperature elevation above 102 F (38.9C), an injection of prednisone or similar steroid should be given.

D) **Elimination of Microfilariae** — no microfilaricide has been developed that will always eliminate the microfilariae at the specific standard dose. All will have to be given to effect.

1) *Dithiazanine iodide* — the only product currently approved by FDA for use as a microfilaricide. It has been used in doses of 2 to 10 mg/lb (0.45 kg) per day, orally. Vomiting and diarrhea often accompany the use of this drug and it is potentially nephrotoxic. To minimize these effects, the lower dose, 2 mg/lb (0.45 kg) is recommended.

To eliminate microfilariae, give dithiazanine iodide at the rate of 2 mg/lb (0.45 kg) daily for 7 days.

If microfilariae are still present and if there has been little or no reaction to the drug, the dose may be increased to 5 mg/lb (0.45 kg). This dose is given daily until the blood is free from microfilariae, but not longer than 10 days.

2) *Fenthion* — an effective microfilaricidal agent, but it is no longer available commercially.

3) *Diethylcarbamazine* (DEC), when given to dogs with microfilariae may cause severe reactions, some of which may be fatal. For this reason, it should not be used as a microfilaricide. At any event, it is at best an indifferent microfilaricide against *D immitis*.

4) *Levamisole* — recently has been successfully used as a microfilaricide. This preparation is sold commercially for use in cattle, sheep and hogs but has not been approved by FDA for use in dogs; therefore, it must be considered an experimental drug.

It has been reported that 5 mg/lb (0.45 kg) of the active ingredient given orally each day without interruption, will usually eliminate all microfilariae within 6 to 12 days. The course of treatment evidently should not exceed 15 days. The blood is examined for microfilariae daily, starting after the 6th treatment, and treatment is terminated when the blood is free of microfilariae. The vomiting which frequently accompanies the use of this drug may be controlled by the administration of an anticholinergic agent such as atropine sulfate shortly before the levamisole is given. Occasionally, signs of restlessness or nervousness develop after a dose of levamisole. When this occurs, treatment should be discontinued.

Fewer undesirable reactions will occur in connection with the use of any microfilaricidal agent if at least 6 weeks have elapsed since thiacetarsamide was given to kill adult worms.

Occasionally, it is impossible to free a dog from microfilariae due to the fact that drug reactions may be severe enough to suspend treatment of to the fact that a particular dog may be refractory to the treatment. When this occurs, the blood should be examined 1 year later. If microfilariae are still present, the blood should be re-examined in another 3 months. If microfilariae are still present and more than 18 months have passed since thiacetarsamide therapy was given, reinfection may be assumed.

E) **Preventive Medication** — two methods of prevention have been shown to be effective.

1) *Diethylcarbamazine citrate* or *styrylpyridinium-diethylcarbamazine* administered orally — at the rate of 2.5 mg DEC citrate/lb (0.45 kg), which equals 1.25 mg DEC base/lb (0.45 kg) of body weight. To prevent heartworm infection, treatment must be started by the beginning of the mosquito season — preferable a little earlier — continued through the mosquito season and for two months thereafter. In places where mosquitoes may be active all year, medication must be given every day of the year.

a) An infected dog must first be treated with thiacetarsamide. This eliminates adult worms. Six weeks later the patient can be treated with a microfilaricide. After that, the dog can be started on prophylactic treatment with DEC. An adult dog with an unknown history of exposure and which is microfilariae-free may be started immediately on a preventive regimen with DEC. Its blood should be examined 3 months later and 6 months thereafter. A dog on a preventive routine with DEC should be examined for presence of microfilariae every 6 months.

b) Occasionally, in an enzootic area, one treatment may not be sufficient — even though the dog is subjected to the preventive routine with DEC after therapy. Continuous exposure may create a condition wherein all stages of the parasite are present in the dog at the time of treatment. The thiacetarsamide kills the adult worms; the microfilaricide eliminates the microfilarial stage. The DEC prevents development of larvae only after administration of the drug has started. Nothing yet known will kill larvae already migrating through the tissues, and some of these larvae may mature. Consequently, in this circumstance, a second treatment with thiacetarsamide may be required some months after the first.

c) Dogs that cannot tolerate DEC but continue to be exposed to mosquitoes in enzootic areas should be treated with thiacetarsamide.

2) *Thiacetarsamide* given in the therapeutic regimen, (*i.e.* 0.1 ml/lb twice a day for 2 or 3 days, at 6-month intervals) is an effective preventive agent — given with this frequency, the drug eliminates the worms before a sufficient number have developed to cause clinical disorders.

a) Many dogs in urban areas have little exposure to mosquitoes therefore, they need not be subjected to a preventive program. Such dogs should be examined for microfilariae when they are 1 year old and every 6 months thereafter. A concentration method (*e.g.* the modified Knott's technique) of microfilariae detection should always be used.

CHAPTER
# 12

# Insecticides

**History:** 1000 BC — sulfur was used for fumigation.
1300 AD — Marco Polo used oil to treat mange in camels.
1942 — DDT was marketed in the United States.
1950 s — organic phosphates were introduced.
1980 s — synthetic pyrethroids became available.

## Chlorinated Hydrocarbons

These compounds are poisonous to insects on contact, have good knock-down capacity, and kill quickly. They are absorbed through the chitinous cuticle of the insect, their residual effect is long-lasting everywhere, including in the environment. Many chlorinated hydrocarbons are known or suspected to be carcinogenic.

A. **DDT**
   1. **Chemistry**
      A) Dichloro, diphenyl, trichloro, ethane
      B) Insoluble in water
   2. **Not to be used on livestock or premises where livestock are housed** — complete ban is controversial.
   3. **Metabolism in animals**
      A) Poorly absorbed from the skin as powder or in water suspension
         1) An oily vehicle increases absorption of DDT
         2) Poorly absorbed from the GI tract
         3) Fat or fat solvents in the GI tract increase absorption of DDT
      B) Distribute to all tissues, but selectively distribute to fat. Will store in fat over a period of time and reach levels higher than

the level in the ration. They are cumulative.
C) Partly biotransformed by the liver
D) Excreted by kidney, both free and in metabolites
E) Excreted by mammary gland in the butterfat of milk

4. **Toxicity**
   A) DDT has a relatively wide margin of safety under common uses because little is absorbed into the blood.
   B) Order of decreasing species-susceptibility to DDT toxicity:

   | | | | |
   |---|---|---|---|
   | 1) Rodents | 4) Rabbit | 7) Swine | 10) Sheep |
   | 2) Cat | 5) Guinea pig | 8) Horse | 11) Goat |
   | 3) Dog | 6) Monkey | 9) Cow | |

   C) Large amounts of body fat protect animals.
   D) Young animals are especially susceptible.
   E) Fasted animals are especially susceptible.
   F) Toxic reations
      1) Stimulation of CNS produces tremors, incoordinated walk, convulsions, coma, respiratory failure and eventually death from respiratory paralysis.
      2) High body temperature
      3) Liver damage by high doses
      4) Will sensitize myocardium to epinephrine
   G) Treatment of toxicity
      1) Use a CNS depressant such as barbiturate anesthesia. Use with care.
      2) Remove the source.
   H) To reduce a body load of DDT, which is particularly useful in lactating dairy cows, administer:
      1) Phenobarbital in the feed. This speeds liver biotransformation of DDT via *enzyme induction.*
      2) Activated charcoal traps DDT and its metabolites in the GI tract for excretion with feces. Not greatly effective.

B. **METHOXYCHLOR**
   1. **Least toxic**
   2. **Little tendency to accumulate in body fat**
   3. **Little secretion into milk**

C. **OTHER CHLORINATED HYDROCARBONS**
   1. **Commonly used on livestock, in buildings, or on premises:**
      A) Toxaphene
      B) Lindane (gamma isomer of benzene hexachloride)
      C) Chlordane — used in buildings or on premises only

2. **Used as field sprays** (restricted use or banned):
   A) Aldrin               B) Dieldrin               C) Heptachlor

# Organophosphates and Polyphosphates

A. **HISTORY** — organophosphates resulted from studies of nerve gases in World War II.

B. **GENERAL PRINCIPLES**
   1. **Have good knock-down ability** — little residue. Residual ability depends on vehicles used in application. Organophosphates are noncumulative and do not saturate fat as do the chlorinated hydrocarbons.
   2. **Chemistry**
      A) Esters of phosphoric acid
      B) Highly soluble in water
   3. **Commonly used as worming agents** — alone or in combination with other agents
   4. **May be used on livestock or on buildings and premises as:**
      A) Sprays, dips or fogs
      B) Pour-on. A small amount poured on the back of an animal is absorbed and circulated throughout the body.
      C) Is given orally to dogs to control fleas.
   5. **Metabolism in animals**
      A) May be absorbed from the GI tract
      B) May be absorbed from the skin (some compounds quite quickly)
      C) Biotransformation
         1) Takes place in the liver microsomal systems
         2) The parent drug of some organophosphates is inactive and is quickly biotransformed to the active metabolite, then biotransformed to an inactive metabolite.
         3) Parathion (inactive) to paraoxon (active)
         4) Enzymes involved may be induced
      D) Excreted by kidney
         1) More quickly eliminated than chlorinated hydrocarbons; no tissue saturation
         2) Some are excreted in milk
      E) Distributed to all tissues
   6. **Organophosphates are extremely toxic** — some much more so than others. Some species of animals are especially sensitive to these drugs.

A) Brahman cattle may be more sensitive but this is apparently not a problem in the field.
B) Mechanism of toxicity is the same for insects and mammals.
  1) Organophosphates complex with and tie-up cholinesterases (inhibit cholinesterase), causing a build-up of ACH at the myoneural junction.
     a) Enzyme is phosphorylated and as such is inactive. Organophosphates have the ability to fit and phosphorylate certain specific amino acids (histidine or serine) on the cholinesterase.
     b) Reversal of complex depends on the substituent groups of the specific organophosphate. Some are less easily reversible, thus are more toxic to mammals than others.
     c) Aging of complex
        a) The longer the complex ages, the tighter it becomes.
        b) The older the complex, the more irreversible and more toxic.
  2) Inactive cholinesterases allow acetylcholine to build up and become excessive.
  3) Toxicity is caused by excess acetylcholine and an uncontrolled parasympathetic predominance, which results in:
     a) Poor gaseous exchange in the lungs
        a) Poor blood flow
        b) Constricted bronchioles and excess fluids
        c) Failure of respiratory muscles
     b) Blood pressure falls
        a) Slowed and weakened heart
        b) Vasodilation and decreased peripheral resistance
     c) Skeletal muscles are also affected; muscle-twitching is followed by progressive paralysis, including the respiratory muscles.
     d) Some CNS involvement occurs, such as stimulation, followed by hypoxia caused by depression.
C) Signs of toxicity:

  1) Defecation and urination
  2) Excess salivation (often watery)
  3) Muscle-twitching, then weakness
  4) Difficult and labored breathing
  5) Cyanosis
  6) Weak pulse
  7) Possible convulsions, coma, and death

D) Treatment of toxicity
1) Give large doses of atropine: 1 mg/kg, divided into two equal doses, the first given IV *slowly*, and the second SC.
2) PAM and 2-PAM pyridine-2-aldoxame methiodide:
    a) These are enzyme reactivators that restore free cholinesterase to normal levels.
    b) They complex with an organophosphate by pulling it off the enzyme, thus freeing the enzyme to act on the excess acetylcholine.
3) Remove the source of intoxication as soon as feasible.
    a) Wash skin.
    b) Empty GI tract.

## C. ORGANOPHOSPHATES USED ON LIVESTOCK AND BUILDINGS

1. **Coumaphos** — Co-Ral® (Haver-Lockhart)
2. **Ronnel** — Ectoral™ (Pitman-Moore), Korlan®, Trolene®, Steer Kleer®
3. **Crufomate** — Ruelene®
4. **Trichlorfon** — Neguvon® (Haver-Lockhart)
5. **Famphur** — Bo-Ana® (American Cyanamid)
6. **Dioxathion** — Co-Nav® (Wellcome/Jen-Sal)
7. **Malathion**
8. **Dichlorvos, DDVP** — Vapona® (Shell)
9. **Fenthion** — Tiguvon® (Haver-Lockhart), Lysoff® (Haver-Lockhart)
10. **Diazinon**
11. **Crotoxyphos** — Ciodrin®

## D. ORAL ORGANOPHOSPHATES — cythioate, (Proban® — (American Cyanamid), Ectoral™ (Pitman-Moore)

1. **For control of fleas in dogs; efficacy is not well documented.**
2. **Ingested organophosphates are absorbed by body fluids.** Fleas are killed when they ingest the dogs body fluids. The flea has already inflicted the damage.
3. **Not for use in Greyhounds** — they are extremely sensitive to organophosphates.
4. **Not for use in animals that are:**
    A) Pregnant     C) Under stress
    B) Sick         D) Recovering from surgery

E. **OTHER ORGANOPHOSPHATES**
1. **Field sprays** — parathion, EPN, systox
2. **Nerve gases** — tabun, sarin, soman

F. **ORGANOCARBAMATES**
1. **Action is similar to that of the organosphophates** — atropine is the antidote.
2. **Do not use 2-PAM to treat**
3. **Used on livestock:** Carbaryl (Sevin® — many manufacturers).
4. **Used in tick and flea collars for dogs:** Sendran® (Haver-Lockhart) and others.

G. **DRUGS TO BE AVOIDED OR USED WITH EXTREME CARE** — either simultaneously with, immediately before, or during an intoxication with organophosphates and carbamates.
1. **Morphine**
2. **Succinylcholine chloride**
3. **Phenothiazine-derivative tranquilizers**
4. **Thiobarbiturates**
5. **Neostigmine**
6. **Carbachol**

# Pyrethrins

A. **BOTANICAL ORIGIN**
1. **Quick kill** — no residue
2. **Use twice a day**
3. **Nontoxic to mammals**

# Rotenone - Derris Powder

A. **BOTANICAL ORIGIN**
1. **Used as fish poison**
2. **Not absorbed through the skin**
3. **Poorly absorbed through the GI tract**
4. **Toxic to mammals if systemic**

# Miscellaneous Insecticides

A. NICOTINE SULFATE — Black Leaf-40®
B. THIOCYANATES
C. BENZYL BENZOATE
D. SULFUR
E. PETROLEUM PRODUCTS
F. ARSENICALS

CHAPTER

# 13

# Histamines and Antihistamines

## Histamine

A. **BIOSYNTHESIZED FROM AND CLOSELY RELATED TO THE AMINO ACID, HISTIDINE**
   1. **Exists in a bound, inactive form** — a complex within the cell
   2. **Found in many tissues** — both plant and animal
      A) Exceptionally high levels are found in skin, intestinal mucosae, lungs, and smooth muscle of vessels.
      B) Exceptionally high concentrations are found in mast cells and in the basophil.
   3. **There is no evidence that histamine plays a physiological role in the normal body processes.**
   4. **Histamine is formed by bacterial action** — takes place in the intestine and in putrefaction.

B. **RELEASE OF HISTAMINE**
   1. **Histamine** — is released from its bound or complexed form within the cell by any form of insult to that cell.
   2. **After release** — the histamine diffuses out of the cell into the surrounding tissue.
   3. **Certain tissues in the body are more prone than others to release their histamine** — these tissues include:
      A) Histamine-releasing cells
      B) Allergic tissue cells
      C) Shock tissue cells

4. **Released histamine** — brings about a toxic reaction in the sensitive tissues.

5. **The toxic reaction** — may localize in single or multiple tissue sites or may be systemic (shock).

6. **Insults to the cells that have been implicated as being capable of causing the release of histamine:**
   A) Physical agents such as heat and cold
   B) Tissue trauma, crush
   C) Anoxia
   D) Toxins, including bacterial toxins and venoms
   E) Drugs such as morphine, procaine, amphetamine, curare, atropine, dextrans, surface-active agents and proteolytic enzymes
   F) Antigen-antibody reaction, such as occurs in an allergic reaction

## SUMMARY OF ALLERGIC REACTION

Initial Exposure · Antigen ⟶ Specific Antibody Production

Subsequent Exposure · Antigen + Specific Antibody ⟶ Antigen · Antibody Reaction

Antigen · Antibody Reaction Releases Toxic Substances:

Histamine and Serotonin, acetylcholine, heparin, kinins,

SRS (slow-reacting substance), and possibly others

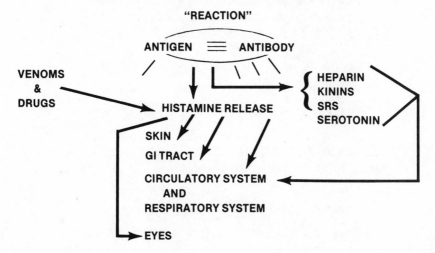

C. **RESPONSES TO HISTAMINE** — many of the disease conditions, such as allergy, are also manifestations of the concurrent responses to the other released toxins.

  1. **Skin**
    A) Pruritus (itching)
    B) Triple response
      1) Reddening caused by capillary dilation
      2) Blister formation caused by leaking of plasma from capillaries
      3) Flare, which is an extension of redness

  2. **Gastrointestinal tract**
    A) Edema of mucosa resulting from erosion and ulceration, which may lead to watery and then bloody diarrhea
    B) Stimulates secretion of HCl
    C) May inhibit functions of the ruminant stomach

  3. **Eye**
    A) Possible itching and swelling of conjunctivae
    B) Increased lacrimal secretions

  4. **Respiratory**
    A) Constricted bronchioles
    B) Edematous mucosa
    C) Increased secretions
    D) Itching of upper respiratory tract; coughing, sneezing, and nasal discharge

  5. **Cardiovascular**
    A) Dilation of arterioles and capillaries
    B) Spasm of the hepatic vein (in the dog), this results in stasis and pooling of blood in the liver.
    C) Increased permeability of capillaries
    D) Fall in mean blood pressure

  6. **Uterus**
    A) Stimulates smooth muscle contractions in most species
    B) Not in the rat

D. **DESTROYED IN TISSUES BY HISTAMINASE** — not a therapeutic tool

E. **THERAPEUTIC PRINCIPLES** for conditions involving the release of histamine and/or other cell toxins:

| | |
|---|---|
| **Allergy** | **Crush syndrome** |
| **Anaphylactic shock** | **Drug hypersensitivity** |
| **Endotoxic shock** | **Inflammatory response** |

1. An emergency antidote for anaphylactic shock is epinephrine — causes a physiological antagonism and opposite effect.
2. Antihistamines — receptor blockade is the mechanism; specific for histamine.
3. Corticosteroids — protect cells from insult due to released toxins.
4. Tranquilizers—Phenergan® (Wyeth), Temaril® (Norden); these tranquilizers belong also to the antihistamine group.

# Antihistamines

A. **GENERAL FORMULA**

1. **Antihistamines are substituted ethyl amines**

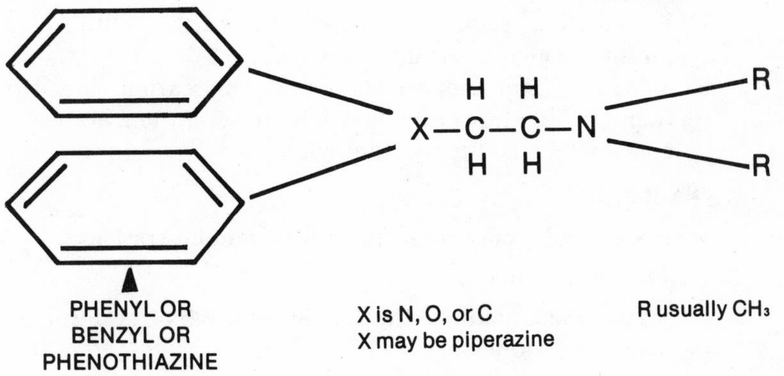

PHENYL OR
BENZYL OR
PHENOTHIAZINE

X is N, O, or C
X may be piperazine

R usually $CH_3$

B. **RESPONSES**

1. **Related to histamine antagonism**

A) This is a *competitive antagonism;* the antihistamines compete for receptor sites.

B) They *do not* interfere with synthesis, storage or release of histamine.

C) Therapeutic implications of this concept:

1) The actions relate to keeping histamine off of the cell receptors.

      2) They do not alleviate results of cell damage caused by histamine.

      3) Antihistamines are more effective in prophylaxis or as early therapy than after histamine has done its damage.

      4) They do not alter responses of the cells to other released cell toxins.

    D) Antagonize the histamine actions to varying degrees

  **2. Organ system responses are caused by the antihistamine itself — not by histamine antagonism.**

    A) Central nervous system

      1) Most antihistamines are CNS depressants. Some are more potent than others.

      2) CNS response depends upon the drug, the dose, and the individual patient.

      3) Large doses may stimulate the CNS.

    B) Local anesthesia may occur in varying degrees.

    C) Heart

      1) Anti-arrythmia effect

      2) Decreased contractile force

    D) Vasodilation. Rapid IV injection may cause a fall in blood pressure which is usually transient.

    E) Some antihistamines are cholinergic, muscarinic, blockers.

    F) Rapid IV administration may inhibit respiration, even cause apnea which is usually transient.

## C. METABOLISM

  **1. Well absorbed from oral or parenteral administration**

  **2. Uniformly distributed**

  **3. Biotransformed mainly in the liver** — some is biotransformed in the lungs and kidneys.

  **4. Excreted by kidney**

  **5. Duration of action up to six hours**

## D. THERAPEUTIC PRINCIPLES

  **1. Indicated in all types of allergic diseases**

      A) Urticaria      C) Stomatitis

      B) Asthma        D) Edemas

  **2. Indicated where the disease is accompanied by death of cells and/or release of toxins** — such as in excessive tissue destruction, gangrenous mastitis, or retained placenta

  **3. Indicated in cases where drugs or venoms have released histamine:**

      A) Insect stings     B) Snake bites

  **4. Indicated in respiratory conditions such as emphysema**

5. Use IV with great care — use part dose and give slowly

6. May be indicated in early inflammatory conditions

7. May be indicated to dry up secretions of respiratory tract. Antihistamines aid breathing and improve sense of smell in respiratory diseases.

E. **FORMULARY**

1. **Diphenhydramine** — Benadryl® (Parke-Davis)

2. **Dimenhydrinate** — Dramamine® (Searle)

3. **Meclizine** — Bonine® (Pfizer), Antivert® (Roerig)

4. **Cyclizine** — Marezine® (Burroughs Wellcome)

5. **Promethazine** — Phenergan® (Wyeth)

6. **Tripelennamine** — Pyribenzamine® (Ciba), Re-covr® (Squibb)

7. **Chlorpheniramine** — Chlor-trimeton® (Schering), Teldrin® (SmithKline French)

8. **Pyrilamine** — Histavet-P (Burns-Biotec), Anti-Tuss with Antihistamine (Med-Tech)

9. **Methapyrilene**

10. **Antihistamine with adrenergic: pyrilamine plus ephedrine** (many manufacturers)

11. **Antihistamine with corticosteroid: chlorpheniramine plus prednisone**

12. **Antihistamine with steroid and antibiotic** (penicillin and streptomycin) chlorpheniramine is the antihistamine used in Azimycin® (Schering), and Combisteroid® (Pfizer).

CHAPTER

# 14

# Drugs Acting Upon the Uterus

## Ergot

Ergot is a fungus (*claviceps purpurea*) that grows on grain of cereals (rye) and on some pasture grasses. Officially ergot for commercial use is from rye.

A. **HISTORY**
1. **Ergotism** — plague that affected people who consumed rye that had been parasitized with ergot

   A) Gangrenous — known as *St. Anthony's Fire*
   B) Convulsive type
2. **Used by midwives in obstetric work**

B. **ASSAY** — by the cock's comb test
1. **Ergot alkaloids produce cyanosis in the comb of birds** — due to vasoconstriction of small arterioles, which causes thrombosis.
2. **The degree of cyanosis is proportionate to the alkaloid concentration.**

C. **CHEMISTRY** — ergot contains many substances.
1. **Important alkaloids of ergot:**
   A) Ergotamine    B) Ergonovine    C) Ergotoxine
2. **All are derivatives of lysergic acid.**
3. **Ergot contains amines and other nitrogen compounds:**
   A) Acetylcholine    B) Choline    C) Histamine

D. **RESPONSES**

1. **Action groups of ergot alkaloids cause:**
   A) Smooth-muscle contraction of the
      1) Uterus                    2) Blood vessels
   B) Alpha adrenergic blockade
   C) CNS stimulation

2. **Ergotamine tartrate** — not used in veterinary medicine.
   A) It is a potent vasoconstrictor and adrenergic blocking agent which was used to first demonstrate "epi-reversal".
   B) Uterine action is less potent.
   C) CNS is first stimulated, then depressed.
   D) Cardiovascular response is an increase in blood pressure. In human medicine it is used as a vasoconstrictor for treatment of migraine headache.
   E) It is effective only when given orally.

3. **Ergonovine maleate** — Ergonil™ (Pitman-Moore)
   A) It is the principal alkaloid from ergot for uterine use.
   B) It has almost an exclusive oxytocic action.
   C) Causes less vasoconstriction
   D) More easily absorpted from IM or SC routes
   E) Uterine responses to ergonovine:
      1) Prompt and powerful contractions
      2) Activity related to the physiological status of the uterus. It is most efficient at parturition and immediately post-partum.
      3) Estrogen renders the myometrium more sensitive to ergonovine. (Progesterone renders the myometrium less sensitive to ergonovine.)
   F) Small doses of ergonovine have no effect on blood pressure.
   G) Methyl ergonovine maleate is formed by adding a $CH_3$ on the alkyl side chain.
      1) Fewer adrenergic effects  2) More-potent uterine activity

E. **TOXICITY OF ERGOT**

1. **Acute** CNS system stimulation and convulsions
2. **Chronic**
   A) Abortion
   B) Lameness; extremities may slough off as a result of vasoconstriction.

   Stiffness ➝ Lameness ➝ Gangrene ➝ Sloughing

   C) Diarrhea

# Drugs Derived from the
# Posterior Pituitary

A. **CHEMISTRY** (polypeptides) — species differences occur.

B. **ACTIVE PRINCIPLES FROM POSTERIOR PITUITARY**
  1. **Oxytocin**
     A) Uterine contractions
     B) Myoepithelial contraction occurs in the mammary gland
  2. **Antidiuretic hormone (ADH)** — Pitressin® (Parke-Davis)
     A) Increases arterial pressure by vasconstriction
     B) Reduces urine formation — useful in certain types of diabetes insipidus

C. **RESPONSES**
  1. **Antidiuretic hormone (ADH)**
     A) Contraction of smooth muscles in the arterioles
     B) Contraction of smooth muscles in the gastrointestinal tract
     C) Contractility from the heart is weakened and cardiac output is decreased if ADH is given in large amounts. Hypoxia of the heart may result from constriction of the coronary artery.
     D) Increases tubular resorption of water. This action is on the kidney tubule cells, thus reducing urine formation.

  2. **Oxytocin**
     A) Causes a contraction of the smooth muscles of the uterus
        1) Varies with species, stage of pregnancy, and the amount of stress on the animal
        2) Enhanced by estrogen
        3) Inhibited by progesterone
     B) Causes a contraction of the myoepithelium of the mammary gland. May increase cistern pressure in the udder by 10 to 15 mmHg.
     C) Action on the smooth muscles of the arterioles is usually vasodilation.
        1) Causes a tendency toward hypotension
     D) Formulary
        1) Pitocin® (Parke-Davis), P.O.P.® (Burns-Biotec), Uteracon® , Vetocin®
        2) Generic oxytocin
        3) Most contain 20 units/ml
     E) Indications
        1) Induces and aids in labor
        2) Control of postpartum hemorrhage

3) Aids in removal of retained fetal membranes
4) Stimulates milk let-down as a therapeutic aid in:
   a) Mastitis in cattle, sheep and goats
   b) Mastitis - metritis - agalactia syndrome (MMA) in sows
5) Pyometra

# Other Uterine
# Smooth-Muscle Stimulators

A. **CARBACHOL** — has been used in sows.

B. **SPARTEINE**, an alkaloid, has a quinidine-like effect on the heart.

C. **QUININE SULFATE** — has been used in treatment for postpartum discharge in the bitch.

D. **PROSTAGLANDINS** — presently used in human medicine.

1. **$E_2$ and $F_2$ alpha**

2. **Administered orally or by IV**

CHAPTER

# 15

# Local Anesthetics

A.  **REVERSIBLE BLOCK** — conduction of nerve impulses is blocked and/or propagation of impulses is prevented.

B.  **METHODS OF PRODUCING LOCAL ANESTHESIA**
    1. **Physical**
       A) *Thermal* — cold or ice applied directly to the area. Ice or a highly volatile spray such as ethyl chloride is used.
       B) *Mechanical* — pressure is applied to the area.
    2. **Chemical**
       A) *Permanent* — may last for weeks, months or years. Ethyl alcohol or quinine is injected into the nerve proper.
       B) *Transient* — reversible within a few minutes — common local anesthetics.

C.  **LOCAL ANESTHETICS** — may provide 3 of the 4 basic components of balanced anesthesia. The animal remains awake. Neither mental block nor hypnosis is achieved.

    1. **Analgesia**     2. **Relaxation**          3. **Hyporeflexia**

D.  **PROPERTIES OF AN IDEAL LOCAL ANESTHETIC**
    1. **Soluble in water** — should be stable and almost neutral in pH
    2. **Produces minimal irritation at the site of injection**
    3. **Specific effect** — on sensory nerve endings and/or nerve fibers
    4. **Poor absorption from injection site** — provides longer-lasting local action, and less drug enters the systemic circulation
    5. **Minimal systemic toxicity**
    6. **Duration of effect and recovery** — should be predictable and controllable
    7. **Should not be addictive**
    8. **Produces a reversible local anesthesia**

## E. CHEMISTRY

1. **Prototype** — procaine

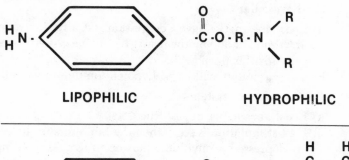

**LIPOPHILIC**

**HYDROPHILIC**

**PROCAINE**

2. **Weak bases** — slightly soluble and unstable in solution

3. **Acid salts are used** — usually hydrochlorides, because they are water-soluble and stable

## F. MECHANISM OF ACTION

1. **Prevents both generation and conduction of the nerve impulse**

2. **Will prevent passage of the impulse at:**
   A) Sensory-nerve endings
   B) Nerve trunk
   C) Gap transmission. Interferes with the depolarization of the postjunctional membrane.

3. **Acts on membranes** — principal action site
   A) Interferes with generation and propagation of the nerve-action potential
   B) Inhibits the large transient increase in the permeability of the membrane to sodium ions
   C) Threshold for electrical excitability is increased
   D) May be related to competition with the calcium ion
   E) Membranes cannot be depolarized

4. **Must penetrate nerve fibers**
   A) Injected as acid salts
   B) Must be neutralized in the tissues with free base liberated
   C) Free base penetrates the tissues
   D) Acid tissue media such as pus or infections may inhibit activity

G. **ORGAN SYSTEM RESPONSES** — absorption of a local anesthetic could affect other organ systems.

    1. **Cardiovascular**

        A) Local anesthetics have a depressant, negative inotrope, anti-arrythmia action on the heart. Lidocaine is used therapeutically for this purpose.

        B) Toxic amounts will cause hypotension due to vasodilation.

    2. **Central nervous system**

        A) Local anesthetics depress the CNS.

        B) First stimulation is seen, then the inhibitors in the synapses are depressed. Convulsions may occur as a result of high systemic levels.

        C) Depression follows.

H. **METABOLISM**

    1. **Absorption from the injection site is fairly rapid** — occurs in minutes.

    2. **Fate**

        A) Hydrolysis of esters produces inactive metabolites; occurs in the plasma.

        B) Hepatic biotransformation

        C) Species variability in the rate of inactivation

        D) Urinary excretion of free drug and metabolites

        E) A metabolite, para amino benzoic acid, antagonizes the action of sulfonamides. This occurs with procaine but not with lidocaine.

I. **Toxicity**

    1. **Hypersensitivity may occur** — results in allergy, asthma or anaphylactic shock.

    2. **Central nervous system**

        A) Restlessness, excitement, tremors, clonic convulsions occur initially.

        B) Depression of the vital centers, principally the respiratory tract, follows.

    3. **Cardiovascular collapse results in death.**

    4. **Treatment**

        A) Oxygen and artificial respiration

        B) Convulsive state responds to:

            1) Succinylcholine given IV. Administer carefully.

            2) Light doses of ultra-short-acting barbiturates

        C) Respiratory analeptics are contraindicated.

## J.  FORMULARY

1. **Procaine** — Novocain® (Winthrop)
   A) Poor topically     B) Lethal to parakeets

2. **Lidocaine** — Xylocaine® (Astra)
   A) Topical or injected; systemically as an antiarrhythmia agent
   B) More potent than procaine

3. **Hexylcaine**
   A) Topical and injected     B) More potent than procaine

4. **Mepivacaine** — Carbocaine-V® (Winthrop)
   A) More potent than procaine     B) Injection

5. **Tetracaine** — Pontocaine® (Winthrop); topical and injection

6. **Dibucaine** — Nupercaine® (Ciba); topical

7. **Butacaine sulfate** — Butyn® (Abbott); topical, insoluble

8. **Dyclonine** — Dyclone® (Dow); topical

9. **Proparacaine** — Ophthaine® (Squibb); topical (eye)

10. **Ethyl aminobenzoate** — Benzocaine® (many manufacturers); topical

11. **Ethyl aminobenzoate with butyl aminobenzoate and tetracaine** — Cetacaine® (Haver-Lockhart); topical

## K.  CLINICAL APPLICATIONS

1. **Topical**
   A) Mucous membranes of the ear, eye, mouth and urethra
   B) Not effective on unbroken skin
   C) Ointment form has slight effect

2. **Infiltration to anesthetize nerve endings**
   A) Intradermal route gives an immediate response.
   B) Subcutaneous route results in rapid onset with diffusion, leakage, and absorption.

3. **Conduction block** — local injection into the immediate area of nerve(s) to be blocked.
   A) Nerve block to relieve pain for diagnosis
   B) Paravertebral block — injection into an area where spinal nerves leave the intervertebral foramina
   C) Epidural — injection into the eqidural space of the spinal canal. Useful in:
   1) Cesarean section 2) Obstetric-gynecologic manipulations
   3) Caudectomy     4) Mammectomy

4. **Drug combinations sometimes used with local anesthetics:**
   A) Vasoconstrictors are used to increase duration of action.
   1) Reduce chances of systemic reactions

2) Epinephrine, ephedrine, Neo-Synephrine® (Winthrop)

B) Hyaluronidase is used to enlarge the area of anesthesia — increases chance of systemic reactions.

## L. COCAINE

1. **An alkaloid from the leaves of the coca tree**
2. **An ester of benzoic acid**
3. **Actions**
   A) Blocks generation and conduction of nerve impulses. It is an excellent local anesthetic.
   B) CNS stimulant (depression of inhibitory neurons)
      1) It acts from the cortex downward.
      2) Some evidence exists that mental powers are improved.
      3) May increase capacity for muscular work, probably because of a lessened sense of fatigue.
      4) Convulsions may follow.
      5) Is followed by depression which occurs via neuronal fatigue.
   C) Cardiovascular
      1) Vasoconstriction, tachycardia, increased blood pressure
      2) Cardiovascular collapse occurs later.
      3) Potentiates adrenergic response. Prevents re-entry of norepinephrine into the nerve ending.
   D) Increases body temperature
4. **Death from respiratory paralysis** — central in origin
5. **Too toxic to use therapeutically by injection**
6. **Psychological dependence may develop in man**
7. **Widely abused as a street drug**

# 16
# Locally Acting External Medications

## Demulcents

A. **CHEMISTRY**
   1. **Water-soluble** — substances of high molecular weight
   2. **Gums, starches, mucilages are examples**

B. **ACTIONS**
   1. **Alleviate irritations** — have a soothing effect
   2. **Form protective coatings** — protect underlying tissues

C. **DRUGS**
   1. **Acacia** (gum arabic)
   2. **Tragacanth** (gum tragacanth)
   3. **Glycerin** (glycerol) — absorbs water. In high concentration it is somewhat dehydrating and irritating.
   4. **Propylene glycol**
   5. **Polyethylene glycols**

## Emollients

A. **FATS AND OILS**

B. **ACTIONS**
   1. **Protectant**
   2. **Soften the skin** — makes it more pliable
   3. **Used as drug vehicles**

C.  **DRUGS**

    1. **Vegetable oils**

        A)  Olive oil        C)  Corn oil        E)  Peanut oil

        B)  Cottonseed oil    D)  Almond oil    F)  Theobroma oil

                                                      (cocoa butter)

    2. **Animal fats**

        A)  Lanolin (wool fat) — contains 25-30% water

        B)  Lard

    3. **Hydrocarbons**

        A)  Paraffin        C)  White petrolatum (Vaseline®)

        B)  Petrolatum    D)  Mineral oil

    4. **Waxes**

        A)  White wax (bleached beeswax)    B)  Yellow wax (beeswax)

# Protectants and Adsorbents

A.  **INSOLUBLE AND INERT SUBSTANCES**

B.  **ACTIONS**

    1. **Cover the skin** — protect it

    2. **Form an adherent,** continuous, flexible or semi-rigid coating

    3. **Some adsorb foreign material** such as gases, toxins or bacteria

C.  **DRUGS**

    1. **Dusting powders**

        A)  Talc, zinc oxide, boric acid, starch

        B)  Zinc stearate and magnesium stearate are not wetted by moisture and will not form a crust.

        C)  Calamine — zinc oxide with ferric oxide

    2. **Mechanical protectants**

        A)  Collodion. Flexible collodion seals the surface against air, which is not always desirable.

        B)  Petrolatum gauze

        C)  Zinc gelatin (zinc oxide plus gelatin)

        D)  Dimethicone (Silicote® — Arnar-Stone) — a silicone oil

# Astrigents

A. **LOCALLY PRECIPITATE PROTEINS** — little penetration. Only the surface of cells is affected.

B. **DRUGS**
   1. **Metallic ions**
      A) Silver      C) Mercury
      B) Zinc        D) Aluminum
   2. **Tannic acid** (tannin, gallotannic acid)
      A) Toughens intact skin
      B) Forms a film when applied to abraded tissue
      C) Used orally as an antidote to certain chemical poisons. It forms an insoluble complex with many heavy metals, alkaloids, and glycosides, inhibiting their absorption.
      D) Are hepatotoxic if absorbed

# Irritants — Inflammatory Agents

Intended to produce a local, acute inflammatory response

A. **ACTIONS**
   1. **Increased circulation** — causes vasodilation, which increases blood flow to the area.
   2. **Movement of more leukocytes to an area**
   3. **Increased nutrient supply to a given area**
   4. **Improved venous and lymphatic drainage from an area**
   5. **Counterirritant**
      A) Irritates the surface of the skin
      B) Irritates afferent nerve impulses from the skin to the CNS
      C) Efferent vasomotor fibers will carry impulses to the deeper structures and visceral organs, causing vasodilation and increased blood flow.

B. **THERAPEUTIC RESPONSES**
   1. **Relief of pain**
   2. **Relief of muscle spasms**
   3. **Restoration of integrity and function to chronically insulted tissues**

C. **SUMMARY OF AGENTS THAT MAY BE USED**
   1. **Physical**
      A) Heat       C) Ultrasound
      B) Radiation    D) Diathermy

2. **Chemical** (drugs used as local irritants)
    A) Terms
        1) *Rubefacient* — causes mild local hyperemia
            a) Liniments       c) Braces
            b) Sweats          d) Paints
        2) *Blisterer or vesicant* — causes a more severe reaction. Plasma escapes and collects under skin to form blisters.
    B) Drugs usually found in combinations:

    | | |
    |---|---|
    | 1) Camphor | 6) Oil of wintergreen (methyl salicylate) |
    | 2) Alcohol | 7) Capsicum (cayenne and red pepper) |
    | 3) Iodine | 8) Cantharides (Spanish fly and Russian fly) |
    | 4) Chloroform | 9) Black mustard |
    | 5) Menthol | 10) Red iodide of mercury |

D. **SODIUM OLEATE** — Osteum® (Schering)

1. **For parenteral use as a sterile solution**

2. **Stimulates formation of fibrous and fibrocartilagenous tissue**

# Anti-Seborrheics

A. **REDUCES SEBUM** — especially in seborrheic dermatitis, which may be "cleaned up".

B. **DRUGS**

1. **Salicylates, benzoic acid, resorcinol**

2. **Sulfur**

3. **Selenium sulfide** — Seleen® (Abbott)

4. **Potassium tetrathionate** — Thionium® (Wellcome/Jen-Sal)

5. **Cadmium sulfide**

# Keratolytics

A. **ACTIONS**

1. **Cause desquamation of epithelium**

2. **Mechanically rid the area of invading microorganisms**

3. **Make underlying layers more accessible to medication**

B.  DRUGS
    1.  Benzoic acid
    2.  Salicylic acid, sodium salicylate

# Caustics, Escharotics

A.  ACTIONS
    1.  Cause destruction of tissue at the site of application
    2.  Inhibit formation of excessive granulation tissue

B.  DRUGS
    1.  Silver nitrate          4.  Phenol
    2.  Alum                    5.  Podophyllum resin
    3.  Glacial acetic acid     6.  Trichloracetic acid

# Enzymes

A.  ACTIONS
    1.  Liquefy purulent debris and exudates — proteolytic effect
    2.  Break down inflammatory barriers
    3.  Fibrinolysis — dissolve blood clots
    4.  Debride wounds
    5.  Do not affect living cells

B.  APPLICATIONS
    1.  Cuts, wounds, abrasions, and burns
    2.  Intratracheally
    3.  Intramammary
    4.  Fistulous tracts — abscesses
    5.  As solution, aerosol, or ointment

C.  DRUGS
    1.  Pancreatic dornase — Dornavac® (Merck, Sharp & Dohme)
        A) Desoxyribonuclease is the enzyme.
        B) Beef pancreas is the source.
    2.  Kymar® (Burns-Biotec) — pancreatic enzymes
    3.  Streptokinase and streptodornase — Varidase® (Lilley)
        A) Streptokinase with streptodornase and human plasminogen
        B) Bacterial origin

    C) Streptokinase plus plasminogen (plasmin). Plasmin is a proteolytic enzyme.

    D) Local or parenteral use

4. **Elase®** (Parke-Davis)

    A) Combination of fibrinolysin of bovine serum origin and desoxyribonuclease

    B) Bovine pancreas origin

5. **Trypsin Granulex®** (Hickam)

    A) Metrizyme® — uterine medication

    B) Tryptar-Vet®

    C) Trypzyme® (Burns-Biotec)

6. **Collagenase** — Sanytl® (Knoll) — digests denatured collagen

7. **Travase®** (Flint) — sutilains; proteolytic enzymes elaborated with *Bacillus subtilis*

CHAPTER

# 17

# Expectorants
# and
# Cough Medicines

## Expectorants

A.  **ACTIONS**
1.  **Local effect on mucous membranes**
2.  **Increase secretions of upper respiratory tract** — make exudate more watery and less viscous
3.  **Promote removal of exudate and mucus from respiratory tract**
4.  **Some act directly on the cells of the respiratory tract**
5.  **Some act by reflex stimulation** — reflex irritation stimulates cells of the respiratory tract. Many expectorants are sub-threshold emetics and gastric irritants.

B.  **MOST ARE GIVEN ORALLY**
1.  **May be applied by inhalation**
2.  **May be given parenterally**

C.  **DRUGS THAT MAY BE USED AS EXPECTORANTS**
1.  **Volatile organic oils**
    A) Terpin hydrate       D) Eucalyptus
    B) Anise                E) Menthol
    C) Pine
2.  **Ammonium chloride**
3.  **Ipecac**
4.  **Guaiacol or guaifenesin**
5.  **Iodides** (sodium, potassium, and organic)
6.  **Chloroform** — no longer a legal ingredient in animal drugs
7.  **Sodium and potassium citrates**

8. **Proteolytic enzymes**
9. **Sulfonamides**
10. **Paregoric**
11. **Cholinergics**
12. **Mucolytics** — Allevaire®, Tergemist®

# Antitussives

A. **COUGHING**
1. **A reflex action** — the cough center in the brain controls coughing.
2. **Irritation in the upper respiratory tract signals the brain** — initiates coughing.

B. **ACTIONS OF COUGH MEDICATIONS**
1. **Suppress coughing**
2. **Relieve symptoms**
3. **Have no curative powers** — they may mask signs; therefore, the primary cause must be diagnosed and treated..

C. **DRUGS** — by type of mechanism:
1. **Expectorants** — make the cough more productive; hence removing the offending material and lessening the stimulation for further coughing.
2. **Bronchodilators** — reduce bronchospasm
 A) Aminophylline B) Isoproterenol, epinephrine, ephedrine
3. **Antihistamines** — Phenergan® (Wyeth), Benadryl® (Parke-Davis)
 A) Reduce bronchospasm
 B) Exert some central action on the cough center
4. **Corticosteroids** — reduce inflammatory stimuli if the tissue is involved
5. **CNS depressants** — inhibit the cough center
 A) *Opiate group* — codeine and codeine derivatives
 B) *Dextromethorphan*
 C) *Noscapine* — Vetinol® (Summit Hill).
 D) Many synthetics
6. **Temaril-P®** (Norden) — trimeprazine (phenothiazine derivative tranquilizer) plus prednisolone (glucocorticosteroid)
7. **Benylin®** (Parke-Davis) — Benadryl® with ammonium

chloride, menthol, and sodium citrate

8. **Levopropoxyphene** — Respireze®

9. **Butorphanol** (Torbutrol® — Beecham) for SC injection in dogs
   A) A synthetic opiate (narcotic type)
   B) A potent inhibitor of the cough center
   C) Has additive action with other CNS depressants
   D) Large doses may cause respiratory depression
   E) Action is reversed by Nalline® or Naloxone®

# Hyaluronidase

A. **A MUCOLYTIC ENZYME**
   1. **Produced from bovine testes**
   2. **Actions**
      A) Hydrolyzes and depolymerizes hyaluronic acid
      B) Hyaluronic acid (a mucopolysaccharide) is an essential component of an intercellular ground substance, intercellular "cement". It is a tissue barrier to fluid diffusion.
      C) Hyaluronidase breaks down the barriers and dramatically increases diffusion of fluids.

B. **CLINICAL APPLICATION**
   1. **Used as a "spreading factor"**
   2. **Increases tissue penetration and absorption into blood of fluids injected SC**
   3. **Fluid therapy by hypodermoclysis**
   4. **Local anesthesia — to enlarge the area anesthetized**
   5. **Enhances removal of exudates**

C. **DRUGS**
   1. **Haglodase®**
      A) Wydase® (Wyeth), Alidase® (Searle), Hyazyme® (Abbott)
   2. **Assay**
      A) Turbidity Reducing Units (TR) = USP Units

CHAPTER

# 18

# Chemotherapy of Cancer

## Principles of Cancer or Neoplasia

A. **CANCER IS A DISEASE OF CELLS.** It is characterized by inhibition or loss of normal cellular control and the maturation mechanism that regulates multiplication.

B. **CELL MULTIPLICATION** is controlled by DNA and RNA.

1. **Disruption in the biochemical make-up or control schemes of DNA and RNA may result in neoplastic growth or tumors.**

2. **Some investigators feel that cells are restrained from becoming cancerous (no control of multiplication) by several independent genes and tumors develop only when mutations accumulate in all of those genes within a single line of cells.** The mutations are seldom spontaneous but are apparently caused by carcinogenic factors such as certain chemicals or possibly certain viruses.

C. **THE ROLE OF BODY DEFENSE MECHANISM** as a means of limiting cancer growth is not clear, but evidently is a major one.

D. **THE GOAL OF ANY CANCER TREATMENT** must be to kill 100% of the neoplastic cells.

E. **CANCER TREATMENT METHODS**

1. Surgery
2. Ionizing radiation
3. Immunotherapy
4. Chemotherapy

# Principles of
# Cancer Chemotherapy

A. **DIAGNOSIS AND PATIENT SELECTION**
  1. Not all animals with cancer can be treated with drugs.
  2. The nature of the neoplasm must be determined.
     A) All cancers are not equally sensitive to drugs.
     B) Certain drugs are best suited for certain cancers.
     C) Sometimes the therapy is worse than the disease.
  3. The stage and spread of the neoplasm must be determined.
  4. The patient's clinical condition must be evaluated.
  5. Chemotherapy of a severely debilitated animal is usually not effective and often dangerous.

B. **CHEMOTHERAPY IS USUALLY PALLIATIVE RATHER THAN CURATIVE;** it may extend life for a few months.

C. **THE LIFE CYCLE OF THE CELL**
  1. Chromosome replication occurs during the period of DNA synthesis or S-Phase.
  2. Period of RNA sythesis is the period of protein synthesis.
  3. Mitotic phase is the period of cell division.
  4. Period of resting (gap period) this varies in duration.
  5. Daughter cells may repeat the cycle, beginning at phase 1.

D. **CANCER DRUGS ARE MOST EFFECTIVE DURING THE S-PHASE OF THE CELL CYCLE.** They are also effective during the RNA synthesis phase.

E. **COMBINATIONS ARE USED AND MAY BE EFFECTIVE**
  1. **Drug plus drug** — by attacking at different stages of the cell cycle, the two drugs may have greatly increased efficacy.
  2. **Ionizing radiation plus drug**

F. **SUPPORTIVE THERAPY**
  1. **Proper hydration**
  2. **Transfusions of blood and erythrocytes or platelets may be necessary.**
  3. **Monitoring of uric acid levels may be needed. If levels are high, allopurinol (Zyloprim® —Burroughs Wellcome) is given. This enhances the excretion of uric acid.**

G.  **TOXICITY OF CANCER DRUGS**

1.  Most drugs used in cancer chemotherapy lack specificity for tumor tissue — depression of normal cells may be difficult to prevent.

2.  Normal cells are affected to varying degrees.

3.  Most treatments require an intoxicating dose of the drug.

4.  Risk *versus* benefit must be evaluated.

5.  The death rate as a result of treatment is estimated to be 10%.

6.  Most common and earliest toxic reactions are manifested in the bone marrow and the epithelial lining of the mouth and GI tract. Cells in these areas reproduce rapidly and are highly susceptible to the toxic, suppressive action of anticancer drugs.
    A) Bone marrow depression
       1) Depressed production of platelets
       2) Depressed production of WBCs
       3) Depressed production of RBCs
    B) Alimentary tract
       1) Lesions and hemorrhage of gums and mouth
       2) Nausea and vomiting
       3) Diarrhea

7.  Other adverse effects:
    A) Severe immunosuppression and increased susceptibility to infections
    B) Alopecia
    C) Cystitis
    D) Chromosomal damage
    E) Teratogenicity
    F) Hepatotoxicity
    G) Hyperpigmentation
    H) Anorexia
    I) Neurotoxicity (5-fluorouracil)
       1) Hyperexcitability, tremors, ataxia
       2) Loss of consciousness and motor seizures

8.  Must constantly evaluate the patient and watch for signs of toxicity, then adjust the dosage regimen accordingly by giving less drug or administering the drug less often.

## H. DOSAGE SHOULD BE BASED UPON SURFACE AREA OF BODY

1. Square meters ($m^2$) is the unit of measurement — said to be more accurate because it reduces the likelihood of toxic reactions.

### Conversion Table of Weight to Body-Surface Area in Meters for Dogs

| Kg | $M^2$ | Kg | $M^2$ |
|------|------|------|------|
| 0.5 | 0.06 | 26.0 | 0.88 |
| 1.0 | 0.10 | 27.0 | 0.90 |
| 2.0 | 0.15 | 28.0 | 0.92 |
| 3.0 | 0.20 | 29.0 | 0.94 |
| 4.0 | 0.25 | 30.0 | 0.96 |
| 5.0 | 0.29 | 31.0 | 0.99 |
| 6.0 | 0.33 | 32.0 | 1.01 |
| 7.0 | 0.36 | 33.0 | 1.03 |
| 8.0 | 0.40 | 34.0 | 1.05 |
| 9.0 | 0.43 | 35.0 | 1.07 |
| 10.0 | 0.46 | 36.0 | 1.09 |
| 11.0 | 0.49 | 37.0 | 1.11 |
| 12.0 | 0.52 | 38.0 | 1.13 |
| 13.0 | 0.55 | 39.0 | 1.15 |
| 14.0 | 0.58 | 40.0 | 1.17 |
| 15.0 | 0.60 | 41.0 | 1.19 |
| 16.0 | 0.63 | 42.0 | 1.21 |
| 17.0 | 0.66 | 43.0 | 1.23 |
| 18.0 | 0.69 | 44.0 | 1.25 |
| 19.0 | 0.71 | 45.0 | 1.26 |
| 20.0 | 0.74 | 46.0 | 1.28 |
| 21.0 | 0.76 | 47.0 | 1.30 |
| 22.0 | 0.78 | 48.0 | 1.32 |
| 23.0 | 0.81 | 49.0 | 1.34 |
| 24.0 | 0.83 | 50.0 | 1.36 |
| 25.0 | 0.85 | | |

The conversion table is based upon the following formula:

$$\frac{Kg\ 0.67}{10} = M^2$$

REFERENCE: Ettinger, S.J.: *Textbook of Veterinary Internal Medicine,* Vol. 1, W.B. Saunders, Philadelphia, Pa., 1975.

2. **As weight increases,** body surface increases to a lesser degree. The more the animal weighs, the greater the difference between its weight and its body surface. The required dose is less, compared to a dose based strictly on body weight. This explains the reduced likelihood of toxicity but with efficacy retained.

## GRAPHIC RELATIONSHIP OF WEIGHT TO WEIGHT RAISED TO A POWER

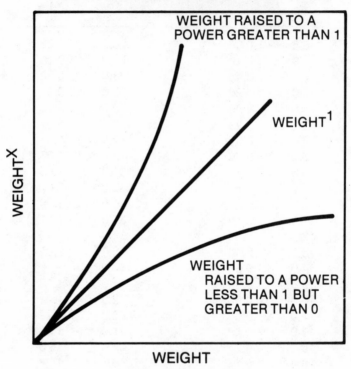

# Chemotherapeutic Agents

## A. POLYFUNCTIONAL ALKYLATING AGENTS

1. **Mechanism of action** — Contain highly reactive groups such as carbonium ions which join and cross-link parallel strands of DNA at the guanine residues. This inactivates or denatures the DNA.

2. **Drugs**

   A) Nitrogen mustard — Mustargen® (Merck)
   B) Cyclophosphamide — Cytoxan® (Mead Johnson)
   C) Chlorambucil — Leukeran® (Burroughs Wellcome)
   D) Bisulfan — Myleran® (Burroughs Wellcome)
   E) Triethylenethiophosphoramide — Thio-TEPA® (Lederle)
   F) Melphalan — Alkeran® (Burroughs Wellcome)
   G) Uracil mustard

## B. ANTIMETABOLITES

1. **Mechanism of action**

   A) They are structural analogues of some substance normally utilized by multiplying cells.
   B) Analogues may:
      1) Act by competitive interference with a normal substrate
      2) Be incorporated into a molecule to produce an abnormal substance
      3) Bind an enzyme and block an important biosynthetic step
   C) The major effect is interference with the biosynthesis of nucleic acids, thus preventing proliferation of cells.

2. **Drugs**

   A) Amethopterin — Methotrexate® (Lederle); folinic acid injections are a specific antidote for host intoxications.
   B) 5-fluorouracil — 5-FU, fluorouracil
   C) 6-mercaptopurine — Purinethol® (Burroughs Wellcome)
   D) 6-thioguanine — Tabloid® (Burroughs Wellcome)
   E) Cytarabine, cytosine arabinoside — Cytosar® (Upjohn)

## C. HORMONES

1. **Corticosteroids** — prednisone, prednisolone; inhibit protein synthesis

2. **Androgens**
   A) Testosterone propionate
   B) Fluoxymesterone — Halotestin® (Upjohn)

3. Estrogens
   A) Diethylstilbestrol
   B) Tace® (Merrell-National)
   C) Ethinyl estradiol
4. Progestins
   A) Medroxyprogesterone — Provera® (Upjohn)
   B) Hydroxyprogesterone caproate — Delalutin® (Squibb)

D. **ANTIBIOTICS** — inhibit RNA synthesis.
   1. **Dactinomycin, actinomycin D** — Cosmegen® (Merck, Sharp & Dohme)
   2. **Mithramycin** — Mithracin® (Dome)
   3. **Bleomycin** — Blenoxane® (Bristol)
   4. **Doxorubicin** — Adriamycin® (Adria)

E. **PLANT ALKALOIDS**
   1. **Vinblastine** — Velban® (Lilly)
   2. **Vincristine** — Oncovin® (Lilly)

F. **MISCELLANEOUS**
   1. **Procarbazine** — Matulane® (Roche), depolymerizes DNA
   2. **Hydroxyurea** — Hydrea® (Squibb)
   3. **Mitotane (O,P¹DDD)** — Lysodren® (Bristol)
      A) Related chemically to DDT
      B) Relatively specific for adrenal carcinomas

G. **LEVAMISOLE**
   1. **Being investigated for anticancer activity**
   2. **Theories of beneficial action:**
      A) Stimulation of immune responses
      B) Suppression of the carcinogenic etiologic mechanisms
      C) Reduction of metastasis to other tissue areas
      D) Prevention of relapses after remission
   3. **Patient not as susceptible to infectious processes**

CHAPTER

# 19

# Antimicrobial Drugs

Since the first recorded history, man has sought means, knowingly or unknowingly, to kill, control, inhibit, prevent spread of, reduce numbers of, or otherwise do away with troublesome microorganisms. Short historical outlines are included in later sections.

Many terms are used to describe these actions and uses, but they can best be summarized as *local* and *systemic*.

Antimicrobial drugs are intended to kill or inhibit the multiplication of pathogenic bacteria, viruses or fungi. There is a considerable degree of overlap within the various drug groups, but their uses can be summarized.

A. **LOCALLY APPLIED DRUGS**
  1. **Intact skin** — skin preparations for use before surgery, and teat dips for prevention of mastitis
  2. **Wound and burn treatment**
     A) Need to clean area, remove debris, provide drainage
     B) Need to rid area of microorganisms
     C) Should not interfere with physiological processes involved in healing or irritate the tissues
     D) Should not interfere with the host factors of body defense via phagocytic cells and/or the immune response
  3. **Mucous membrane surfaces to which drugs are applied:**
     A) GI, reproductive, urinary, and respiratory tracts
     B) Eye and ear
     C) Intramammary

B. **DRUGS INTENDED TO BE ABSORBED** act systemically.

C. **DRUGS APPLIED LOCALLY TO NON-LIVING SURFACES:**
  1. **May disinfect** — kill the microorganisms.
  2. **May sanitize** — reduce the population of microorganisms to an acceptable level.

# Antiseptics and Disinfectants

A. **TERMINOLOGY**
   1. **Inhibit or kill microorganisms:** bacteriostatic, bactericidal, virucidal, fungicidal
   2. **Applied topically**
   3. **Antiseptic** — if applied to living tissue
   4. **Disinfectant** — if applied to nonliving surfaces

B. **HISTORY**
   1. **Ancient Egypt** — wines, vinegar, volatile oils, myrrh were used for embalming.
   2. **Ignaz Semmelweis (1847)** — A Hungarian obstetrician who instigated washing hands with soap plus a chlorine rinse before aiding in deliveries. This resulted in a reduced death loss from childbirth.
   3. **Pasteur (1850s)** — Germ theory
   4. **Lister (1867)** — Chemical sterilization with carbolic acid

C. **MECHANISMS OF ANTIMICROBIAL ACTION**
   1. **Coagulation of the protein of bacterial cells** — denaturation of protein
   2. **Changes permeability of cell membranes** — causes a loss of essential substances from the cell and/or entry of unwanted substances into the cell.
   3. **Interferes with enzyme systems**
      A) Inactivate enzymes — through the SH group
      B) Competitive and noncompetitive inhibition by chemical analogues
      C) Oxidation and reduction reactions

D. **FACTORS INFLUENCING THE ACTION OF ANTISEPTICS AND DISINFECTANTS**
   1. **Potency related to:**
      A) Concentration of the agent
         1) *Bacteriostatic* in weak concentration
         2) *Bactericidal* in higher concentration
      B) Duration of contact with the organism
   2. **Temperature**
      A) Heat increases efficacy
      B) Cold reduces efficacy
   3. **Nature of medium** — a clean surface is ideal.
      A) Organic matter tends to protect microorganisms.

B) Disinfectants have poor penetrating power.

C) Hardness of water for solution; dissolved mineral may inhibit activity of drug.

D) pH of medium will be optimal, depending on the microorganism.
1) May affect bacteria
2) May affect disinfectant

4. **Type of microorganism involved**

A) Viruses, fungi, or bacteria

B) Vegetative or spore forms of bacteria

C) Acid-fast and non acid-fast

D) Populations of microorganisms

5. **Agent antagonisms** — there usually is physical or chemical incompatability between the drug and the environment and/or between two or more drugs used concurrently.

E. **PROPERTIES OF AN IDEAL ANTISEPTIC**

1. **High antimicrobial potency**—preferably a killing action

2. **Wide chemotherapeutic spectrum**

3. **Safe**
A) No adverse effects
B) Does not harm living tissues

4. **Fast-acting, with prolonged action**

5. **Not inhibited by extraneous substances**

6. **Odorless, nonstaining, stable, noncorrosive, and inexpensive**

7. **Not absorbed into the animal's system in amounts that may have adverse effects**

F. **CHEMICAL AGENTS**

1. **Acids and alkalies**

A) Alter pH and enzyme activity

B) Benzoic acid, boric acid, acetic acid, salicylic acid, nalidixic acid

C) Sodium hydroxide, borax, sodium borate, potassium hydroxide

2. **Phenols**

A) Protein coagulation

B) Cresol (Lysol® — Lehn & Fink) — an emulsion of cresol, soap and water
| | |
|---|---|
| 1) Phenol | 3) Resorcinol |
| 2) Thymol | 4) Menthol |

   C) Hexachlorophene (a bi-phenolic) — slow acting
      1) G-11®
      2) Gamophen® (Arbrook)
      3) pHisohex® (Winthrop)
      4) Septisol®
      5) Alcohol denatures and inactivates hexachlorophene
   D) Pine tar, creosote — irritating
   E) Substituted phenols
      1) Staphene®            4) Lph®
      2) Amphyl®             5) Tergisyl®
      3) Hil-phene®

3. **Surface-active agents**

   A) Effects on membranes are caused by decreased surface tension and/or metabolic effects.
   B) Anionics are fatty-acid soaps.
   C) Cationics are quaternary ammonium compounds:
      1) Roccal® (Winthrop)
      2) Zephiran® (Winthrop)
      3) Phemerol® (Parke-Davis)
   D) Non-ionics: polysorbate — Tween 80® (City Chemical) and Cerumex®

4. **Halogens**

   A) Interfere with enzyme systems and coagulate proteins
   B) Iodine
      1) *Tincture* = 2% iodine, 2.3% sodium iodide, 40% alcohol
      2) *Strong tincture* = 7% iodine, 5% potassium iodide, 80% alcohol
      3) *Lugol's solution* = 5% iodine, 10% potassium iodide, water
   C) Organic iodines — "tamed iodines"; iodophores are iodine combined with a surface-active agent. Loosely-bound iodine is complexed with PVP.
      1) Weladol® (Pitman-Moore)
      2) Povidol®
      3) Betadine® (Purdue-Frederick)
      4) Iosan®
      5) Wescodyne® (West Chemical)
   D) Chlorine
      1) Hypochlorous acid — Warexin®.
      2) Sodium hypochlorite — Clorox® or Purex®. Clorox is a 5.6% solution. When diluted 1:32 (0.175% solution) it is an excellent virucidal agent.
      3) Chlolramine T

5. **Heavy metals**
   A) Protein denaturation, causing inactivation of sulfhydryl groups on bacterial enzymes
   B) Mercury
      1) Mercuric oxide, chloride, and nitrate
      2) Merbromin — Mercurochrome® (Hynson, Wescott & Dunning)
      3) Thiomersol — Merthiolate® (Lilly)
      4) Nitromersol — Metaphen® (Abbott)
   C) Silver
      1) Silver nitrate
      2) Silver protein — Argyrol® (Cooper)
      3) Silver picrate
   D) Zinc
      1) Zinc oxide      3) Zinc chloride
      2) Zinc sulfate    4) Zinc stearate
   E) Copper sulfate
   F) Bismuth tribromphenate — Xeroform® (Day-Baldwin)
6. **Dyes**
   A) Enzyme inhibition
   B) Acridines
      1) Acriflavin    2) Proflavin    3) Monoflavin
   C) Triphenylmethanes
      1) Methyl rosaniline (gentian violet, crystal violet, and pyoktannin blue)
      2) Brilliant green
      3) Methyl violet
   D) Azo
      1) Scarlet Red® (Lilly)
      2) Dimazon
      3) Piridium®
7. **Oxidizing agents**
   A) Hydrogen peroxide      C) Zinc peroxide
   B) Sodium perborate       D) Potassium permanganate
8. **Alcohols and aldehydes**
   A) Coagulate protein and enzyme inhibition
   B) Alcohols
      1) Ethyl — 70%    2) Isopropyl — 50%
   C) Aldehydes
      1) Formaldehyde — formalin 40%.
      2) Methenamine liberates formaldehyde
   D) Glycols
      1) Propylene glycol    3) Polypropylene glycol
      2) Triethylene glycol

9. **Chlorhexidine** — Nolvasan® (Fort Dodge), Hibitane® (Ayerst)
   A) Ear ointment, skin ointment, shampoo
   B) Suspension and tablets for reproductive tracts
   C) Disinfecting solution

10. **Glutaraldehyde** — Cidex® (Arbrook)
    A) Supplied in acid form. Is activated by the addition of sodium bicarbonate.
    B) Irritating. For disinfectant use only.

11. **Kopertox®** (Ayerst) — Forms coating

12. **Mycodex®** (Beecham) — Forms coating

13. **Nitrofurans** (Furacin® — Norden)

14. **Sani-Squad®** — A disinfectant combining formaldehyde, quaternary ammonium, alcohols, and substituted phenol

15. **Environ®** — Combination of substituted phenols

16. **Glutaraldehyde** — Sonacide®
    A) **Potentiated acid form. Buffers need not be added.**
    B) **Complete sterilization if heated (140 F) and exposed for one hour**
    C) **Irritating to eyes**
    D) **Avoid prolonged contact with skin**

17. **A summary of the properties of the common classes of disinfectants**

See summary on facing page.

# Antimicrobial Chemotherapy

"In order to pursue chemotherapy, we must look for substances which possess a high *affinity* and high *lethal potency*. In other words, we must learn to aim and to aim in a chemical sense" — Paul Ehrlich, 1909

A. **CHEMOTHERAPEUTIC DRUGS**
   1. **Chemicals that selectively inhibit specific causative agents of disease**
   2. **Ideal drug**
      A) Very specific and highly lethal to agents of disease
      B) No adverse reaction in the animal
         1) The inhibited reaction must not exist in animal cells.
         2) The inhibited reaction follows a different scheme in the animal cells.
         3) If the drug is reactive in the animal, the small concentrations used have "slight" effects upon the animal cells.

# A SUMMARY OF THE COMMON CLASSES OF DISINFECTANTS

| Disinfectant Class → | Quaternary Ammonium Compound | Phenolics | Sodium Hypochlorite | Iodophore | Glutaraldehyde | Chlorhexidine |
|---|---|---|---|---|---|---|
| Example → | (Roccal) | (Staphene) | (Clorox) | (Betadine) | | (Nolvasan) |
| **Property** | | | | | | |
| Relative cost per gallon of disinfectant at recommended use — dilution | $0.03 | $0.06 | $0.02 | $0.15 | $9.00 | $0.24 |
| Bactericidal | + + | + + | + + | + + + | + + + | + + |
| General virucide | – | – | + + + | + + + | + + + | – |
| Lipophilic or lipophilic-like viruses | + + + | + + + | + + + | + + | + + + | + + + |
| Sporocidal at room temperature | – | – | – | + | + + | – |
| Fungicidal | + + | + + + | + + + | + + + | + + + | + + |
| Effective in the presence of organic material | + + | + + + | + | + + | + + + | + + |
| Effective in the presence of soaps, amonidet | – | + + + | + + | + + | + + + | – |
| Effective in hard water | + | + + + | + + | + + | + + + | + + |
| Most effective pH range | alkaline | neutral | acid | neutral | alkaline | alkaline |

3. **Chemotherapeutic drugs (antimicrobials) are either**
   A) Of natural origin (*e.g.* antibiotics)
   B) Synthetic substances such as sulfonamides or nitrofurans
   C) Definitions:
      1) *Antibiosis* occurs when two populations of microorganisms exist together; one has an inhibitive influence upon the other.
      2) *Symbiosis* occurs when two organisms exist together and have a mutually favorable influence.
      3) *An antibiotic* is a substance produced by a growing microorganism (fungi, bacteria, and actinomycetes) that inhibits and/or destroys other microorganisms.
   D) Antibiotic-producing microorganisms, usually soil-borne, are gathered from all over the world.

4. **Antibacterial drugs are either:**
   A) *Bacteriostatic* — inhibit multiplication of bacterial cells.
   B) *Bactericidal* — kill bacteria.

5. **The four principal mechanisms of action:**
   A) Cause the rupture of the cell wall
   B) Alter the lipoprotein in the cell membrane, which increases the permeability, thus permitting vital metabolites to escape or foreign materials to enter the cell
   C) Interfere with nucleic acid (RNA and DNA) metabolism, thus inhibiting synthesis of cell protein
   D) Interfere with intermediary metabolism of the cells

6. **All antimicrobial drugs rely heavily on the defense mechanisms of the animal's body to bring about a cure.** The bacteriostatic drugs rely most heavily on these mechanisms.
   A) *Phagocytosis* — occurs when phagocytes (white blood cells) engulf the microorganism.
   B) *Immune response* is the mechanism by which antibodies neutralize the microorganism.
   C) *Interferon* inhibits viruses.

B. **HISTORY** — Since ancient times, molds have been used empirically in medicine for the treatment of infections. Curative poultices of mosses and molds have been described in Greek, Roman, and Arabic medical writings, and in the medical writings of medieval monasteries.

1633 — Cinchona bark — used to treat "the fever" (malaria)
1820 — Quinine — malaria treatment
1877 — Pasteur observed and recorded the phenomenon of antibiosis. He observed that contaminant microorganisms in his anthrax cultures markedly inhibited survival of the anthrax bacilli.

1907 — Arsphenamine — syphilis
1929 — Penicillin — description of its antibacterial properties
1932 — Sulfonamides (Prontosil)
1938 - 1941 — Penicillin, clinical use
1944 — Streptomycin
1945 — Isoniazid — tuberculosis.
1947 — Chloramphenicol
1948 — Aureomycin® (Lederle)
1950 — Terramycin® (Pfizer)
1959 — Synthetic penicillins

C. **RESISTANCE OF ORGANISMS TO ANTIMICROBIAL AGENTS**
  1. **Two general types**
     A) Natural resistance
        1) Considered by species. Bacteria are susceptible to some antibacterial drugs and resistant to others.
        2) Basis of the effective spectrum of antibacterial drugs
     B) Acquired resistance
        1) Sensitive strains become resistant after they are exposed to the drug.
        2) Alterations in the microorganisms allow them to survive in the presence of an increased concentration of the antibacterial drug in question.
  2. **Mechanisms of resistance**
     A) Microorganisms tolerate the drug.
        1) There may be a change in cell permeability that interferes with the drug entering the organism.
        2) Modifications in the organism may occur which prevent attachment of the drug to the inhibition site in the cell.
        3) The organism develops an alternate metabolic pathway, thereby circumventing the inhibition site of the drug.
        4) The organism increases the biosynthesis of the metabolite being competitively antagonized by the drug.
     B) Microorganisms are capable of destroying the antibacterial drug — some organisms produce enzymes that inactivate the drug (*e.g.* organisms that produce penicillinase).
  3. **Cross-resistance** — organisms that become resistant to one antibacterial drug may also exhibit resistance to related drugs to which they have not been previously exposed. *Example*: an organism that develops resistance to oxytetracycline usually becomes resistant to chlortetracycline and tetracycline.
  4. **Passage of resistance from organism to organism**
     A) Microorganisms can pass drug resistance to their daughter

cells. This is true of most all types of bacteria, both Gram-positive and Gram-negative.

B) Transferable resistance

    1) Resistance can be transmitted from one cell to another that is not a daughter cell.

    2) Resistance can be transmitted between organisms not necessarily of the same species.

    3) Transfer is carried out by a complex mechanism involving R factors or plasmids (transfer of genetic material).

    4) Resistance may be transferred to more than one antibiotic at one time. Exposure to therapeutic levels of one antibiotic may bring about (through transfer) a population of pathogens resistant to several unrelated antibiotics.

    5) Involves primarily Gram-negative bacteria (*e.g. Escherichia coli* and *Salmonella*)

5. **Important clinically to recognize that:**

A) Bacteria are not all sensitive to all antibacterial drugs. Know the drug spectrum.

B) Bacteria that were once sensitive may become resistant — sometimes quickly. Sensitivity testing is a valuable tool.

C) The pressure of increased antibacterial drug therapy has brought about many changes in the susceptibility of bacteria. Changes of spectrum will continue to occur.

D) Indiscriminate use of antibacterial drugs definitely plays a role in increasing the problem of bacterial resistance.

E) Inadequate dosage (amount and/or duration) of antibacterial drugs can promote bacterial resistance.

F) Bacterial resistance may differ from one geographic area to another.

# Sulfonamides

A. **CHEMISTRY**

1. **Basic chemical group** — an amino benzene sulfonamido. Sulfonamides are weak acids.

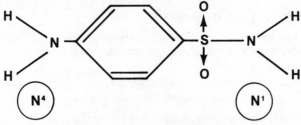

**SULFANILAMIDE**

A) $N^4$ substitutions (*See* previous page)
   1) Inactivate unless removed in body
   2) May delay absorption from the intestine
B) $N^1$ substitutions (*See* previous page)
   1) Form salts with strong bases

$$-\!\!-\!N\!\!<^{\displaystyle H}_{\displaystyle Na}$$

   2) Increase solubility
   3) Alter absorption, biotransformation and excretion
2. **Historically derived from prontosil, which is inactive** *in vitro.*

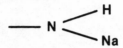

PRONTOSIL

IN VIVO

Sulfanilamide (active)

3. **Sodium salts are strongly alkaline (pH 9 to 11), therefore irritating. Parenterally, they should be given IV only.**
4. **They are slightly more soluble in plasma than in water or urine.**

A. **MECHANISM OF ACTION** (*See* schematic on following page.)
   1. **Sulfonamides are bacteriostatic.**
   2. **Sulfonamides inhibit multiplication of bacteria.**
   3. **Summary of the Fildes-Woods theory of sulfonamide mechanism of action:**
      A) The sulfa drug competes with para-aminobenzoic acid (PABA). The competition is for incorporation into the scheme for the biosynethsis of bacterial folic acid.

      PABA + pteridines + glutamic acid $\longrightarrow$ folic acid.
      B) Folic acid (dihydrofolic acid) is converted to tetrahydrofolic acid (THFA).
      C) THFA is the active form of folic acid. It is a vital cofactor for amino acid metabolism relative to purine synthesis and hence the formation of RNA.
      D) Metabolic mistake (biological antagonism) inhibits the biosynthesis of folic acid — inhibits the formation of RNA.
      E) Reduced RNA synthesis leads to inhibition of bacterial protein synthesis; multiplication of bacteria is arrested.

## Sulfonamides: Mechanism of Action

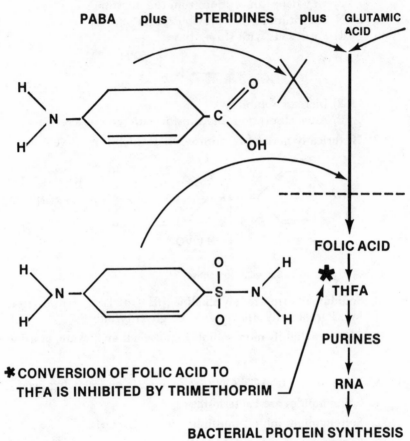

PABA    plus    PTERIDINES    plus    GLUTAMIC ACID

FOLIC ACID

THFA

PURINES

RNA

**✱ CONVERSION OF FOLIC ACID TO
THFA IS INHIBITED BY TRIMETHOPRIM**

**BACTERIAL PROTEIN SYNTHESIS
+
BACTERIAL MULTIPLICATION**

4. **An aid to the reticuloendothelial system** — sulfonamides prevent the rapid growth of bacteria populations in a disease but the body defense mechanisms must overcome the disease by phagocytosis of bacteria.

5. **Sulfonamides are not active in the presence of pus and cellular debris from necrotizing tissue;** folic acid and purines are already available for use by bacterial cells and they skip the spot of sulfonamide antagonism and inhibition.

6. **Do not interfere with the protein synthesis scheme in the**

animal's body; the animal supplies the animal cells with folic acid from the diet.

C. **BEST THERAPEUTIC EFFICACY IS ACHIEVED IN THE EARLY STAGES OF BACTERIAL INFECTION.**

1. **Sulfonamides** are of questionable value in treatment for chronic infections.

2. **Basic principles** — that support the superior efficacy of sulfonamides when they are used early in the course of disease:

   A) Bacteria have a high metabolic level; they readily pick up and mistakenly incorporate sulfonamides into cellular biosynthetic schemes.

   B) The animal has an active reticuloendothelial system; capability for phagocytosis is high.

   C) Inflammatory reactions have not yet produced tissue barriers to hinder diffusion of the drug into infection sites.

   D) There is no cellular debris to limit drug action.

D. **BACTERIAL RESISTANCE** — adaption of bacteria to a sulfonamide that was once toxic to them.

1. **May develop rapidly and persist over many generations.**

2. **Cross-resistance** — resistance is not limited to one sulfonamide.

3. **Resistance** — based upon changes in the requirement of the bacterial cell for PABA.

   A) Requirement for PABA is circumvented.

   B) Bacteria increase their production of PABA. Intracellular concentrations in resistant bacteria have been shown to increase to 100 times normal.

   C) Bacteria develop systems that can use the sulfonamide in place of PABA. Some bacteria may even become dependent on a sulfonamide.

E. **METABOLISM**

1. **Most sulfonamides (intestinal sulfonamides excepted) are readily absorbed** from the GI tract.

   A) Degrees and rates of absorption vary, depending upon the sulfonamide and species of animal.

   B) Water solubility does not affect absorption.

   C) Some sustained-release sulfonamides are poorly absorbed when given orally to sick animals with atonic rumens. These drugs do not reach therapeutic blood levels.

   D) Sulfaethoxypyridazine (S.E.Z.® —American Cyanamid) — concentrations in blood during the absorption phase have been shown to be less in water-deprived calves than in control animals.

2. **Sulfonamides are well distributed to all tissues,** except to the brain. The amount in cerebrospinal fluid depends on the sulfonamide used, the dosage, and duration of treatment. Sulfadiazine may be the best (based upon data from human medicine).

3. **Well absorbed from most tissues** — including the uterus and denuded areas resulting from burns and wounds.
   A) 250 ml of 25% Sulmet® (American Cyanamid) infused in the uterus gave a sulfonamide level of 20mg/100ml in in blood in two hours.
   B) Uterine sulfonamides are carried to the blood and into the milk.

4. **Readily pass the placental barrier** — concentration in fetal blood approaches that in maternal blood.

5. **Plasma binding**
   A) Sulfonamides are bound to plasma proteins, chiefly albumin.
   B) Bound form is inactive. It acts as a depot. The greater the percent of free drug, the greater the potency.
   C) Sulfonamides with a lower binding power diffuse more readily to extravascular space and give higher concentrations in the lymph, synovial fluid, peritoneal fluid, pleural fluid, and cerebrospinal fluid.

6. **Distribution between blood and milk:**
   A) The ratio of sulfonamide concentration in milk to plasma is based on the Henderson-Hasselbach prediction for weak-acid ionization ratios.
   B) Distribution of sulfonamide between the blood and milk depends on:
      1) pH of milk (normal 6.6.) and pKa of drug
      2) pH of plasma (assumed constant at 7.4)
   C) Based on equilibrium conditions and a constant plasma level — clinically not likely to reach equilibrium conditions.
   D) Clinically important inferences:
      1) The greater the pKa values, the greater the sulfonamide concentration in the milk. The greater the pKa of the drug, the weaker the drug is as an acid. It is less able to ionize at pH 7.4 in the blood, thus increasing its ability to move from blood into milk.
      2) The greater the pH of milk the greater the sulfa concentration in the milk. The more alkaline the milk, the

greater the ionization of the sulfonamide (weak acid) and the greater the trapping of the ionized sulfa in the milk.
E) Systemic sulfonamides do reach significant amounts in milk.
F) Intramammary infusion gives significant systemic levels by back-diffusion. With mastitis, less back-diffusion occurs. If one quarter is infused, milk should be discarded from all quarters for the proper withdrawal time.

**SULFA IN QUARTER 1** → **SULFA IN BLOOD** → **SULFA IN QUARTERS 2, 3, 4**

7. **Biotransformation mechanisms**

A) Acetylation — occurs primarily in the liver.
   1) Acetylated sulfonamide is inactive.
   2) Extent of acetylation differs with animal species and with the sulfonamide.
      a) *Dog* — no significant acetylation
      b) *Most domestic animals* — moderate acetylation
      c) *Man* — considerable acetylation
B) Glucuronic acid conjugation and sulfate conjugation: renal clearance of glucuronides is greater than that of free sulfonamides.

8. **Excretion**

A) Primarily by the urinary system
   1) Excreted as conjugates and some as free drug
   2) Water-deprivation slows the urinary excretion (S.E.Z.® — American Cyanamid) and gives higher blood levels during the excretory phase.
B) Poorly absorbed sulfonamides are excreted in the feces.
C) Small amounts of sulfonamide are excreted in bile, pancreatic juice, intestinal juice, saliva, and milk.

9. **Urinary excretion problems:**

A) Fluid balance
   1) Dehydration and limited intake of water increase the resorption of water and increase the resorption of absorbable sulfonamides from the filtrate. Dehydration also reduces excretion of sulfonamides and prolongs blood levels.
   2) Excessive excretion of water increases the excretion of sulfonamides.

B) Solubility of sulfonamides
   1) The greater the solubility of the sulfonamide, the more easily it is excreted.
   2) Sulfonamides are more concentrated in the glomerular filtrate than in the blood.
   3) If the concentration of sulfonamide in the glomerular filtrate exceeds the limit of saturation, crystals develop and are deposited in the urinary system, usually in the renal pelvis.
   4) The pH of the filtrate fluid influences the solubility of sulfonamides. An increase in acidity decreases the solubility of the sulfonamide.
   5) In animals that have acidic urine (carnivora), the use of sodium bicarbonate increases urinary pH and increases the solubility of most sulfonamides, thus inhibiting precipitation of crystals.
   6) In herbivores, the urine is normally pH 8 or more. There is no indication for alkaline therapy under usual conditions of sulfonamide therapy.
C) Incidence of crystal formation depends upon:
   1) Solubility of the sulfonamide
   2) Volume of urine
   3) Amount of sulfonamide excreted; this is a function of plasma level, which in turn is a function of the route of administration, dose, and frequency of administration.
   4) pH of urine
   5) Individual susceptibility
D) Combination of sulfonamides and the *law of independent solubility:*
   1) Solution of one compound is not affected by the presence in the solution of another compound.
   2) Urine saturated with sulfanilamide will dissolve sulfathiazole to the point of normal saturation as though no other sulfonamide were present.
   3) Other sulfonamide combinations act similarly.
E) Advantages of different sulfonamides given simultaneously:
   1) Broader antibacterial spectrum
   2) Greater safety from urinary toxicity because the dose is based upon total drug in the combination; hence lesser concentrations of each sulfonamide in the glomerular filtrate and urine occur at one time.

F. **TOXICITY**
   1. **Acute toxicity** is not seen frequently in veterinary therapy. The nervous system may be affected if levels are high.

   A) Stimulation of the CNS causes:
   1) Emesis                     3) Ataxia
   2) Running movements      4) Convulsions
   B) Degeneration of myelin has been noted.
2. **Chronic toxicity** (more likely than acute toxicity)
   A) May be renal, due to formation of sulfonamide crystals. Irritation of mucosa may lead to calculi and obstructions.
   B) Neuritis in chickens
   C) Blood dyscrasias, (leukopenia, granulocytopenia and hemolytic anemia) have been demonstrated in human medicine. This has not been shown to be a problem in veterinary therapy.
   D) Capable of oxidizing hemoglobin to methemoglobin
   E) Inhibition of the enzyme, carbonic anhydrase, causes a tendency toward acidosis via an increased loss of bicarbonate and a loss of buffering ability of plasma. This is not a clinical problem under normal use.
   F) Supression of egg production in chickens
   G) Inhibition of bacteria in digestive tract of ruminants and single-stomached animals
   H) Hypersensitivity — due to drug allergy. Light-skinned animals are more prone to skin reactions.
   I) Sulfonamides inhibit production of vitamin K in the gut, resulting in hypoprothrombinemia.
      1) Vitamin K is a necessary metabolite for the biosynthesis of prothrombin.
      2) May lead to problems in blood clotting
   J) Have been shown to be teratogenic in some laboratory animals
   K) Drug eruption — in the dog causes a pruritic, eczematous dermatitis.
      1) Sulfisoxazole — after several months of therapy.
      2) Triple sulfa has caused drug eruption.
   L) Reported to cause kerätoconjunctivitis in dogs, with onset within 18 hours to several months after administration.

G. **SPECTRUM OF SUSCEPTIBLE MICROORGANISMS**
   1. **These are broad-spectrum antibacterial agents.**
   2. **Gram-positive and Gram-negative bacteria**
      A) Certain streptococci and staphylococci     B) *Actinomyces*
      C) *Pasteurella*     D) Certain strains of *Escherichia coli*
      E) *Nocardia*   F) *Proteus*     G) *Hemophilus*
      H) *Fusobacterium*
   3. **Coccidia**

## H.  PRINCIPLES OF PROPER THERAPY

1. **Proper diagnosis is mandatory.** Is the disease causing the presence of organism(s) that are susceptible to sulfonamides?

2. **Choose the right sulfonamide or combination.** Which will be most effective?

3. **Treat early.**
   A) Bacteria are metabolically more active; they take up sulfonamides more rapidly.
   B) Body defense systems are not worn out.

4. **Value in treatment for chronic disease is questionable.**

5. **Use proper dose and dosage schedule.**
   A) Vary sulfonamides used, depending on absorption and excretion patterns of individual sulfonamides.
   B) Quickly establish a therapeutic blood level.
      1) First dose may require IV administration.
      2) 5 mg/100 ml is a minimum concentration in blood.

6. **Continue therapy for proper period** — at least 5 to 6 days. For actinomycotic peritonitis in the dog, use triple sulfa for three months.

7. **Administer ample amounts of fluids.**

8. **Sulfonamides are not active in the presence of pus or cellular debris.**

9. **Be alert for toxic reactions.** It is helpful to monitor urine sample for formation of crystals in animals with acid urine.

## I.  FORMULARY

1. **Dosage forms available**
   A) Oral
      1) Tablets              4) Feed additive
      2) Oblets               5) Solutions for drench and
      3) Powder for drench         drinking water
   B) Topical
      1) Skin
         a) Ointments   b) Sprays
      2) Uterine bolus
      3) Intramammary infusions
   C) Parenteral solutions: IV only (intraperitoneally?)

2. **Sulfonamides**
   A) Sulfamerazine
   B) Sulfadimethoxine

      1) Bactrovet™ (Pitman-Moore)    2) Sudine® (Beecham)
      3) Albon® (Roche)   4) Medacide SDM® (Medico)

C) Sulfamethazine
1) AS 250® (American Cyanamid)
2) SM-15® (Med-Tech)
3) Spanbolet II® (Norden)
4) Veta-Meth® (Vet-A-Mix)
5) Hava-Span® (Haver-Lockhart)
6) Sulfachel® (Rachelle)
D) Sulfanilamide
1) Duatok® (American Cyanamid)
2) Sul-Trol® (Hess & Clark)
3) Sul-Thi-Zol® (Merck)
E) Sulfathiazole
1) Morumide® (Beecham)
2) Thiuramide (Med-Tech)
F) Sulfapyridine
G) Sulfadiazine
H) Sulfamethoxypyridazine — Midicel® (Parke-Davis)
I) Sulfabromomethazine — Sulfabrom® (Merck)
J) Sulfabenzamide — Sulben® (Haver-Lockhart)
K) Sulfamethizole
L) Sulfacetamide — Sulamyd® (Schering)
M) Azosulfamide — Neoprontosil® (Winthrop)
N) Sulfaethoxypyridazine — S.E.Z.® (American Cyanamid)
O) Sulfisoxazole
1) Gantrisin® (Roche)
2) Soxisol® (Fort Dodge)
P) Sulfachlorpyridazine
1) Vetisulid® (Squibb)
2) Prinzone®
Q) Sulfamethoxazole (Wellcome)(Roche)

3. **Combination sulfonamide solutions**
A) Tri-Sulfa-G® (Norden) — sulfamethazine, sulfathiazole, and sulfapyridine glucosides (12.5%).
B) Sulfatose® (Norden) — sulfamethazine (7%), sulfathiazole (6.5%).
C) Tri-Vet-Sul® (Haver-Lockhart) — sulfathiazole, sulfamethazine, sulfamerazine (10%).
D) Soxifour® (Fort Dodge) — sulfamethazine, sulfathiazole, sulfamerazine.
E) Sulfa 24® (Bio-Ceutic) — sulfamethazine (8%), sulfapyridine (8%), and sulfathiazole (8%).

4. **Intestinal sulfonamides**
A) Sulfaguanidine

B) Phthalylsulfathiazole — Sulfathalidine® (Merck, Sharp & Dohme).

C) Sulfaquinoxaline

D) Succinylsulfathiazole

E) Phthalysulfacetamide

## J. SPECIFIC SULFONAMIDES

### 1. Sulfanilamide

A) Historically important; chemically, it is the simplest sulfon-amide.

B) Not widely used

### 2. Sulfathiazole

A) Rapidly excreted

B) Potent *in vitro*

C) Not used alone

D) Used orally — every 6 to 8 hours

E) Found in sulfonamide combinations

### 3. Sulfadiazine

A) Short-acting

B) Used in therapy of meningitis — better penetration of CNS.

C) Used in Tribrissen® (Wellcome/Jen-Sal) and Di-Trim® (Diamond)

### 4. Sulfamerazine, sulfamethazine — both are methylated diazine sulfonamides. They give longer duration of action and are more slowly excreted than other sulfonamides.

A) Sulfamethazine

  1) *Large animals* — gives 24-hour blood levels

    a) Withdrawal

      (1) Milk — 96 hours

      (2) Slaughter — 10 days

    b) Aureo-700® (American Cyanamid) — aureomycin plus methazine; a feed additive.

  2) *Small animals* — gives 12-hour blood levels.

B) Spanbolet II® (Norden) — sulfamethazine in a layered bolus.

  1) Quick-release layer dissolves rapidly into solution

  2) Sustained-release layer prolongs the blood level

  3) Therapeutic blood level is reached in 2 to 6 hours after oral administration

  4) Gives 5-day blood level

  5) Withdrawal before slaughter: 28 days

  6) Is used prophylactically

C) Hava-Span® (Haver-Lockhart) — sulfamethazine

  1) Achieves therapeutic blood levels in 14 to 18 hours

2) Blood level is maintained 3 to 5 days, depending on dose

5. **Sulfapyridine**
   A) Used in combinations
   B) Gives 12-hour blood levels

6. **Sulfisoxazole** — Soxisol® (Fort Dodge)
   A) High concentrations in urine
   B) Gives 8-hour blood levels

7. **Sulfachlorpyridazine** — Vetisulid® (Squibb)
   A) Gives 8-hour blood levels
   B) Withdrawal before slaughter: calves, 7 days; pigs, 4 days

8. **Sulfacetamide**
   A) Topical — eye and ear ointment
   B) Available in combination with neomycin and prednisolone

9. **Sulfabromomethazine** — Sulfabrom® (Merck)
   A) Oral administration — cattle
   B) Effective blood levels
      1) Established in 3 to 5 hours     2) Last 48 to 72 hours
   C) Withdrawal
      1) Milk — 4 days        2) Slaughter — 10 days

10. **Sulfadimethoxine**
    A) Gives 24-hour blood levels
       1) Reduce daily dose by one-half after the first day
       2) Withdrawal
          a) Milk — 60 hours
          b) Slaughter — 7 days
    B) Bactrovet™ (Pitman-Moore); Sudine® (Beecham)—small animals only
    C) Albon® (Hoffmann-LaRoche)
       1) For large and small animals; give orally or IV
          a) Agribon® — for poultry
          b) Albon-SR® — gives blood levels for 4 days

11. **Sulfamethoxypyradazine** — Midicel® (Parke-Davis); give orally; gives 24-hour blood levels

12. **Sulfamethizole with methenamine** — Mesulfin® (Ayerst)
    A) Orally — small animals
    B) Gives 8-hour blood levels
    C) Concentrates in and is extremely soluble in urine

13. **Sulfaethoxypyridazine** — S.E.Z.® (American Cyanamid)
    A) Oral
       1) Cattle (controlled-release oblets)
          a) Effective blood levels
             (1) Established in 4 hours
             (2) Last 72 hours

2) Swine (24-hour blood levels)
    a) Withdrawal
       (1) Milk — 72 hours
       (2) Slaughter — 16 days

14. **Sulfabenzamide** — Sulben® (Haver-Lockhart)
    A) Oral — 24-hour blood levels
    B) Withdrawal — milk, 72 hours

15. **Sulfadiazine plus trimethoprim** — Tribrissen® (Wellcome/Jen-Sal), Di-Trim® (Diamond)
    A) This attacks the metabolism of the bacteria, relative to protein synthesis, at two points.
       1) Sulfadiazine inhibits biosynthesis of dihydrofolic acid.
       2) Trimethoprim inhibits conversion of dihydrofolic acid to tetrahydrofolic acid (the active form); is an antimetabolite of folic acid.
    B) Broader spectrum
    C) Combination exhibits potentiation
    D) Combination is bactericidal
    E) Widely used in Europe. Large animals: 15 mg/kg, IM, twice a day

16. **CSP-250®** (Diamond Shamrock)
    A) Feed additive (swine)
    B) Chlortetracycline with sulfathiazole and procaine penicillin

# Antibiotics

## A. PENICILLINS

### 1. Description

A) Produced by the mold, *penicillium*

B) Chemical formula — an organic acid

---

SITE OF SALT FORMATION:
$H^+$ — ACID
$Na^+$ OR $K^+$
PROCAINE

PENICILLIN G·R* =

PENICILLIN V·R* =

AMPICILLIN·R* =

---

C) Sodium and potassium salts of penicillin G are:
   1) Crystalline
   2) Highly soluble in water
   3) Unstable in solution; available only as powder and should be reconstituted as needed.

D) Penicillin G
   1) Procaine salts of penicillin G are not soluble in water.
   2) Suspensions of procaine penicillin G are stable in water.

E) Benzathine penicillin G
    1) A large complex molecule made up of:

An organic bridge

A molecule of                              A molecule of
penicillin G                                  penicillin G

    2) Not soluble in water
    3) Suspensions are stable
F) Synthetic penicillins
    1) Basic penicillin nucleus is the same
    2) Side chains are added

2. **General Principles**
  A) The first antibiotic — may still be *safest and best.*
  B) Oral administration of penicillin G is not feasible; it is degraded by stomach acid.
  C) SC route of administration for procaine penicillin G is as effective as IM route and is preferable in some instances.
  D) Formulations for oral administration should be given before the patient is fed.
  E) Advantages of semisynthetic penicillins:
    1) Increased resistance to acid degradation in stomach, thus allowing administration *per orum*
    2) Longer action because of slower biotransformation and excretion
    3) Resistance to penicillinase, which enhances treatment against penicillin G-resistant staphylococci (exception: ampicillin is not penicillinase-stable).
    4) Wider spectrum of activity; includes more Gram-negative organisms
    5) Most semisynthetic penicillins give quicker and higher blood levels as compared to those attained with penicillin G or even penicillin V.

3. **Metabolism**
  A) Absorption
    1) Sodium or potassium salts of penicillin G are rapidly absorbed from an intramuscular site, reaching therapeutic blood levels in 30 minutes. They are poorly absorbed after oral administration.
    2) Procaine penicillin G is well absorbed from intramuscular or subcutaneous sites. It reaches therapeutic blood levels in 2 to 3 hours.
    3) Benzathine penicillin G is well absorbed from intramuscular sites, but more slowly than procaine penicillin G.

4) Synthetic penicillins are rapidly absorbed.
   a) *Oral*
      (1) Therapeutic blood levels are reached at 1 hour.
      (2) Food retards development of blood levels.
   b) *Intramuscular* — therapeutic blood levels are reached in ½ to 1 hour.
5) Penicillin diffuses from milk (intramammary infusion) back into plasma.
6) Differences in absorption of penicillin G and dicloxacillin between male and female have been shown in dogs (Beagles) after oral administration. Absorption is greater in females.

B) Distribution
   1) All penicllins are protein-bound in plasma, but the extent of binding varies greatly.
      a) *High* — oxacillin and cloxacillin............80%
      b) *Intermediate* — penicillin G...............50%
      c) *Low* — ampicillin.......................20%
   2) Rapid but uneven distribution to various tissues
      a) High concentrations in:
         (1) Kidney    (4) Skin
         (2) Lung      (5) Intestines
         (3) Liver
      b) Lesser concentrations in:
         (1) Bone marrow
         (2) Central nervous system (greater if inflamed)
         (3) Eye
         (4) Muscle
      c) Low concentration in:
         (1) Joints    (2) Pleural fluid    (3) Milk
   3) Pass into fetal circulation
C) Biotransformation and excretion
   1) Penicillin is excreted unchanged, predominately in the urine.
   2) Synthetic penicillins are excreted chiefly in the urine, but large amounts are also excreted in the bile.
   3) Excretion of penicillin from the plasma is rapid. Synthetics may be excreted somewhat more slowly.
   4) Excretion in the kidney is predominately (80%) by active tubular secretion.
D) Duration of action after IM or SC injection: penicillin is rapidly eliminated from plasma and tissues. There, the most practical way to increase the duration and cut the number of doses is to delay absorption of the drug into plasma.

1) Alter the vehicle (oil *vs* aqueous). An oil vehicle slows the absorption.
2) Change the salt form (procaine salt). The procaine is now a part of the penicillin molecule, which delays absorption.
3) Alter the molecular structure (benzathine). Benzathine penicillin is two molecules of penicillin G joined with an organic bridge. It is a large and slowly absorbed molecule.

4. **Mechanism of action**
   A) Penicillins are *bactericidal*.
   B) Inhibit the construction of the bacterial cell wall
      1) The underlying cell membrane is not properly protected.
      2) The cell membrane is damaged. It is not able to withstand the osmotic pressure gradient.
      3) Lysis and cell death ensue.

5. **Spectrum**
   A) Relatively narrow (Gram-positive)
      1) *Streptococcus*           7) *Bacillus anthracis*
      2) *Staphylococcus*          8) *Proteus*
      3) *Clostridium*             9) *Fusobacterium*
      4) *Erysipelothrix*         10) *Actinomyces*
      5) *Klebsiella*             11) *Leptospira*
      6) *Pasteurella multocida*

6. **Adverse reactions**
   A) One of the safest antibiotics with respect to organ toxicity.
   B) Hypersensitivity (drug allergy) may be encountered.
      1) Skin reactions, pharyngitis, salivation
      2) Anaphylactic shock may occur (incidence estimated at less than 0.5% in veterinary medicine).
   C) Capable of producing CNS stimulation — with very high doses or direct injection into cerebrospinal fluid.
   D) Procaine penicillin G is toxic to parakeets.
   E) Procaine penicillin G is toxic to snakes and turtles.

7. **Interactions**
   A) Penicillin may be displaced from plasma protein-binding sites by aspirin or phenylbutazone — gives more free penicillin and greater activity.
   B) Phenylbutazone competes with penicillin for active secretion sites in kidney; excretion of penicillin is slowed, giving higher plasma levels and longer duration.

8. **Formulary**
   A) Penicillin G (sodium or potassium salts
      1) Administer IV, SC, IM or by intramammary infusion.

2) Administer every 4-6 hours.
B) Procaine penicillin G
   1) Administer SC or IM
   2) Administer every 24 hours (horses every 12 hours)
C) Benzathine penicillin G
   1) Bicillin® (Wyeth)
   2) Longicil® (Fort Dodge)
   3) Slow onset of action due to slow absorption
D) Benzathine penicillin G plus procaine penicillin G — equal parts in the fixed drug combination.
   1) Bicillin® fortified (Wyeth)
   2) Longicil® fortified (Fort Dodge)
   3) Flocillin® (Bristol)
   4) Benza-Pen® (Beecham)
   5) Pen B and G (Pitman-Moore
   6) Depo® Penicillin (Upjohn)
   7) Administer SC or IM
   8) Fast blood levels from procaine penicillin G
   9) Longer duration from benzathine penicillin G
  10) Administer every 48 hours
E) Phenoxymethyl penicillin, penicillin V
   1) Available as generic
   2) Administer orally
   3) Administer every 4 to 6 hours
F) Ampicillin
   1) Princillin® (Squibb)
   2) Polyflex® (Bristol)
   3) Amcill® (Parke-Davis)
   4) Ampi-Tab® (Beecham)
   5) Omnipen® (Wyeth)
   6) Rea-Cil®
   7) Totacillin® (Beecham-Massengill)
   8) Amp-Equine® (Beecham)
   9) Broader spectrum, includes *E. coli* and *Salmonella spp*
  10) Administer orally, SC or IM
  11) Administer every 8 to 12 hours (every 24 hours to cattle and swine).
G) Phenethicillin K
   1) Darcil® (Wyeth)
   2) Alpen® (Lederle)
   3) Administer orally
   4) Administer every 4 hours
H) Hetacillin
   1) Hetacin-K® (Bristol)
   2) Chemically related to ampicillin

          3) Hydrolyzed in blood to ampicillin
          4) Administer orally or by intramammary infusion
          5) Administer every 12 hours
     I) Nafcillin
          1) Unipen® (Wyeth)
            a) *Oral* — administer every 6 hours
            b) *Intramuscular* — administer every 12 hours
   J) Dicloxacillin sodium
          1) Prostaphlin® (Bristol)
          2) Dariclox® (Beecham)
          3) Dicloxin® (Bristol)
          4) Penicillinase-resistant
          5) Administer orally
          6) Administer every 8 hours
   K) Benzathine cloxacillin
          1) Orbenin-DC® (Beecham)
          2) Boviclox®
          3) Administer via intramammary infusion
          4) Dry cow treatment only
   L) Methicillin
          1) Staphcillin® (Bristol)
          2) Administer IV or IM
          3) Administer every 6 hours
   M) Amoxicillin
          1) Amoxi-tabs® (Beecham)
          2) Dogs — orally
          3) Administer dosage of 5 mg/lb every 12 hours

## B. STREPTOMYCIN

   1. **Description**
     A) Produced by the actinomycete *Streptomyces griseus*
     B) Is an organic base
     C) Forms highly soluble salts, both hydrochloride and sulfate
     D) Dihydrostreptomycin — has two hydrogens added to strep-
        tomycin. Changes an aldehyde group to an alcohol group.
     E) Dihydrostreptomycin is more stable in solution.

   2. **General principles**
     A) Streptomycin and dihydrostreptomycin have basically the
        same antibacterial and pharmacological effects.
     B) First introduced in human medicine for the treatment of tu-
        berculosis

   3. **Metabolism**
     A) Absorption
          1) Rapidly absorbed from IM or SC injection. Therapeutic

levels are reached in 60 to 90 minutes.

2) Not absorbed from GI tract in sufficient amounts to reach a therapeutic level in the plasma

3) Remains *active* in the GI tract

4) After intramammary infusion, diffuses back into the plasma

B) Distribution

1) Rapidly distributes to most tissues

2) High concentrations in:
   a) Kidney        b) Muscle      c) Bile
   d) Peritoneal fluids            e) Eye

3) Lesser concentrations in:
   a) Pleural fluid
   b) Synovial fluid and pericardial fluid
   c) Milk

4) Poorly distributed to cerebrospinal fluid

5) Readily crosses into fetal circulation

6) Will penetrate acute abscesses

7) Residue persists in kidneys of cattle for at least 60 days

C) Biotransformation and excretion

1) Is excreted, predominately unchanged, by the kidney via glomerular filtration.

2) Streptomycin levels fall rapidly in plasma.

D) Duration of action: in most species, parenteral administration of streptomycin will give therapeutic action for 12 hours.

4. **Mechanism of action**

A) Is *bactericidal*

B) Modifies permeability of the cell membrane

C) Interferes with protein synthesis and cellular respiration

5. **Spectrum**

A) Relatively narrow (basically Gram-negative)

| | |
|---|---|
| 1) *Actinomyces* | 5) *Leptospira* |
| 2) *Brucella* | 6) *Pasteurella* |
| 3) *Salmonella* | 7) *Vibrio* |
| 4) *Escherichia coli (?)* | 8) *Mycobacteria* |

B) Resistance develops rapidly

6. **Adverse reactions**

A) Acute (caused by large parenteral doses)

1) A seemingly irreversible drop in blood pressure is caused by inhibition of the vasomotor center in the brain.

2) Respiratory depression and paralysis may occur.

3) Early signs are nausea, vomiting, ataxia, restlessness and

labored breathing.
4) Causes paralysis of skeletal muscle. It acts at the myo-neural junction to give a curare-like action.
5) Nephrotoxicity has been reported.

B) Chronic (caused by large doses given for extended periods [20 days])
1) Neurotoxicity
2) Impairment of hearing
3) Impairment of the vestibular apparatus, loss of balance
4) Possibly irreversible
5) Cat is the most sensitive of the domestic animals

7. **Interactions**
   A) Potentiates neuromuscular paralysis and respiratory depression caused by:
   1) Anesthetics     2) Curare     3) Succinylcholine chloride

8. **Formulary**
   A) Streptomycin — oral and injectable
   B) Dihydrostreptomycin — oral and injectable
   C) Available in combination with penicillin — usually dihydro-streptomycin; for IM or SC administration. May also contain a local anesthetic (procaine or lidocaine). Combiotic® (Pfizer), Penstrep® (Merck), Distrycillin® (Squibb) and many generics are available.

## C. CHLORAMPHENICOL

1. **Description**
   A) Originally produced from the actinomycete, *Streptomyces venezuela*
   B) Is now produced synthetically
   C) Chemical formula
   1) A nitro-benzene group is present.
   2) It is an organic base.

D) Base is very bitter — relatively insoluble in water.

E) Forms salts (palmitate and succinate)

1) *Palmitate* is more palatable; is used as an oral form.

2) *Succinate* is more soluble in water; is available as a powder for injection.

F) Chloramphenicol base is the active form.

G) Chloramphenicol base in propylene glycol is available for oral and parenteral use.

2. **General principles**

A) First of the broad-spectrum antibiotics

B) Stormy history in human medicine because of its ability to produce serious blood dyscrasias in man

C) Discrepancies have been shown between the bioavailability of the marketed preparations. These differences are in the plasma concentrations reached and the duration of therapeutic plasma levels.

3. **Metabolism**

A) Absorption

1) Is rapidly absorbed after oral administration. Peak levels are reached in 1 to 2 hours.

2) Rapidly absorbed from IM site. Therapeutic blood levels are reached in less than one hour.

B) Distribution

1) Is *very* rapidly distributed from plasma into the tissues

2) Large concentrations in the cerebrospinal fluid, liver, bile and kidney

3) Somewhat lesser concentrations in the eye, muscle, pleural fluid, peritoneal fluid, lungs and heart

4) Diffuses into the cerebrospinal fluid better than any antibiotic

5) Highly bound to protein in plasma (up to 45%)

6) Crosses readily into fetal circulation

C) Biotransformation and excretion

1) Chloramphenicol is biotransformed by the liver.

2) The principal metabolite is the glucuronide conjugate.

3) Glucuronide is inactive.

4) The glucuronide is excreted chiefly by the kidney.

5) Some glucuronide appears in bile. It goes to the intestine, where it may be hydrolyzed back into the active form and resorbed into the plasma.

6) Small amounts (10%) of free chloramphenicol appear in the urine.

7) Some chloramphenicol is biotransformed into an inactive reduced nitroderivative.

   D) Duration of action
     1) Varies somewhat with the different species
     2) After oral, IV or IM administration, therapeutic levels remain for 6 to 8 hours in most species (12 hours in cats).

4. **Mechanism of action**
   A) Bacteriostatic
   B) Large concentrations may be bactericidal under clinical conditions.
   C) Interferes with protein synthesis in bacteria

5. **Spectrum**
   A) Broad-spectrum (Gram-positive and Gram-negative)

| | |
|---|---|
| 1) *Staphylococcus* | 6) *Salmonella* |
| 2) *Streptococcus* | 7) *Proteus* |
| 3) *Brucella* | 8) *Klebsiella* |
| 4) *Pseudomonas* | 9) *Nocardia* |
| 5) *Escherichia coli* | 10) *Corynebacterium* |

   A) Rickettsia
   B) Large viruses — psittacosis

6. **Adverse reactions**
   A) Has produced aplastic anemia and fatal myeloblastic leukemia. It also has caused gray syndrome of newborn human infants.
   B) Extensively used therapeutically — large doses tested in animals; blood dycrasias have not been shown to occur when the drug is used at recommended dosages.
   C) Vomiting and diarrhea have been noted.
   D) Anorexia and depression were observed in cats treated for longer than 7 days.
   E) Severe shock-like reactions have occurred in young kittens.
   F) Chloramphenicol is relatively safe for use in veterinary medicine, *if used properly*.
     1) Reduce dosage for the newborn.
     2) Do not overdose.
     3) Do not treat for more than 7 days.
     4) Reduce dosage for animals with impaired kidney or liver function.
     5) Administer with care to animals with depressed bone marrow function.
   G) Chloramphenicol inhibits certain enzyme systems — primarily those enzymes in the liver involved with drug biotransformation.
   H) May inhibit antibody production if given for long periods.
   I) May inhibit wound healing if given for long periods.
   J) May interfere with protein synthesis of villi in the small in-

testine thus inhibiting the absorption of glucose and possibly other substances. This reaction was seen in rats given repeated large doses. The rats returned to normal in 10 days.

7. **Interactions**
   A) Chloramphenicol inhibits the inactivation of and increases plasma levels of:
      1) Pentobarbital
      2) Codeine
      3) Diphenylhydantoin sodium
      4) Analgesic-antipyretic drugs
      5) Anticoagulants given *per orum*

8. **Formulary**
   A) Chloramphenicol
      1) *Oral* — base and palmitate
      2) *Intravenous and intramuscular* — base and succinate
   B) Chloromycetin® (Parke-Davis)
   C) Tevcocin® (Tevco)
   D) Amphicol-V® (McKesson)
   E) Bemacol® (Beecham)
   F) Mychel-Vet® (Rachelle)
   G) Anacetin® (Bio-Ceutic)

D. **TETRACYCLINES**

1. **Description**
   A) Organic bases
   B) Produced by:
      1) *Streptomyces aureofaciens* (chlortetracycline)
      2) *Streptomyces rimosus* (oxytetracycline)
      3) Synthetic alteration of either of the above produces tetracycline.

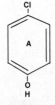

Chlortetracycline

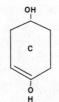

Oxytetracycline

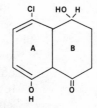

Demethylchlortetracycline

C) Chemically, they are all closely related.

D) Are sparingly soluble in water.

E) Acid salts (HCl) are more soluble in water.

F) Aqueous solutions are not stable.

G) Solutions containing propylene glycol are relatively stable.

H) Solutions containing polyvinylpyrollidone (PVP or povidone) are relatively stable.

2. **General principles**

   A) The tetracyclines differ slightly in spectrum and activity.

   B) Basic pharmacology of the group is similar.

   C) Cross-resistance — an organism that is resistant to one tetracycline is likely to be resistant to the other tetracyclines.

3. **Metabolism**

   A) Absorption

      1) Rapidly absorbed after oral administration. Effective blood levels are reached within 2 to 4 hours.

      2) Absorption of tetracyclines after oral administration is inhibited by presence of food, calcium, magnesium, iron and aluminum salts and (slightly) by milk. A poorly absorbed chelate is formed.

      3) Tetracyclines are absorbed from the uterus into the blood.

      4) After intramammary infusion, tetracyclines are absorbed, by back diffusion, into plasma.

   B) Distribution

      1) Tetracyclines vary in their protein-binding ability.

         a) Aureomycin® (American Cyanamid) has the greatest ability (65% in man).

         b) Oxytetracycline and tetracycline have the least ability (25% and 20%, respectively).

      2) Rapidly distributed to body tissues

      3) Large concentrations in liver, bile, kidney, urine, bone and lungs

      4) Passage of tetracyclines into the cerebrospinal fluid is good; it depends on dose and duration of therapy.

      5) Pass from plasma into milk

      6) Readily cross into fetal circulation

      7) Lesser concentrations in pleural fluid, peritoneal fluid, pericardial fluid, and eye

   C) Biotransformation and excretion

      1) Excretion is principally by the kidney via glomerular filtration.

      2) Most is excreted unchanged.

      3) Considerable free tetracycline is excreted via bile. Some is

resorbed; the rest appears in feces.

D) Duration of action

1) After oral, IV, or IM administration, therapeutic levels are maintained for more than 12 hours, but not longer than 24 hours.

2) An exception is concentrations of tetracyclines in the urine, where therapeutic levels are easily maintained for 24 hours.

3) In horses, the IV route of administration is superior to the IM route. Intravenous injection gives higher plasma levels of longer duration. Intravenous injection gives a 24-hour level; IM does not.

4) Oxytetracycline products with polyvinylpyrollidone (PVP) as a vehicle appear to give greater and somewhat longer-lasting blood levels after IM injection

4. **Mechanism of action**

A) Tetracyclines are bacteriostatic.

B) Large concentrations may be bactericidal under clinical conditions.

C) Tetracyclines interfere with protein synthesis in bacteria.

5. **Spectrum**

A) Broad-spectrum (Gram-positive and, to a lesser extent, Gram-negative)

| | |
|---|---|
| 1) *Fusobacterium* | 6) *Clostridium* |
| 2) *Brucella* | 7) *Pasteurella* |
| 3) *Streptococcus* | 8) *Escherichia coli* |
| 4) *Hemophilus* | 9) *Salmonella* |
| 5) *Klebsiella* | 10) *Nocardia* |

B) Coccidia

C) Rickettsia

D) Large viruses, psittacosis

E) Mycoplasma

6. **Adverse reactions**

A) Administration by mouth inhibits bacterial digestion in ruminants.

B) May exert an antianabolic effect

C) Drug allergy reactions, including anaphylactic shock, have been observed but are rare.

D) Hepatotoxicity in man has been reported (not a reported problem in animals).

E) Photosensitization may occur in man, especially from Declomycin® (Lederle).

F) Will stain teeth of neonates, or the fetus if given to pregnant females. The tetracyclines are incorporated into the enamel because of their affinity for and chelation with calcium.

G) Shock reactions when given IV.

H) Intravenous tetracyclines can precipitate milk fever in a pre-disposed animal; they are strong chelators of calcium.

I) May inhibit enzymes in the liver that biotransform the drug.

J) Renal toxicity; impair ability to concentrate urine in dogs given 20 mg/lb/day for 14 days. When given together to man, the tetracyclines and halothane or methoxyflurane can cause renal failure. This reaction has been studied in dogs and apparently is not a problem in that species.

K) May induce uremia or exacerbate uremia in patients with renal insufficiency

L) May cause severe diarrhea in horses under stress, as by surgery and anesthesia, usually when given orally.

7. **Formulary**
A) Oral, IV, and IM
B) Chlortetracycline — Aureomycin® (American Cyanamid)
C) Oxytetracycline — Terramycin® (Pfizer), generics
D) Injectable oxytetracycline
 1) *Propylene glycol vehicle* — IV and IM administration
  a) Liquamycin® (Pfizer)
  b) Terramycin® (Pfizer)    d) Aquachel® (Rachelle)
  c) Biocycline® (Upjohn)    e) Oxyject®
 2) PVP vehicle — IM administration
  a) Liquamycin-100® (Pfizer)   b) Oxybiotic®
  c) Bio-Mycin® (Bio-Ceutic)    d) Oxysteclin® (Squibb)
 3) Two concentrations are available: 50 and 100 mg/ml
E) Demethylchlortetracycline (Declomycin® —Lederle)
F) Tetracycline
 1) Polyotic® (American Cyanamid)
 2) Achromycin® (Lederle)
 3) Panmycin® (Upjohn)    5) Tetracyn® (Pfizer)
 4) Steclin® (Squibb)    6) Tetrachel-Vet® (Rachelle)
G) Methacycline (Rondomycin® —Wallace)
H) Doxycycline (Vibramycin® —Pfizer)
I) Minocycline (Minocin® —Lederle)
J) Oxytetracycline (Liquamycin LA-200® —Pfizer)
 1) Long-acting injectable; an injection of 9 mg/lb body-weight given IM gives blood levels for three days. A special vehicle is used for slow, controlled absorption into the blood.
 2) Approved for use in beef and nonlactating dairy cattle, and swine. Withdrawal time is 28 days.

## E. ERYTHROMYCIN

1. **Description**
   A) Produced from *Streptomyces erythreus*
   B) Is an organic base
   C) Forms acid salts
   D) Moderately soluble in water
   E) Powders are stable. Solutions are stable if refrigerated, but they are not stable at room temperature.

2. **General principles** — resistance develops rapidly.

3. **Metabolism**
   A) Absorption
      1) Absorption varies after *oral* administration, depending upon the salt form. Therapeutic blood levels are reached in 2 to 3 hours.
      2) After IM administration, peak blood levels are reached in 1 to 2 hours.
   B) Distribution
      1) Leaves plasma and enters tissues readily.
      2) Large concentrations in:
         a) Lungs          c) Liver
         b) Kidney         d) Salivary glands
      3) Lesser concentrations in:
         a) Pleural fluid   b) Peritoneal fluid   c) Seminal fluids
      4) Traces in the cerebrospinal fluid
      5) After intramammary infusion, diffuses back into plasma
   C) Biotransformation and excretion
      1) Biotransformed by liver
      2) Excreted primarily in bile. Large concentrations of active drug are present.
      3) Excreted in the urine. Large concentrations of active drug are present.
   D) Duration of action
      1) Recommendations concerning frequency of administration are conflicting.
      2) Duration varies with species.
      3) Duration of action is from 8 to 12 hours.

4. **Mechanism of action**
   A) Erythromycin is bacteriostatic.
   B) High concentrations may be bactericidal to highly susceptible organisms.
   C) Inhibits protein synthesis

5. **Spectrum**
   A) Acts chiefly on Gram-positive, but some Gram-negative,

organisms.

1) *Staphylococcus*  4) *Vibrio*
2) *Streptococcus*  5) *Pasteurella*
3) *Clostridium*   6) *Fusobacterium*

B) Resembles penicillin
C) Penicillin-resistant bacteria may be sensitive to erythromycin.

6. **Adverse reactions**
   A) Relatively nontoxic
   B) Local use may produce skin reaction
   C) Nausea and vomiting (rare)
   D) Under clinical use, no organ toxicity

7. **Interactions** — none recorded

8. **Formulary**
   A) Erythro-100® (CEVA)
   B) Erythro-200® (CEVA)
   C) Erythrocin® (Abbott)
   D) Ilotycin® (Lilly)
   E) E-Mycin® (Upjohn)

## F. LINCOMYCIN

1. **Description**
   A) Produced from *Streptomyces lincolnensis*
   B) Is an organic acid
   C) Readily forms salts — hydrochloride.
   D) Soluble in water
   E) Stable in powder and solution

2. **General principles**
   A) Clindamycin is a derivative of lincomycin.
   B) Cross-resistance with other antibiotics has not been demonstrated *in vivo* (erythromycin, *in vitro*).
   C) Resistance does not develop rapidly.
   D) It is approved for use in dogs, cats, and swine.

3. **Metabolism**
   A) Absorption
      1) Is rapid after oral administration. Peak blood levels are reached in 2 to 4 hours.
      2) Is rapid after IM administration. Therapeutic blood levels are reached within 10 minutes to 2 hours.
   B) Distribution
      1) Rapid diffusion into tissues
      2) Large concentrations in:
         a) Bone  b) Peritoneal fluid  c) Pericardial fluid
         d) Bile  e) Heart     f) Skin

3) Poor distribution to CNS

C) Biotransformation and excretion

1) Excreted in:

    a) Bile       b) Urine       c) Milk

D) Duration of action

1) After *oral* administration — 8 hours

2) IM or IV administration — 12 hours

## 4. Mechanism of action

A) Lincomycin may be bacteriostatic or bactericidal, depending upon sensitivity of the organism and concentration of the drug.

B) Inhibits protein synthesis

C) Presence of erythromycin in the body reduces or eliminates the action of lincomycin and vice versa.

## 5. Spectrum

A) Acts chiefly on Gram-positive bacteria:

| | |
|---|---|
| 1) *Staphylococcus* | 4) *Clostridium* |
| 2) *Streptococcus* | 5) *Corynebacterium* |
| 3) *Erysipelothrix* | 6) *Mycoplasma* |

## 6. Adverse reactions

A) Oral dosage

1) Loose stools

2) Vomiting (cats)

B) Serious gastrointestinal problems if given to horses

1) Profuse diarrhea

2) Dehydration and death

C) No reported organ toxicity

D) Skeletal-muscle paralysis with heavy concentrations

## 7. Interactions — additive effect upon respiratory depression when used with anesthetics and skeletal-muscle paralyzing agents

## 8. Formulary — Lincocin® (Upjohn)

# G. GENTAMICIN

## 1. Description

A) Produced by *Micromonaspora purpurea*

B) Is an organic base

C) Readily soluble in water

D) Stable in solution

## 2. General principles

A) Has been shown to exhibit cross-resistance with:

1) Neomycin     2) Kanamycin     3) Streptomycin

B) Resistance does develop

C) Approved for parenteral use in dogs and cats and intra-uterine use in horses.

3. **Metabolism**
   A) Absorption
      1) *Oral* — poor absorption
      2) *Intramuscular* — rapid absorption. Peak blood levels are reached at 1 hour.
   B) Distribution
      1) Plasma-protein bound (40% in man)
      2) Evidence suggests selective accumulation occurs initially somewhere in the body.
      3) Distribution to the CNS is moderate.
   C) Biotransformation and excretion
      1) It is excreted almost entirely unchanged in the urine.
      2) The kidney excretes gentamicin by glomerular filtration.
   D) Duration of action
      1) Initially therapeutic blood levels may be maintained for 12 hours with a single dose.
      2) After 1 to 2 days, therapeutic blood levels may be maintained for 24 hours with a single dose.

4. **Mechanism of action**
   A) Gentamicin is *bactericidal.*
   B) It interferes with protein synthesis of cell membranes.

5. **Spectrum**
   A) Broad (Gram-positive and Gram-negative bacteria)
      1) *Pseudomonas*      5) *Staphylococcus*
      2) *Proteus*      6) *Streptococcus*
      3) *Escherichia coli*   7) *Aerobacter*
      4) *Klebsiella*      8) *Neisseria*

6. **Adverse reactions**
   A) In man: disturbances of balance and ototoxicity.
   B) Large concentrations are toxic to the kidney; two to three times the normal dose will cause nephrotoxicity in dogs.
   C) Paralysis of skeletal muscle with high concentrations.

7. **Interactions**
   A) Additive effect upon respiratory depression with:
      1) Anesthetics      2) Skeletal-muscle paralyzing agents

8. **Formulary**
   A) Gentocin® (Schering)
   B) Garamycin® (Schering)
   C) Gentavet® (Burns-Biotec)

## H.  KANAMYCIN

### 1.  Description
A) Produced from *Streptomyces kanamyceticus*
B) Chemically similar to streptomycin and neomycin
C) Is an organic base
D) Soluble in water
E) Stable in solution

### 2.  General principles
A) Resistance develops slowly.
B) It is approved for use in dogs and cats.

### 3.  Metabolism
A) Absorption
    1) Poorly absorbed after oral administration
    2) Well absorbed from IM or SC sites. Peak blood levels are reached in 1 hour.
B) Distribution
    1) Diffuses readily into most body fluids. Highly concentrated in:
        a) Bile           d) Pleural fluid
        b) Synovial fluid    e) Kidney
        c) Peritoneal fluid
    2) Poor passage into CNS. Higher levels are present in the cerebrospinal fluid in the young (human).
    3) Poor passage into fetal circulation
C) Biotransformation and excretion
    1) Excreted almost entirely unchanged in the urine
    2) Kidney excretes kanamycin by glomerular filtration
D) Duration of action — therapeutic blood levels last for 12 hours.

### 4.  Mechanism of action
A) Kanamycin is *bactericidal*
B) Inhibits protein synthesis

### 5.  Spectrum
A) Broad (Gram-positive and Gram-negative bacteria)
    1) *Aerobacter*    5) *Corynebacterium*
    2) *Salmonella*    6) *Staphylococcus*
    3) *Proteus*    7) *Escherichia coli*
    4) *Pasteurella*

### 6.  Adverse reactions
A) Weight loss (cats)
B) Ototoxicity
C) Potential for toxicity to kidney
D) Paralysis of skeletal muscle with high concentration

7. **Interactions**

A) Strong binding affinity for free calcium — large concentrations of calcium inhibit the activity of kanamycin.

B) Additive effect upon respiratory depression with:

    1) Anesthetics    2) Skeletal-muscle paralyzing agents

8. **Formulary**

A) Kantrim® (Bristol)    B) Kantrex® (Bristol)

I. **NEOMYCIN**

1. **Description**

A) Produced from *Streptomyces fradiae*

B) Chemically similar to streptomycin

C) Soluble in water

D) Stable in solution

2. **General principles:** resistance develops slowly.

3. **Metabolism**

A) Absorption

    1) Poorly absorbed when given orally. Absorbed to a greater degree than is streptomycin.

    2) It remains active in the GI tract.

    3) It is absorbed from IP or IM injection sites. Therapeutic blood levels are reached in 1 hour.

B) Distribution

    1) Will diffuse into pleural and peritoneal fluids

    2) Will pass into the cerebrospinal fluid

    3) Residues may persist in the kidneys of cattle for at least 90 days.

C) Biotransformation and excretion

    1) Is excreted, unchanged, in the urine

D) Duration of action

    1) *Oral* — 4 to 6 hours

    2) *Intramuscular* — 8 to 12 hours

4. **Mechanism of action**

A) Is *bactericidal* at high concentrations

B) Inhibits protein synthesis

5. **Spectrum**

A) Broad (Gram-positive and Gram-negative bacteria)

    1) *Staphylococcus*    6) *Proteus*

    2) *Corynebacterium*    7) *Klebsiella*

    3) *Bacillus anthracis*    8) *Escherichia coli*

    4) *Listeria*    9) *Neisseria*

    5) *Aerobacter*

6. **Adverse reactions**
   A) Ototoxicity
   B) Potential for toxicity to kidney
   C) Administer to postpartum cows systemically with great caution; may trigger milk fever.
   D) Paralysis of skeletal muscle with large concentrations. The antidote is neostigmine.

7. **Interactions**
   A) Additive effect upon respiratory depression with:
      1) Anesthetics
      2) Skeletal-muscle paralyzing agents

8. **Formulary**
   A) Biosol® (Upjohn)   B) Generics

J. **TYLOSIN**

   1. **Description**
      A) Produced from *Streptomyces fradiae*, (a strain different from the producer of neomycin)
      B) Chemically related to erythromycin
      C) Is an organic base
      D) Slightly soluble in water (salts are soluble)
      E) Unstable in acid media (less than pH 4)

   2. **General principles**
      A) Used in veterinary medicine, not in human medicine.
      B) Resistance to tylosin develops rather slowly.
      C) Cross-resistance with erythromycin has been shown.
      D) Not to be mixed with other drugs administered by parenteral routes.

   3. **Metabolism**
      A) Absorption
         1) *Oral* — well absorbed, mainly from intestine
         2) *Intramuscular* — rapid absorption
      B) Distribution
         1) Well distributed to most tissues
         2) Apparently not well distributed to CNS
         3) Passes readily into milk (greater concentrations than in plasma)
      C) Biotransformation and excretion: tylosin is excreted in the bile and urine, apparently unchanged.
      D) Duration of action
         1) *Oral* — 8 hours
         2) *Intramuscular* — 12-24 hours

   4. **Mechanism of action:** tylosin is *bacteriostatic*.

5. **Spectrum**

   A) Is essentially active against Gram-positive bacteria — some Gram-negative.

      1) Spirochetes (*Leptospira*)   4) *Campylobacter*
      2) Large viruses              5) PPLO—*Corynebacterium*
      3) *Mycoplasma*               6) *Fusobacterium—Moraxella*

6. **Adverse reactions**

   A) Relatively safe; wide margin of safety
   B) Reactions have been noted in swine:
      1) Edema and erythema of rectal mucosa
      2) Anal protrusion     3) Pruritus     4) Diarrhea

7. **Reported to cause severe diarrhea in horses.** In some cases the diarrhea has been irreversible and led to death.

8. **Interactions:** may increase the toxicity of digitalis.

9. **Formulary** — Tylan® (Elanco)


K. **SPECTINOMYCIN**

   1. **Description**

      A) Produced from *Streptomyces flavopersicus*
      B) Is an organic base
      C) Highly soluble in water (both base and salts)
      D) Highly stable in solution

   2. **General principles**

      A) Approved for oral administration to pigs less than 4 weeks old
      B) Approved for oral and IM administration to dogs
      C) Approved for SC administration to poultry
      D) Resistance develops slowly

   3. **Metabolism**

      A) Absorption
         1) *Oral* — poorly absorbed from GI tract (7% absorbed). Remains active in the GI tract.
         2) Readily absorbed from IM and SC injection sites
      B) Distribution — (data not available)
      C) Biotransformation and excretion
         1) Excreted via the kidney, apparently unchanged.
      D) Duration of action
         1) *Oral* — 12 hours
         2) *Parenteral* — 8 to 12 hours in man; duration in animals has not been established.

4. **Mechanism of action**
   A) Is *bacteriostatic*
   B) Inhibits protein synthesis

5. **Spectrum**
   A) Relatively broad spectrum (Gram-positive and Gram-negative bacteria)

   | | |
   |---|---|
   | 1) *Staphylococcus* | 7) *Aerobacter* |
   | 2) *Streptococcus* | 8) *Klebsiella* |
   | 3) *Pasteurella* | 9) *Salmonella* |
   | 4) *Proteus* | 10) *Pseudomonas* |
   | 5) *Clostridium* | 11) *Campylobacter* |
   | 6) *Escherichia coli* | 12) *Mycoplasma* |

6. **Adverse reactions**
   A) No reported toxic reactions at usual dosages.
   B) Decreases in hematocrit and hemoglobin levels in man

7. **Interactions** — none reported

8. **Formulary**
   A) Spectinomycin — oral and injectable
      1) Spectam® (CEVA)     2) Trobicin® (Upjohn)

L. **CEPHALORIDINE**

1. **Description**
   A) A partially synthetic derivative of cephalosporin C
   B) Cephalosporin C is produced from *Cephalosporium acremonium.*
   C) Organic acids
   D) Related chemically to penicillin
   E) Solutions are stable.
   F) Oily preparation

2. **General principles**
   A) Should be administered in a dry syringe; contact with water may cause loss of potency.
   B) Resembles penicillin pharmacologically

3. **Metabolism**
   A) Absorption
      1) *Oral* — poorly absorbed
      2) *Intramuscular* — rapidly absorbed. Therapeutic blood levels are reached in 1 hour.
      3) *Subcutaneous* — more slowly absorbed and blood levels are not quite as high as those achieved with IM injection.
   B) Distribution
      1) Not significantly bound to plasma proteins
      2) Widely distributed throughout body tissues and fluids

3) Minimal concentrations in CNS

4) Passes through placenta into fetal circulation

5) Passes into milk

C) Biotransformation and excretion

1) Excreted rapidly via the kidney

2) High concentrations are excreted unchanged in urine

D) Duration: therapeutic blood levels exist for 12 hours.

4. **Mechanism of action**

A) Is *bactericidal*

B) Antimicrobial action — quantitatively and qualitatively similar to penicillin

C) Interferes with cell-wall synthesis

5. **Spectrum**

A) Active against both Gram-positive and Gram-negative bacteria. Gram-positive are highly sensitive; Gram-negative are slightly less sensitive.

1) *Staphylococcus*     6) *Klebsiella*

2) *Streptococcus*     7) *Salmonella*

3) *Proteus*     8) *Escherichia coli*

4) *Pneumococcus*     9) *Clostridium*

5) *Corynebacterium*

6. **Adverse reactions**

A) Relatively low order of toxicity

B) Chronic use in cats depresses hemoglobin, hematocrit, and RBC values.

C) Excessively large doses (200 mg/kg) in rabbits have caused nephrotoxicity.

D) Evidence exists of partial cross-allergenicity with penicillin. Must be used with extreme caution in animals that have shown hypersensitivity to penicillin.

E) Safety in pregnant animals has not been established.

7. **Interactions** — none reported

8. **Formulary**

A) Loridine® (Lilly) — a former trade name (not available)

B) Keflodin™ (Pitman-Moore) (no longer available)

## M. NOVOBIOCIN

1. **Description**

A) Produced from *Streptomyces niveus*

B) An organic acid

2. **General principles**

A) Not extensively used in human medicine

B) Available in veterinary medicine in combination with tetracycline (Albaplex® — Upjohn).

3. **Metabolism**

A) Absorption

1) Rapidly absorbed from gastrointestinal tract

2) Peak blood levels are reached in 2 to 3 hours after oral administration.

B) Distribution

1) Diffuses readily into most tissues. It is absorbed to a lesser extent into the pleural, ascitic, and joint fluids.

2) Greatly concentrated in the liver

3) No appreciable concentrations in the CNS

C) Biotransformation and excretion

1) Some biotransformed to a yellow pigment

2) Small amounts excreted in the urine

3) Primarily excreted via the bile and feces

D) Duration of action: *orally* — 12 hours

4. **Mechanism of action**

A) Novobiocin is both *bacteriostatic* and *bactericidal.*

B) It complexes magnesium within the cell of the bacterium; inhibits protein synthesis.

5. **Spectrum**

A) Active against Gram-positive and Gram-negative bacteria

1) *Staphylococcus*          4) *Proteus* (some strains)

2) *Streptococcus*          5) *Leptospira* (canine)

3) *Pneumococcus*          6) *Coccidium* (canine)

6. **Adverse reactions**

A) May cause allergic reactions

B) Has produced jaundice in man; inhibits the enzyme (glucuronyl transferase) that conjugates bilirubin to prepare it for excretion.

7. **Interactions** — none found

8. **Formulary**

A) Albamycin® (Upjohn)

B) Cathomycin® (Merck, Sharp & Dohme)

C) Albaplex® (Upjohn) — novobiocin with tetracycline

D) Delta Albaplex® (Upjohn) — Albaplex plus prednisolone

N. **BACITRACIN**

1. **Description**

A) Produced from a strain of *Bacillus subtilis*

B) A polypeptide organic acid

C) Soluble in water (except zinc bacitracin)

D) Stable

2. **General principles**
   A) Almost exclusively used topically
   B) Not used systemically in human medicine

3. **Metabolism**
   A) Not absorbed from the skin
   B) Not absorbed from the GI tract

4. **Mechanism of action**
   A) Bacitracin is *bactericidal*.
   B) It interferes with cell-wall formation.

5. **Spectrum**
   A) Narrow; chiefly Gram-positive bacteria
   B) Similar to penicillin
      1) *Streptococcus*   2) *Clostridium*   3) *Staphylococcus*

6. **Adverse reactions**
   A) Topically — none reported
   B) Systemically is somewhat toxic (nephrotoxic)

7. **Interactions** — none found

8. **Formulary**
   A) Bacitracin (generic)
   B) Feed additive

O. **POLYMYXIN B**

1. **Description**
   A) Produced from *Bacillus polymyxa*
   B) Many different compounds (polymyxins A, B, C, D and E)
   C) Soluble in water
   D) Stable

2. **General principles** — primarily used topically

3. **Metabolism**
   A) Not absorbed from the skin
   B) Not absorbed from the GI tract

4. **Mechanism of action**
   A) Polymyxin B is *bactericidal*.
   B) It disrupts integrity of the cell wall, alters permeability of the cell membrane and interferes with maintenance of proper osmotic equilibrium in the cell.

5. **Spectrum**
   A) Narrow — chiefly Gram-negative bacteria.
      1) *Aerobacter*          5) *Shigella*
      2) *Escherichia coli*    6) *Pseudomonas*
      3) *Salmonella*          7) *Brucella*
      4) *Campylobacter*

6. **Adverse reactions**
   A) Topically — none
   B) Systemically — somewhat toxic, nephrotoxic, neurotoxic
7. **Interactions:** antagonized by quaternary ammonium compounds
8. **Formulary:** polymyxin B (generic)

P. **VIRGINIAMYCIN**
   1. **Description**
      A) Produced by *Streptomyces virginiae*
      B) Soluble in water
      C) Composed of several factors
   2. **General principles** — used orally only; administered as a feed-additive or in the drinking water.
   3. **Metabolism** — no information found
   4. **Mechanism of action** — no information found
   5. **Spectrum**
      A) Several factors; they act independently and are reported to be synergistic.
      B) Active primarily against Gram-positive bacteria
      C) Reported to be specific for swine dysentery
   6. **Nontoxic**
   7. **Interactions** — none found
   8. **Formulary** — Stafac®

Q. **SODIUM CEPHAPIRIN**
   1. **Cefa-Lak®** (Bristol)
   2. **Intramammary infusion** for lactating cows
   3. **Withdrawal**
      A) Milk — 96 hours, 8 milkings
      B) Slaughter — 4 days

R. **CUPRIMYXIN**
   1. **Unitop® topical cream** (Hoffmann-LaRoche)
      A) A cupric complex of the antibiotic, myxin
      B) Broad sprectrum
      C) Topical use only
      D) Antibacterial, antifungal, and anti-yeast activity

S. **LS$^{50}$** — A powder for oral administration to chickens in their drinking water. Each package contains 16.7 g lincomycin and 33.3 g spectinomycin.

# Nitrofurans

A. **DESCRIPTION**

　1. **Completely synthetic** — derivatives of furan

　2. **Chemical formula** — from the basic nitrofuran group:

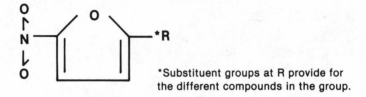

　　*Substituent groups at R provide for the different compounds in the group.

B. **GENERAL PRINCIPLES**

　1. No evidence of cross-resistance with other antimicrobial drugs

　2. Resistance develops slowly.

C. **METABOLISM**

　1. **Absorption**
　　A) *Nitrofurantoin* (oral) — rapid and complete
　　B) *Nitrofurazone* (oral) — variable

　2. **Distribution**
　　A) High levels of free drug are found in the urine and also in the interstitial fluid and lymph of the kidney. The drug is especially effective in many urinary infections.
　　B) Acid urine enhances concentration in the kidney.
　　C) Tightly and highly protein-bound in plasma with little free (active) drug in the plasma; not effective against septicemias.

　3. **Biotransformation and excretion**
　　A) Excreted, unchanged, via urine and bile
　　B) Some is biotransformed by liver and excreted in bile

　4. **Duration of action:** *nitrofurantoin* — 8 hours

D. **MECHANISM OF ACTION**

　1. **Nitrofurans may be bacteriostatic or bactericidal,** depending on the concentration and the nitrofuran used.

　2. **Enzyme inhibition** is possibly related to production of energy by the bacteria.

E. **SPECTRUM**

1. **Antibacterial** (Gram-positive and Gram-negative)
   A) *Escherichia coli*      E) *Pseudomonas* (may be resistant)
   B) *Staphylococcus*        F) *Proteus* (may be resistant)
   C) *Streptococcus*         G) *Aerobacter*
   D) *Salmonella*

2. **Coccidiostatic**

3. **Antifungal**

F. **ADVERSE REACTIONS**

1. **Nausea and emesis**

2. **Diarrhea** — gastrointestinal hemorrhage

3. **Neurotoxicity in calves has been reported**
   A) Head tremors, ataxia, and visual impairment
   B) Fits (climbing-the-wall)

G. **INTERACTIONS** — none found

H. **FORMULARY**

1. **Nitrofurazone**
   A) Furacin® (Norden)
   B) Furadex® (Norden)
   C) Pelizone ointment (National)

2. **Nitrofurantoin**
   A) Furadantin® (Eaton)
   B) Dantafur® (Norden)
   C) Equidantin®

3. **Furazolidone**
   A) Topazone® (Norden)
   B) Furoxone® (Norden)

4. **Nifuraldezone**
   A) Furamazone® (Eaton)
   B) Entefur® (Eaton)

# Antifungal Agents

A. **OBJECTIVES OF TREATMENT**

1. **Eliminate the fungal infection**
   A) Systemic treatment        B) Topical treatment

2. **Prevent spread**
   A) Clip hair, trim toenails, bathe.
   B) Isolate animal.
   C) Clean up contaminated areas.

B. **AGENTS TO TREAT DERMATOMYCOSIS**

1. **Griseofulvin** (Fulvicin U/F® [Schering], Grifungal™[Pitman-Moore])
   A) An antibiotic; no antibacterial activity. Not water-soluble.
   B) Inhibits the growth of dermatophytic fungi of the skin.

Mechanism of action is via interference with biosynthesis of nucleic acid and hence protein synthesis.

C) For oral administration only to:

    1) Dogs        2) Cats        3) Horses

D) Metabolism

    1) Absorption

        a) Depends upon particle size. Micro-size particles are absorbed twice as well.

        b) Feeding of fat enhances absorption.

        c) Administer after meals to enhance absorption.

    2) Selectively distributes to diseased skin

    3) Excreted unchanged, principally in feces.

E) May be embryotoxic and teratogenic

F) Resistance may develop.

G) Topical efficacy is doubtful.

H) Stimulates the hepatic drug biotransformation scheme (enzyme induction)

  2. **Topical agents**

    A) Pimaricin (Myprozine® )

    B) Hexetidine (Sterisil)

    C) Triacetin (Enzactin® —Ayerst), (Fungacetin® —Blair)

    D) Nifuroxime (Mycofur® —N.F.)

    E) Sodium propionate

    F) Undecylenic acid

    G) Salicylanilide

    H) Phenolic compounds (phenol, thymol)

    I) Benzoic acid

    J) Salicylic acid

    K) Potassium permanganate

    L) Rosaniline dyes (gentian violet, basic fuchin)

    M) Nitrofurfuryl methyl ether — Furaspor®

    N) Tolnaftate (Tinactin® —Schering)

    O) Mercaptocaine® a fungicide plus bactericide and topical anesthetic

    P) Thiabendazole (Tresaderm® —Merck)

    Q) Mycodex® (Beecham)

    R) Iodophores

    S) Nystatin (Mycostatin® —Squibb)

C. **SYSTEMIC MYCOSES**

  1. **Amphotericin B** (Fungizone® —Squibb)

    A) An antibiotic; no antibacterial activity.

    B) Used in treatment for blastomycosis, coccidioidomycosis, cryptococcosis and histoplasmosis

    C) Mechanism of action: disturbs the permeability of the cell membrane. This results in loss of intracellular components (cations) and causes irreversible damage.

    D) Administered IV diluted; a colloidal preparation.

    E) Poorly absorbed from GI tract

    F) Highly toxic compound; the following adverse reactions have been reported:

       1) Inhibition of kidney and liver function

       2) Anemia

       3) Decline of blood pressure

       4) Electrolyte disturbances

       5) Disturbances of CNS

2. **Nystatin** (Mycostatin® —Squibb)

    A) An antibiotic; no antibacterial activity.

    B) Used in treatment for candidiasis

    C) Mechanism of action is similar to that of amphotericin B.

    D) Poorly absorbed when given orally; requires large doses.

    E) Relatively nontoxic

3. **Actinophytoses, nocardiosis**

    A) Treat with sulfonamides.

    B) Sulfadiazine is probably the most effective sulfonamide.

# Miscellaneous Antimicrobial Drugs

A. **CARBADOX**

1. **Description**

    A) Not an antibiotic, sulfonamide, or nitrofuran

    B) Chemistry: a quinoxaline-di-N-oxide

    C) Not water-soluble

2. **General principles:** feed-additive for swine

3. **Spectrum:** effective in control of swine dysentery and *Salmonella cholerasuis.*

4. **Adverse reactions** — none found

5. **Interactions** — none found

6. **Formulary:** Mecadox®

B. **ISONIAZID**

1. **Description**

    A) A derivative of isonicotinic acid

    B) A synthetic compound
    C) Soluble in water

2. **General principles**
    A) Developed for use in human medicine for the treatment and control of tuberculosis.
    B) Not available with a veterinary label

3. **Metabolism**
    A) Absorption: rapid after oral administration
    B) Distribution
       1) Diffuses readily into all body fluids and cells
       2) Passes into fetal circulation
       3) Passes into milk
       4) Penetrates well into caseous material
    C) Biotransformation and excretion
       1) Some biotransformed by the liver
       2) Some excreted unchanged in urine
    D) Duration of action
       1) Not well documented for domestic animals
       2) Is recommended for administration twice a day (12-hour duration of activity)

4. **Mechanism of action**
    A) Capable of bactericidal activity
    B) Interferes with cellular intermediary metabolism

5. **Spectrum (most useful in chronic infections)**
    A) *Mycobacterium tuberculosis* — said by some to be the *only* susceptible microorganism.
    B) *Actinomyces (?)*
    C) *Fusobacterium (?)*

6. **Adverse reactions**
    A) Relatively safe in domestic animals
    B) Human
       1) Hypersensitivity    2) Hepatitis    3) Convulsions
    C) Reported to be embryocidal
    D) May inhibit hepatic drug biotransformation system

7. **Interactions:** may lead to a deficiency of pyridoxine

8. **Formulary**
    A) Isoniazid (generic)        C) Niadox®
    B) Nydrazid® (Squibb)         D) INH® (Ciba)

# Principles of Antibiotic
# Use in Chemotherapy

A. **METABOLISM**

1. **Absorption**

   A) Most antibiotics are well absorbed after parenteral and oral administration.

      1) Intestinal antibiotics are the exception. These *are not* absorbed when given orally:

         a) Streptomycin     d) Bacitracin

         b) Neomycin         e) Vancomycin

         c) Kanamycin

   B) Variation of absorption of drugs by sex has been shown.

2. **Distribution**

   A) Passage into the cerebrospinal fluid is facilitated if the meninges are inflamed. Less protein binding occurs in the cerebrospinal fluid; hence antibacterial activity is achieved with lesser concentrations.

   B) Most antibiotics will pass the placental barrier.

3. **Biotransformation and excretion:** decreased in neonates and old animals. Activity is of longer duration.

B. **BASIS FOR CLINICAL EFFICACY**

1. **Narrow spectrum and broad-spectrum drugs are available.** Use the proper drug to combat *sensitive* bacteria.

   A) May be predictable

   B) Sensitivity testing may be a help; however, sensitivity *in vitro* does not guarantee success in treating infectious diseases *in vivo* — usually indicates what *will not* work.

   C) Simple Gram stain may be of help.

2. **Use antibiotics early in disease:** this approach utilizes, to the fullest, the animal's body defense mechanisms, especially when bacteriostatic drugs are used.

3. **Use the most effective drug available.** A single antibiotic chosen on the basis of its spectrum is most desirable.

4. **Avoid using less than the optimal dose for the disease involved.** Large doses, of a well chosen antibiotic, for appropriate periods are usually the most beneficial.

5. **Provide adequate duration** of treatment for effective *in vivo* antibiotic activity — usually at least four days.

6. **Testing for cure may be desirable.**

7. **Change antibiotics if needed,** based upon observations of indi-

vidual cases and past experience. This approach is more logical than shotgun therapy based upon a generalized cook-book type of regimen under which all animals are treated alike.

C. **MECHANISMS OF ANTIBIOTIC ACTION AND COMBINATION THERAPY**
 1. **Bactericidal antibiotics**
    A) Rupture of cell wall; cells must be multiplying rapidly.
    B) Alters permeability of cell membrane and also changes the metabolism of bacteria.
    C)

| | | |
|---|---|---|
| 1) Penicillins G & V | 7) Oxacillin | 13) Kanamycin |
| 2) Bacitracin | 8) Nafcillin | 14) Neomycin |
| 3) Vancomycin | 9) Gentamicin | 15) Cephaloridine |
| 4) Ampicillin | 10) Polymyxin | 16) Tribrissen® |
| 5) Hetacillin | 11) Novobiocin | 17) Nitrofurans |
| 6) Methicillin | 12) Streptomycin | |

    D) High blood levels of tetracyclines, chloramphenicol, and lincomycin.

 2. **Bacteriostatic antibiotics**
    A) Inhibit protein synthesis; also inhibit nucleic acid synthesis and intermediary metabolism of bacterial cells.
    B) Retard multiplication of bacteria
    C) Rely heavily on the host's defense mechanisms
    D)

| | |
|---|---|
| 1) Tetracyclines | 5) Erythromycin |
| 2) Chloramphenicol | 6) Novobiocin |
| 3) Lincomycin | 7) Sulfonamides |
| 4) Tylosin | 8) Nitrofurans |

 3. **Effect of combined antibacterial therapeutic agents** — the action of drugs in combination may be:
    A) *Additive* — two or more drugs interfere with the same constituent in cellular or metabolic processes. The result is an additive effect similar to increased dosage. These combinations are useful when increased dosage of one drug may produce undesirable side effects.
    B) *Synergistic* — this is accomplished when two drugs interfere with different constituents in cellular or metabolic processes. The result is an effect greater than could be attributed to additive action. Organisms surviving the first drug, if susceptible to the second, would succumb. In theory, a drug affecting the permeability of the cell membrane (streptomycin), plus a drug affecting the cell wall (penicillin), when used in combination, may be more effective than either drug used alone.
    C) *Antagonistic* — this effect is produced when the action of

the two drugs in combination is less than could be achieved by the most effective member of the combination acting alone. (*See* graph below.)

Effect of Penicillin, Streptomycin, and Chloromycetin on Enterococcus *in vitro*, (From Jawetz, Gunnison, J.B., and Coleman, V.R.: *Science 111*, 1950.)

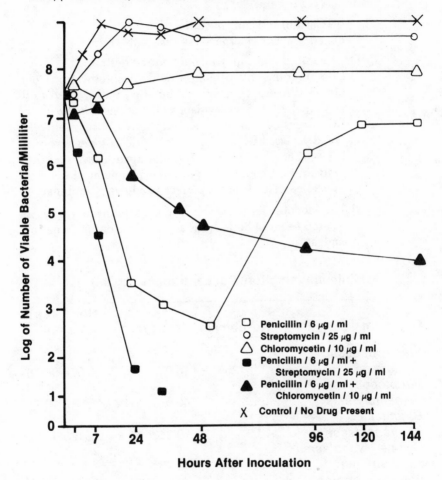

D) *Independent* — this effect occurs when the action of the combined drugs is about equal to the activity of the most effective of the two drugs.

4. **Guidelines for combinations of therapeutic agents**
   A) Bacteriostatic and bactericidal drugs may be antagonistic towards each other.
   B) Antagonism does not occur between members of the same

group (bacteriostatic or bactericidal).

C) Bacteriostatic antibiotics are never synergistic; however, they may be additive.

D) Bactericidal antibiotics also may be synergistic.

E) Combination therapy:

   1) Should be used only when specifically indicated

     a) Mixed infections

     b) Certain resistant bacteria

     c) To prevent emergence of resistant strains

F) Drug combinations may or may not be desirable.

   1) Combinations of penicillin and streptomycin: Combiotic® (Pfizer) is a good combination with regard to its action; there is even evidence of synergism between the two drugs. However, the durations of their effective blood levels differ. When Combiotic is given every 24 hours, there are 12 hours of subtherapeutic levels of streptomycin that could be inviting development of bacterial resistance. This is not a perfect fixed-drug combination.

   2) The novobiocin-tetracycline combination may be indicated because both drugs are bactericidal in large concentrations.

## Minimum Inhibitory Concentrations ($\mu$g/ml)

| Organism | Novobiocin | Tetracycline | Novo./Tetra. 1:1 ratio |
|---|---|---|---|
| Staphylococcus aureus | 0.3125 | 10.0 | 0.078/0.078 |
| Streptococcus hemolyticus | 10.0 | 40.0 | 10.0/10.0 |
| Bordetella bronchiseptica | 10.0 | 0.3125 | 0.3125/0.3125 |
| Canine Mycoplasma (6 strains) | 3.54 | 0.73 | 0.73/0.73 |
| Resistant strains of Mycoplasma | 3/6 | 2/6 | 0/6 |

These data demonstrate that the minimum inhibitory concentration (MIC) of novobiocin against staphylococci and streptococci is less than that of tetracycline. The MIC of the combination against staphylococci is less than that of either component alone. The MIC of tetracycline against *Bordetella* and *Mycoplasma* is less than that of novobiocin, but only the combination of novobiocin and tetracycline was effective against all strains of *Mycoplasma* tested.

3) Tylosin plus oxytetracycline is synergistic *in vivo* and *in vitro* against *Pasteurella multocida*.

4) Gentamicin and semisynthetic penicillins are thought to have synergistic activity against Gram-negative organisms. Both are bactericidal.

5) Antagonistic combinations shown in human medicine:
   a) Lincomycin and erythromycin
   b) Chloramphenicol and gentamicin
   c) Penicillin and aureomycin
   d) Chloramphenicol and ampicillin

6) Favorable combinations, shown in human medicine:
   a) Ampicillin and streptomycin
   b) Lincomycin and streptomycin
   c) Ampicillin and chloramphenicol
   d) Cephaloridine and gentamicin
   e) Ampicillin and gentamicin

## D. REASONS FOR FAILURE OF ANTIBACTERIAL DRUG THERAPY

1. **Incorrect clinical diagnosis or procedures**
   A) Failure to recognize mixed infections
   B) Treatment of fever of undiagnosed origin
   C) Complete reliance on culture and sensitivity reports
   D) Improper dose, duration, or route of administration
   E) Worthless prophylaxis
   F) Concomitant administration of other drugs that interfere with antibacterial drugs (*e.g.* simultaneous chronic use of anti-inflammatory steroids)
   G) Combination of antagonistic antibacterial drugs
   H) Treatment of untreatable infections (*e.g.* viral diseases)

2. **Host factors**
   A) Failure of the host's defense mechanisms
      1) Disease (agammaglobulinemia, lymphoma) and/or debility
      2) Administration of other drugs (corticosteroids or anti-cancer drugs)
      3) See table of experimental data on facing page.

   B) Inaccesibility of drugs to infection (*e.g.* in meninges, bone, skin or urinary tract in a patient with renal insufficiency)
   C) Formation of abscess
   D) Infection incurable because of presence of foreign body, kidney stone, malignancy, or congenital anomaly
   E) Presence of undiagnosed complicating conditions

## Mortality and Postmortem Growth of Infectious Strain Under Different Antibiotic and Immunosuppressive Treatment of Mice

**(All Mice Injected with a Virulent Pathogen)**

| Treatment | Antibiotic employed | Immuno-suppression | Mortality | Postmortal growth of infectious strain |
|---|---|---|---|---|
| None (controls) | None | None | 100% | 100% |
| Bactericidal | Oxacillin Plus Neomycin | None | 0% | 10% |
| | Neomycin | Splenectomy | 5% | 15% |
| | Neomycin | Prednisolone 1 mg | 10% | 30% |
| | Neomycin | Prednisolone 5 mb | 30% | 70% |
| Bacteriostatic | Lincomycin Plus Erythromycin | None | 0% | 30% |
| | Erythromycin | Splenectomy | 15% | 20% |
| | Erythromycin | Prednisolone 1 mg | 30% | 50% |
| | Erythromycin | Prednisolone 5 mg | 70% | 90% |

## E. INFLUENCE OF pH CHANGES IN ENVIRONMENT ON ANTIBACTERIAL ACTIVITY

1. **Increased activity in acid, decreased activity in alkaline**
   A) Nitrofurans     B) Sulfonamides     C) Tetracyclines

2. **Increased activity in alkaline, decreased activity in acid**
   A) Chloramphenicol     D) Kanamycin
   B) Gentamicin     E) Erythromycin
   C) Neomycin     F) Streptomycin

# Biotransformation and Excretion of Antibacterial Agents

Legend: BT = Biotransformed
  B  = Bile
  M  = Metabolite
  *  = Principle form when both occur

|  | LIVER | KIDNEY AND URINE |
|---|---|---|
| Sulfa | BT M & B | M & F* |
| Penicillin | ----- | F |
| Ampicillin | F in B | F |
| Synthetic penicillin | BT M&F in B | F* |
| Tetracyclines | BT M&F* in B | M & F* |
| Chloramphenicol | BT | M* & F |
| Gentamicin | ----- | F |
| Kanamycin | ----- | F |
| Neomycin | ----- | F |
| Erythromycin | BT F* in B | M & F* |
| Bacitracin | ----- | F |
| Novobiocin | BT M* in B | M & F |
| Spectinomycin | ----- | F |
| Lincomycin | F in B | F |
| Tylosin | F in B | F |
| Cephaloridine | ----- | F |
| Nitrofurans | BT M&F in B | F* |

F.  **ADVERSE REACTIONS**
  1. **Causes of toxic manifestations of therapeutic agents:**
    A) Frank overdose
    B) Relative overdose
      1) Failure to reduce dose or frequency of administration when biotransformation and/or excretion are impaired because of the patient's age, the disease, or the administration of other drugs
      2) Improper administration
      3) Extremely hyperreactive animal
    C) Use of antibiotic combinations in which both drugs have the same potential for toxicity.

D) Interactions with other drugs
  1) Neuromuscular blocking antibiotics when used with other muscle-relaxing drugs such as anesthetics, curare, succinylcholine, M-99, or guaifenesin, may cause respiraratory embarrassment or even paralysis.
  2) Nephrotoxic antibiotics used with (Lasix® —American Hoechst) may enhance the potential for nephrotoxicity.
  3) Increased plasma levels caused by competitive displacement from plasma-protein carrier sites, increased toxicity potential:
    a) Methotrexate and sulfonamides increase methotrexate.
    b) Penicillin and phenylbutazone increase penicillin.
    c) Sulfonamides and phenylbutazone increase sulfonamides.
    d) Sulfonamides and aspirin increase sulfonamides.
    e) Penicillin and aspirin increase penicillin.
  4) Increased plasma levels due to competition for active secretion sites in kidney:
    a) Methotrexate and sulfonamides increase methotrexate.
    b) Penicillin and phenylbutazone increase penicillin.
    c) Cephalosporins and phenylbutazone increase cephalosporins.
E) Pre-existing pathology; *e.g.* cardiovascular, renal, hepatic, or severely debilitating conditions.
F) Species idiocyncrasies
  1) Procaine penicillin G is toxic to parakeets, turtles, and snakes.
  2) Cats are highly susceptible to the neurotoxicity of streptomycin.
  3) Horses react adversely to lincomycin and tylosin, and to tetracyclines when stressed.

2. **Adverse reactions** — when drugs are used under usual clinical conditions and under an appropriate regimen, these adverse reactions are rare. When any of the situations or conditions cited as causes of treatment failure exist, toxic reactions may result.
  A) Sterile gut accompanied by diarrhea and impaired biosynthesis of vitamin K and B complex vitamins may result from prolonged oral therapy.
  B) Superinfection — antibiotics given orally inhibit susceptible organisms in the gut and allow the rapid proliferation of resistant bacteria. These resistant organisms are usually harmless because they are kept in check by competition with the susceptible organisms. Without this competition, the resis-

tant organisms rapidly proliferate and may enter the systemic circulation. Septicemias and endotoxin shock may result. When antibiotics with a narrow-spectrum against Gram-positive organisms only are given orally, the result may be superinfection by Gram-negative organisms.

C) Hypersensitivity — drug allergy
1) Penicillin G is most notorious.
2) Many are capable.
3) Allergic reactions range from skin rashes to anaphylactic shock.

D) Inhibition of protein synthesis — anti-anabolic:
1) May inhibit general protein anabolism
2) May inhibit wound healing
3) May inhibit fracture healing
4) May inhibit antibody synthesis
5) Are additive with corticosteroids
6) Tetracyclines, chloramphenicol

E) Inhibition of drug biotransformation systems impairs inactivation of certain other drugs, hence giving them longer duration of action:
1) Chloramphenicol   2) Tetracyclines (?)

F) Paralysis of skeletal muscle:
1) Thought to interfere with the function of free calcium ion and to block acetylcholine at the myoneural junction.
2) Treatment consists of calcium salts and neostigmine.
3) Aminoglycoside antibiotics are the chief offenders:
   a) Neomycin          c) Gentamicin
   b) Streptomycin      d) Kanamycin
4) Tetracyclines and lincomycin have been reported to cause paralysis of skeletal muscle; the reason is unknown.

G) Inhibition of respiration resulting from progressive paralysis of the respiratory muscles.

H) Cardiovascular:
1) Large doses; experimental situations in domestic animals
2) Cardiac depression:
   a) May be related to interference with function of free calcium ion as cited in F) 1) above.
   b) Treat with calcium salts
   c) Aminoglycosides (F) 3) above)
   d) Tetracyclines
3) Vasodilation and drop in blood pressure (from aminoglycosides)
4) Reported cardiovascular depression; cause unknown:
   a) Lincomycin   b) Chloramphenicol

I) Neurotoxicity
   1) Aminoglycosides may produce:
      a) Vestibular inhibition      b) Auditory inhibition
   2) Large concentrations of penicillin will:
      a) Stimulate the CNS      b) Possibly cause convulsions
   3) Nitrofurans
      a) Ataxia          c) Convulsions
      b) Excitement      d) Head-pressing
   4) Tetracyclines and neomycin may possibly trigger milk fever (hypocalcemia).
J) Nephrotoxicity (aminoglycosides)
K) Blood dyscrasias
   1) Reported to occur in many human patients
   2) Not a reported clinical problem in veterinary therapy
L) Miscellaneous
   1) In horses stressed by anesthesia and surgery, tetracyclines may produce a diarrhea and colitis-X.
   2) Tetracyclines may cause shock-like syndrome when given IV especially when given very rapidly to cattle. Occurrence in horses has also been reported.

# Drug Index

**Controlled Substances:** For a separate listing of controlled substances of importance to veterinary medicine, see page 13.

**Veterinary Prescription Drugs:** An alphabetical listing of these drugs begins on page 22.